Natural Healing with Chinese Medicine

Natural Healing
with Chinese Medicine

Edited by Harriet Schmidt

SYRAWOOD
PUBLISHING HOUSE
New York

Published by Syrawood Publishing House,
750 Third Avenue, 9th Floor,
New York, NY 10017, USA
www.syrawoodpublishinghouse.com

Natural Healing with Chinese Medicine
Edited by Harriet Schmidt

International Standard Book Number: 978-1-64740-105-4 (Hardback)

Cataloging-in-Publication Data

Natural healing with chinese medicine / edited by Harriet Schmidt.
      p. cm.
Includes bibliographical references and index.
ISBN 978-1-64740-105-4
1. Medicine, Chinese. 2. Naturopathy. 3. Nature, Healing power of. 4. Alternative medicine. I. Schmidt, Harriet.
R601 .N38 2022
610.951--dc23

TABLE OF CONTENTS

PREFACE

The world is advancing at a fast pace like never before. Therefore, the need is to keep up with the latest developments. This book was an idea that came to fruition when the specialists in the area realized the need to coordinate together and document essential themes in the subject. That's when I was requested to be the editor. Editing this book has been an honour as it brings together diverse authors researching on different streams of the field. The book collates essential materials contributed by veterans in the area which can be utilized by students and researchers alike.

Chinese medicine includes various forms of herbal medicine, acupuncture, exercise and dietary therapy. It utilizes plant elements as well as animal, human and mineral products. One of the basic principles of Chinese medicine is the use of the body's vital energy. It is believed that the body's energy circulates through channels called meridians and it has branches connected to bodily organs and functions. Chinese medicine considers diseases as imbalance in the interactions of yin, yang, qi, meridians, etc. The disharmony in these interactions is diagnosed by measuring the pulse, inspecting the skin, tongue, eyes and observing the eating and sleeping habits of a person. This book traces the progress of this field and highlights some of its key concepts and applications. It presents researches and studies performed by experts across the globe. Those in search of information to further their knowledge will be greatly assisted by this book.

Each chapter is a sole-standing publication that reflects each author's interpretation. Thus, the book displays a multi-facetted picture of our current understanding of application, resources and aspects of the field. I would like to thank the contributors of this book and my family for their endless support.

Editor

The influence of duodenally-delivered Shakuyakukanzoto (*Shao Yao Gan Cao Tang*) on duodenal peristalsis during endoscopic retrograde cholangiopancreatography

Haruka Fujinami[1], Shinya Kajiura[2], Jun Nishikawa[2], Takayuki Ando[2] and Toshiro Sugiyama[2*]

Abstract

Background: Anti-cholinergic agents may be used to inhibit duodenal peristalsis, but they may have adverse effects. Shakuyakukanzoto (*Shao Yao Gan Cao Tang*) has an anti-spasmodic effect and has been used before for oesophagogastroduodenoscopy and colonoscopy. This randomised clinical trial aimed to evaluate the inhibitory effect of Shakuyakukanzoto on duodenal peristalsis, and its usefulness when administered into the duodenum just before endoscopic retrograde cholangiopancreatography (ERCP).

Methods: Participants were recruited between June 2008 and December 2010. All were aged ≥18 years and provided written informed consent. Exclusion criteria were: acute pancreatitis, a history of ischemic heart disease, prostatic hypertrophy or glaucoma, and altered/postsurgical upper gastrointestinal anatomy. The recruited participants were randomly assigned to the Shakuyakukanzoto group and control group. Shakuyakukanzoto 100 mg/mL solution or placebo (warm water) was administered directly as a spray into the duodenum during endoscopy. Efficacy was evaluated by observing the extent of duodenal peristalsis and assessing the difficulty of cannulating the common bile duct, the required time (RT) from administration to inhibition of duodenal peristalsis and the stop duration time (DT, the duration for which peristalsis was inhibited). Side effects were evaluated by measuring serum potassium concentration after ERCP.

Results: Of 28 participants, 15 were assigned to the Shakuyakukanzoto group and 13 to the control group. Duodenal peristalsis was inhibited in eight of the 10 eligible participants (80.0%) in the Shakuyakukanzoto group and none (0%) of the nine eligible participants in the control group ($P = 0.026$). In the Shakuyakukanzoto group, mean RT (±standard deviation) was 76.0 ± 23.9 s and DT was 11.3 ± 4.2 min. No adverse effects were observed in the Shakuyakukanzoto group during or after ERCP.

Conclusion: Duodenal peristalsis can be inhibited by spraying Shakuyakukanzoto solution directly into the duodenum.

*Correspondence: tsugi@med.u-toyama.ac.jp
[2] Department of Gastroenterology, Graduate School of Medicine
and Pharmaceutical Science, University of Toyama, Sugitani 2630, Toyama
City, Toyama 930-0194, Japan

Background

Endoscopic retrograde cholangiopancreatography (ERCP) has become increasingly important in the diagnosis and treatment of pancreatic and biliary diseases [1]. It is important to obtain a clear view, without duodenal peristalsis, to perform ERCP safely and effectively. Antispasmodics such as hyoscine-N-butylbromide or glucagon are often used to inhibit duodenal spasm [2], but their systemic use may cause adverse events, including dry mouth, urinary retention, orthostatic hypotension, palpitations, hyperglycaemia and anaphylaxis. Furthermore, these drugs are contraindicated in participants with ischaemic heart disease, prostatic hypertrophy, glaucoma and diabetes mellitus [3, 4].

Shakuyakukanzoto (*Shao Yao Gan Cao Tang*), an aqueous mixture of extracts of *Paeoniae radix* (*Shakuyaku, Shao Yao*) and *Glycyrrhizae radix* (*Kanzo, Gan Cao*), is reported to rapidly reduce abdominal pain and muscular cramps [5, 6], and suppress contraction of the ileum [7]. We have previously reported the inhibitory effect of Shakuyakukanzoto on duodenal peristalsis during ERCP [8], a finding that was later corroborated by Sakai et al. [9]. This randomised clinical trial aimed to evaluate the inhibitory effect of Shakuyakukanzoto on duodenal peristalsis and its utility when administered directly into the duodenum just before ERCP.

Methods

Study design

This was a prospective, randomised, placebo-controlled trial to investigate the effectiveness of Shakuyakukanzoto solution on intestinal peristalsis. A CONSORT flow diagram of the study protocol is presented in Fig. 1 [10]. The study was approved by the Ethics Committee of the University of Toyama, Toyama, Japan (Additional file 1), and informed consent was obtained from all participants (Additional file 2). Participants scheduled for ERCP at Toyama University Hospital were invited at this study between June 2008 and December 2010. Inclusion criteria were: (1) participants ≥18 years old, with (2) the capacity to provide written informed consent. Exclusion criteria were: (1) acute active pancreatitis; (2) a history of ischemic heart disease, prostatic hypertrophy or glaucoma, and (3) altered or postsurgical upper gastrointestinal anatomy. Randomization was achieved by a computer-generated list of numbers to assign group allocation.

ERCP

Endoscopic retrograde cholangiopancreatography was performed by one of four trained endoscopists, each with at least 5 years of experience (HF, SK, JN and TA). Images of all procedures were recorded digitally. All participants were administered midazolam 5 mg (Astellas

Pharma Inc., Tokyo, Japan) intravenously before the procedure, and heart rate and peripheral oxygen saturation were monitored by pulse oximetry during the procedure. We prepared a 100 mg/mL Shakuyakukanzoto solution by dissolving 5.0 g Shakuyakukanzoto extract (TJ-68; Tsumura Co., Tokyo, Japan) in 50 mL of warm water, while 50 mL of warm water was used as the placebo control. Both solutions were administered at 36 °C by spraying directly towards the major papilla of the duodenum through the endoscope. Those cases with no duodenal peristalsis at the major papilla were excluded from the study, and the study drug was not administered.

Evaluation of duodenal peristalsis

We measured duodenal peristalsis during ERCP using a four-grade scoring system of the degree of peristalsis and the difficulty of cannulation previously described by Niwa et al. [11]. The four scores used were as follows: (+0) no peristalsis of the duodenum during ERCP, cannulation was easy to perform; (+1) slight peristalsis of the duodenum, cannulation was easy to perform; (+2) moderate peristalsis of the duodenum, cannulation was difficult to perform; and (+3) severe peristalsis of the duodenum, cannulation could not be performed.

Efficacy and side effects of Shakuyakukanzoto solution

The primary efficacy was inhibition of duodenal peristalsis, calculated as the proportion of participants scoring either +0 or +1 after treatment. To further assess the effects of Shakuyakukanzoto solution, we reviewed the digital recordings of ERCP to measure the required time (RT) from administration of the study drug until peristalsis was diminished, and the duration time (DT) of inhibition of peristalsis (Fig. 2). As hypokalaemia has been reported as a side effect of Shakuyakukanzoto [12], we measured serum potassium concentration before and 24 h after ERCP.

Statistical analysis

The primary outcome criterion was the efficacy rate of Shakuyakukanzoto compared with placebo. The sample size calculation for this study was based on the effective rate achieved in a previous trial, with the response rates in the Shakuyakukanzoto and control groups expected to be 70 and 10%, respectively. The no-peristalsis rate was expected to be 40% [9, 13]. The target sample size required to detect a difference in the response rate between the groups with a significance level of 5% and a power 90% was 13 per group, including a 40% dropout rate. Data are expressed as mean ± standard deviation (SD). Either Fisher's exact test or Student's t test were used to compare paired data. A P value less than 0.05 was considered statistically significant. All statistical analyses

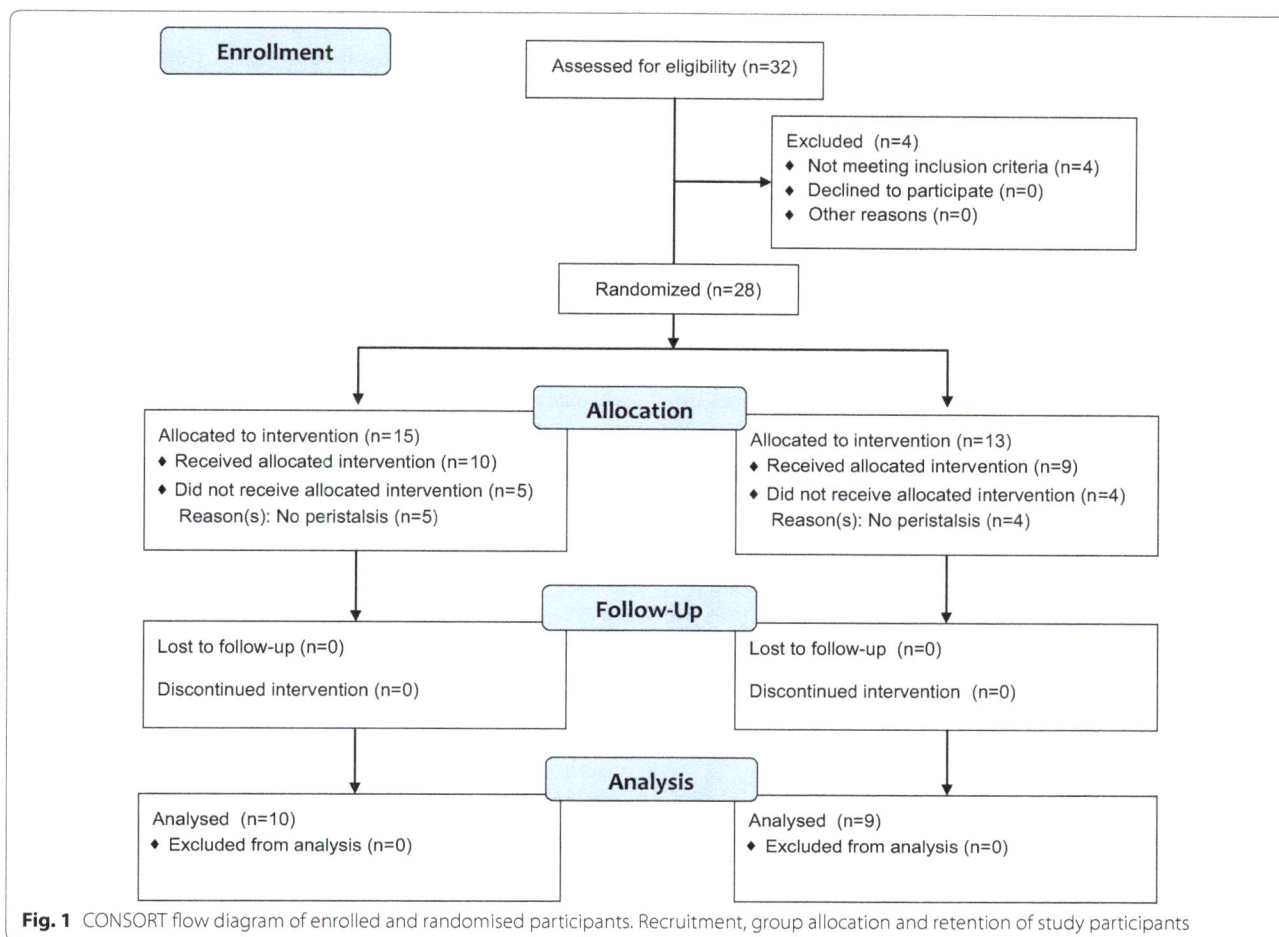

Fig. 1 CONSORT flow diagram of enrolled and randomised participants. Recruitment, group allocation and retention of study participants

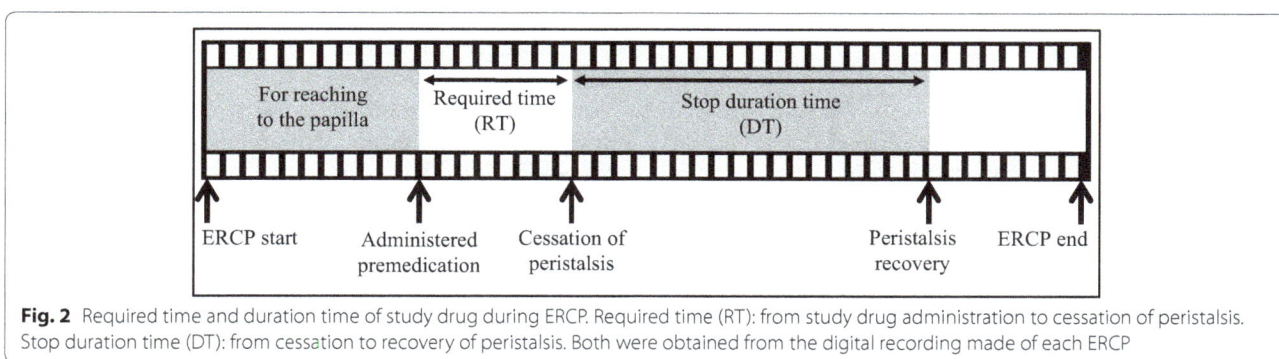

Fig. 2 Required time and duration time of study drug during ERCP. Required time (RT): from study drug administration to cessation of peristalsis. Stop duration time (DT): from cessation to recovery of peristalsis. Both were obtained from the digital recording made of each ERCP

were performed using the Statview 5.0 (Abacus Concepts Inc., Berkeley, CA, USA).

Results

In total, 149 ERCP procedures were performed during the study period, and 32 participants were enrolled into the study. Four were excluded due to exacerbation of acute pancreatitis and/or cholangitis. The remaining 28 participants fulfilled the inclusion criteria and were randomly allocated to one of the two groups: 15 participants to the Shakuyakukanzoto group and 13 to the placebo control group. Five participants in the Shakuyakukanzoto group and four in the control group were excluded as no duodenal peristalsis was evident at duodenoscopy.

Consequently, we subjected the data of 10 and nine participants from the Shakuyakukanzoto and control groups to analysis, respectively. Participants' demographic and clinical characteristics are summarised in Table 1. There was no significant difference in sex, mean age or indication for ERCP between the groups. Duodenal peristalsis was inhibited in eight of the 10 participants (80.0%) in the Shakuyakukanzoto group and none (0%) of the control group ($P = 0.026$; Table 2). Mean RT and DT for Shakuyakukanzoto were 76.0 ± 23.9 s and 12.4 ± 5.0 min, respectively. There was no significant difference in the serum potassium concentration in the Shakuyakukanzoto group before or after the procedure (4.1 ± 0.3 mEq/L versus 4.3 ± 0.3 mEq/L, respectively, $P = 0.192$; Table 2).

Discussion

To the best of our knowledge, this is the first placebo-controlled study that has shown that Shakuyakukanzoto is an effective and safe anti-spasmodic premedication for ERCP. In a previous observational study [9], Shakuyakukanzoto acted as an anti-spasmodic agent and abolished duodenal peristalsis in the majority of participants

Table 1 Participants' demographic and clinical characteristics

	Shakuyakukanzoto group	Control group	P value
Participants	10 (52.6)	9 (47.4)	
Male	7 (70.0)	6 (66.7)	1.000[a]
Age (years old)	69.1	71.2	0.708[b]
Diagnostic ERCP	7 (36.8)	3 (15.8)	0.179[a]
Therapeutic ERCP	3 (15.8)	6 (31.6)	

Data are presented as number (proportion, %) or mean ± standard deviation

[a] Fisher's exact test was used to assess statistical significance

[b] Student's *t* test was used to assess statistical significance

Table 2 Efficacy and safety of *Shakuyakukanzoto*

	Shakuyakukanzoto group	Control group
Ceased peristalsis	8 (80.0)	0 (0)
Required time (s)	76.0 ± 23.9	ND
Stop duration time (min)	11.3 ± 23.9	ND
Potassium concentration (mEq/L)		
Before procedure	4.1 ± 0.3	4.0 ± 0.3
24 h after procedure	4.3 ± 0.3	4.2 ± 0.2

*ND no data. The required time and stop duration time in the control group were not measured because inhibition of duodenal peristalsis was not achieved with the placebo

Data are presented as number (proportion, %) or mean ± standard deviation

to whom it was administered, but this was not a randomised, controlled study and the extent of suppression of peristalsis was not measured. In this study, we excluded participants in whom duodenal peristalsis was not evident at duodenoscopy, and assessed peristalsis and its influence on the technical difficulty of cannulating the common bile duct using the scoring system previously described by Niwa et al. [11].

Gastrointestinal peristalsis may be an impediment to accurate endoscopic examination. Intramuscular or intravenous administration of an anti-cholinergic agent such as hyoscine-N-butyl bromide is generally required to abolish peristalsis [14]. Administration of an anti-cholinergic drug may, however, cause potentially serious complications, including cardiovascular events, urinary retention and ocular hypertension [4]. Glucagon may also be used to reduce peristalsis, but while it has fewer adverse effects on the cardiovascular system, it may induce hyperglycaemia [15]. Therefore, these drugs are not recommended for participants with cardiac disease, glaucoma, prostatic hyperplasia or diabetes mellitus [4, 15].

Shakuyakukanzoto has two active components. Paeoniflorin is a bioactive component of *Paeoniae radix*, and reportedly exhibits anti-coagulant [16], neuromuscular blocking [17–23], immunoregulating [24] and anti-hyperglycaemic effects [25]. Glycyrrhizic acid is a bioactive component of *Glycyrrhizae radix* and is reported to have anti-inflammatory [26] and hepatoprotective activity [27], and inhibit anti-platelet aggregation [28] and formation of peptic ulcers [29, 30]. These two components may exert synergistic effects. Although paeoniflorin is poorly absorbed in the gastrointestinal tract and has low bioavailability [31, 32], its absorption is significantly improved when administered orally in Shakuyakukanzoto solution [33].

Rather than administering standard anti-spasmodic drugs, or administering Shakuyakukanzoto orally, we sprayed Shakuyakukanzoto directly into the duodenum during duodenoscopy, and found that duodenal peristalsis was inhibited in 80% of cases. These effects were likely observed because the *Glycyrrhizae radix* reportedly inhibits acetylcholine-induced contraction and the contractile machinery of smooth muscle, while *Paeoniae radix* inhibits neurogenic contraction in the small bowel (the latter reportedly inhibits peristalsis in guinea pig ileum and in mouse jejunum and ileum) [7, 34]. Although paeoniflorin and glycyrrhizin may be ineffective when applied individually, they are recognised to block neuromuscular synapses when applied in combination in animal models [21].

Peppermint oil, a major constituent of which is menthol, also inhibits the contraction of smooth muscle of the gastrointestinal tract [35–37]. Instillation of peppermint oil into the colon during colonoscopy reduces spasm and reduces the need for intramuscular or intravenous anti-spasmodic agents during endoscopic examination [13, 38, 39]. The mechanism of smooth muscle relaxation brought about by peppermint oil has been investigated in models using the smooth muscle of guinea pigs and mice.

The brown colour of Shakuyakukanzoto solution might affect endoscopic examination by obscuring the entrance to the common bile duct; however, ductal cannulation was possible in all cases in which Shakuyaku-kanzoto was administered. Nevertheless, its distinctive colour made blinding of the study to the endoscopist impractical.

The intraluminal administration of a rapidly acting agent that directly affects smooth muscle has obvious advantages over the systemic administration of an anticholinergic drug. In this study, we evaluated the efficacy of Shakuyakukanzoto administered directly into the duodenum immediately before ERCP. We have also found that Shakuyakukanzoto sprayed directly onto the duodenal papilla significantly reduced serum amylase concentration 1 h and 1 day after ERCP [40]. Although we assessed only ERCP, our findings might also apply to other endoscopic examinations, such as upper endoscopy, balloon endoscopy and colonoscopy.

Conclusion
Duodenal peristalsis can be inhibited by spraying Shakuyakukanzoto solution directly into the duodenum.

Abbreviations
DT: stop duration time; ERCP: endoscopic retrograde cholangiopancreatography; RT: required time.

Authors' contributions
HF, SK, JN, TA and TS conceived and designed the study protocol. HF, SK, JN and TA collected data and endoscopic examination. HF, SK and JN conducted the clinical trial. HF wrote and revised the manuscript. All authors read and approved the final manuscript.

Author details
[1] Department of Endoscopy, Toyama University Hospital, Toyama, Japan.
[2] Department of Gastroenterology, Graduate School of Medicine and Pharmaceutical Science, University of Toyama, Sugitani 2630, Toyama City, Toyama 930-0194, Japan.

Competing interests
The authors declare that they have no competing interests.

References
1. Schofl R, Haefner M. Diagnostic cholangiopancreatography. Endoscopy. 2003;35:145–55.
2. Chang FY, Guo WS, Liao TM, Lee SD. A randomized study comparing glucagon and hyoscine N-butyl bromide before endoscopic retrograde cholangiopancreatography. Scand J Gastroenterol. 1995;30:283–6.
3. Mintzer J, Burns A. Anticholinergic side-effects of drugs in elderly people. J R Soc Med. 2000;93:457–62.
4. Ai M, Yamaguchi T, Odaka T, Mitsuhashi K, Shishido T, Yan J, et al. Objective assessment of the antispasmodic effect of shakuyaku-kanzo-to (TJ-68), a Chinese herbal medicine, on the colonic wall by direct spraying during colonoscopy. World J Gastroenterol. 2006;12:760–4.
5. Hinoshita F, Ogura Y, Suzuki Y, Hara S, Yamada A, Tanaka N, et al. Effect of orally administered shao-yao-gan-cao-tang (Shakuyaku-kanzo-to) on muscle cramps in maintenance hemodialysis patients: a preliminary study. Am J Chin Med. 2003;31:445–53.
6. Hyodo T, Taira T, Kumakura M, Yamamoto S, Yoshida K, Uchida T, et al. The immediate effect of Shakuyaku-kanzo-to, traditional Japanese herbal medicine, for muscular cramps during maintenance hemodialysis. Nephron. 2002;90:240.
7. Maeda T, Shinozuka K, Baba K, Hayashi M, Hayashi E. Effect of shakuyaku-kanzoh-toh, a prescription composed of shakuyaku (Paeoniae Radix) and kanzoh (Glycyrrhizae Radix) on guinea pig ileum. J Pharmacobiodyn. 1983;6:153–60.
8. Fujinami H, Hirano K, Sugiyama T. Assessment of diminished peristalsis using shakuyakukanzoto (TJ-68) as premedication for endoscopic retrograde cholangiopancreatography (ERCP). DDW-Japan. Sapporo; 2006.
9. Sakai Y, Tsuyuguchi T, Ishihara T, Kato K, Tsuboi M, Ooka Y, et al. Confirmation of the antispasmodic effect of shakuyaku-kanzo-to (TJ-68), a Chinese herbal medicine, on the duodenal wall by direct spraying during endoscopic retrograde cholangiopancreatography. J Nat Med. 2009;63:200–3.
10. Schulz KF, Altman DG, Moher D. CONSORT Group: CONSORT 2010 statement: updated guidelines for reporting parallel group randomised trials. Int J Surg. 2011;9:672–7.
11. Niwa H, Nakamura T, Fujino M. Endoscopic observation on gastric peristalsis and pyloric movement (in Japanese with English abstract). Gastroenterol Endosc. 1975;17:236–42.
12. Kinoshita H, Okabayashi M, Kaneko M, Yasuda M, Abe K, Machida A, et al. Shakuyaku-kanzo-to induces pseudoaldosteronism characterized by hypokalemia, rhabdomyolysis, metabolic alkalosis with respiratory compensation, and increased urinary cortisol levels. J Altern Complement Med. 2009;15:439–43.
13. Hiki N, Kaminishi M, Yasuda K, Uedo N, Honjo H, Matsuhashi N, et al. Antiperistaltic effect and safety of L-menthol sprayed on the gastricmucosa for upper GI endoscopy: a phase III, multicenter, randomized, doubleblind, placebo-controlled study. Gastrointest Endosc. 2011;73:932–41.
14. Sissons GR, McQueenie A, Mantle M. The ocular effects of hyoscine-n-butylbromide ("Buscopan") in radiological practice. Br J Radiol. 1991;64:584–6.
15. Mochiki E, Suzuki H, Takenoshita S, Nagamachi Y, Kuwano H, Mizumoto A, et al. Mechanism of inhibitory effect of glucagon on gastrointestinal motility and cause of side effects of glucagon. J Gastroenterol. 1998;33:835–41.
16. Ishida H, Takamatsu M, Tsuji K, Kosuge T. Studies on active substances in herbs used for Oketsu ('stagnant blood') in Chinese medicine. VI. On the anticoagulative principle in Paeoniae Radix. Chem Pharm Bull. 1987;35:849–52.
17. Dezaki K, Kimura I, Miyahara K, Kimura M. Complementary effects of paeoniflorin and glycyrrhizin on intracellular Ca2 + mobilization in the nerve-stimulated skeletal muscle of mice. Jpn J Pharmacol. 1995;69:281–4.
18. Kimura M, Kimura I, Muroi M, Nakamura T, Shibata S. Depolarizing effects of glycyrrhizin-derivatives relating to the blend effects with paeoniflorin in mouse diaphragm muscle. Jpn J Pharmacol. 1986;41:263–5.
19. Kimura M, Kimura I, Kimura M. Decreasing effects by glycyrrhizin and paeoniflorin on intracellular Ca2 + -aequorin luminescence transients with or without caffeine in directly stimulated-diaphragm muscle of mouse. Jpn J Pharmacol. 1985;39:387–90.
20. Kimura M, Kimura I, Nojima H. Depolarizing neuromuscular blocking action induced by electropharmacological coupling in the combined effect of paeoniflorin and glycyrrhizin. Jpn J Pharmacol. 1985;37:395–9.

21. Kimura M, Kimura I, Takahashi K, Muroi M, Yoshizaki M, Kanaoka M, et al. Blocking effects of blended paeoniflorin or its related compounds with glycyrrhizin on neuromuscular junctions in frog and mouse. Jpn J Pharmacol. 1984;36:275–82.

22. Kimura M, Kimura I, Takahashi K. The neuromuscular blocking actions of coclaurine derivatives and of paeoniflorin derivatives. Planta Med. 1982;45:136.

23. Kimura M, Kimura I, Nojima H. The electropharmacological mechanisms of depolarizing neuromuscular blocking effects induced by the combination of paeoniflorin and glycyrrhizin. Jpn J Pharmacol. 1981;31(Suppl):72.

24. Liang J, Zhou A, Chen M, Xu S. Negatively regulatory effects of paeoniflorin on immune cells. Eur J Pharmacol. 1990;183:901–2.

25. Hsu FL, Lai CW, Cheng JT. Antihyperglycemic effects of paeoniflorin and 8-debenzoylpaeoniflorin, glucosides from the root of Paeonia lactiflora. Planta Med. 1997;63:323–5.

26. Inoue H, Mori T, Shibata S, Koshihara Y. Modulation by glycyrrhetinic acid derivatives of TPA-induced mouse ear oedema. Br J Pharmacol. 1989;96:204–10.

27. van Rossum TG, Vulto AG, de Man RA, Brouwer JT, Schalm SW. Review article: glycyrrhizin as a potential treatment for chronic hepatitis C. Aliment Pharmacol Ther. 1998;12:199–205.

28. Tawata M, Aida K, Noguchi T, Ozaki Y, Kume S, Sasaki H, et al. Anti-platelet action of isoliquiritigenin, an aldose reductase inhibitor in licorice. Eur J Pharmacol. 1992;212:87–92.

29. van Marle J, Aarsen PN, Lind A, van Weeren-Kramer J. Deglycyrrhizinised liquorice (DGL) and the renewal of rat stomach epithelium. Eur J Pharmacol. 1891;72:219–25.

30. Baker ME. Licorice and enzymes other than 11 betahydroxysteroid dehydrogenase: an evolutionary perspective. Steroids. 1994;59:136–41.

31. Xu S, Chen C, Chen G. The pharmacokinetics of paeoniflorin. Eur J Pharmacol. 1990;183:2390.

32. Takeda S, Isono T, Wakui Y, Matsuzaki Y, Sasaki H, Amagaya S, et al. Absorption and excretion of paeoniflorin in rats. J Pharm Pharmacol. 1995;47:1036–40.

33. Chen LC, Chou MH, Lin MF, Yang LL. Pharmacokinetics of paeoniflorin after oral administration of Shao-yao Gan-chao Tang in mice. Jpn J Pharmacol. 2002;88:250–5.

34. Sato Y, Akao T, He JX, Nojima H, Kuraishi Y, Morota T, et al. Glycycoumarin from Glycyrrhizae Radix acts as a potent antispasmodic through inhibition of phosphodiesterase 3. J Ethnopharmacol. 2006;105:409–14.

35. Nair B. Final report on the safety assessment of Mentha piperita (peppermint) oil, Mentha piperita (peppermint) leaf extract, Mentha piperita (peppermint) leaf, and Mentha piperita (peppermint) leaf water. Int J Toxicol. 2001;20:61–73.

36. Hills JM, Aaronson PI. The mechanism of action of peppermint oil on gastrointestinal smooth muscle. An analysis using patch clamp electrophysiology and isolated tissue pharmacology in rabbit and guinea pig. Gastroenterology. 1991;101:55–65.

37. Micklefield G, Jung O, Greving I, May B. Effects of intraduodenal application of peppermint oil (WS (R) 1340) and caraway oil (WS (R) 1520) on gastroduodenal motility in healthy volunteers. Phytother Res. 2003;17:135–40.

38. Asao T, Mochiki E, Suzuki H, Nakamura J, Hirayama I, Morinaga N, et al. An easy method for the intraluminal administration of peppermint oil before colonoscopy and its effectiveness in reducing colonic spasm. Gastrointest Endosc. 2001;53:172–7.

39. Imagawa A, Hata H, Nakatsu M, Yoshida Y, Takeuchi K, Inokuchi T, et al. Peppermint oil solution is useful as an antispasmodic drug for esophagogastroduodenoscopy, especially for elderly patients. Dig Dis Sci. 2012;57:2379–84.

40. Fujinami H, Kajiura S, Ando T, Mihara H, Hosokawa A, Sugiyama T. Direct spraying of shakuyakukanzoto onto the duodenal papilla: a novel method for preventing pancreatitis following endoscopic retrograde cholangiopancreatography. Digestion. 2015;91:42–5.

2

Diversity and composition of bacterial endophytes among plant parts of *Panax notoginseng*

Linlin Dong[1], Ruiyang Cheng[1], Lina Xiao[1], Fugang Wei[2], Guangfei Wei[1], Jiang Xu[1], Yong Wang[3], Xiaotong Guo[4], Zhongjian Chen[3] and Shilin Chen[1*]

Abstract

Background: Bacterial endophytes are widespread inhabitants inside plant tissues that play crucial roles in plant growth and biotransformation. This study aimed to offer information for the exploitation of endophytes by analyzing the bacterial endophytes in different parts of *Panax notoginseng*.

Methods: We used high-throughput sequencing methods to analyze the diversity and composition of bacterial endophytes from different parts of *P. notoginseng*.

Results: A total of 174,761 classified sequences were obtained from the analysis of 16S ribosomal RNA in different parts of *P. notoginseng*. Its fibril displayed the highest diversity of bacterial endophytes. Principal coordinate analysis revealed that the compositions of the bacterial endophytes from aboveground parts (flower, leaf, and stem) differed from that of underground parts (root and fibril). The abundances of *Conexibacter*, *Gemmatimonas*, *Holophaga*, *Luteolibacter*, *Methylophilus*, *Prosthecobacter*, and *Solirubrobacter* were significantly higher in the aboveground parts than in the underground parts, whereas the abundances of *Bradyrhizobium*, *Novosphingobium*, *Phenylobacterium*, *Sphingobium*, and *Steroidobacter* were markedly lower in the aboveground parts.

Conclusions: Our results elucidated the comprehensive diversity and composition profiles of bacterial endophytes in different parts of 3-year-old *P. notoginseng*. Our data offered pivotal information to clarify the role of endophytes in the production of *P. notoginseng* and its important metabolites.

Keywords: *Panax notoginseng*, Endophytes, Plant parts, High-throughput sequencing, 16S ribosomal RNA

Background

Panax notoginseng is renowned for its remarkable antihypertensive, antithrombotic, anti-atherosclerotic, and neuroprotective bioactivities, making it one of the most valuable ingredients in staple household medicines [1–3]. Protopanaxadiol and protopanaxatriol saponins are the main active compounds detected in the different parts of *P. notoginseng* [4, 5]. *P. notoginseng* is a perennial plant cultivated in fixed plots, and continuous cropping leads to decreased productivity, reduced tuber quality, and

even seedling death [6, 7]. Approximately 8–10 years of crop rotation are necessary for improving the soil conditions for planted *P. notoginseng* [8]. *P. notoginseng* has a narrow ecological range, and its production mainly occurs in Wenshan, Yunnan Province, where the climatic and soil conditions are optimal for its cultivation. Nevertheless, arable soils available for *P. notoginseng* cultivation are becoming scarce.

Endophytic bacteria localized inside plant tissues have shown no negative effect on their host plants [9]. Bacteria inhabit different plant tissues, including rhizosphere, root, leaf, and stem [10]. Bacterial endophytes play key roles in improving plant growth, increasing tolerance against biotic factors, and producing secondary metabolites [11, 12]. Song et al. reported that

*Correspondence: slchen@icmm.ac.cn
[1] Institute of Chinese Materia Medica, China Academy of Chinese Medical Sciences, Beijing 100700, China

endophytic *Bacillus altitudinis* isolated from *Panax ginseng* enhanced ginsenoside accumulation [13]. Gao et al. reported that *Paenibacillus polymyxa* isolated from *P. ginseng* leaves improved plant growth, increased ginsenoside concentration, and reduced morbidity [14]. Endophytes stimulated secondary metabolites and enhanced plant growth. Numerous works highlighted that the composition of the bacterial endophytes were influenced by plant species, parts, and growth stage [11, 15]. Analysis of the diversity and composition of endophytes in plant parts could provide valuable resources for plant growth promotion and biotransformation [16]. Although the diversity and composition of root endogenous bacteria in *P. notoginseng* have been described [17], limited information is available on the endophytic community in different parts of *P. notoginseng*. Thus, the diversity and composition of bacterial endophytes must be investigated to exploit the agronomical and metabolic potential of *P. notoginseng*.

Cultivation-independent methods can facilitate a rapid analysis of vast samples and provide reliable information on the diversity and composition of endophytic bacteria [18]. Many studies have explored rhizosphere and plant-associated bacterial communities by using high-throughput sequencing analysis [19–21]. Metagenetic methods for analyzing endophyte communities would provide deeper insight into the diversity and composition of bacterial endophytes, thereby leading to the potential discovery of new endophytes [22, 23]. Checcucci et al. reported the high taxonomic diversity of bacterial endophytes in the leaves of *Thymus* spp. by using 16S rRNA gene metagenomic sequencing [24]. A total of 29 culturable bacterial endophytes have been identified in the tissues of *Aloe vera* and characterized to 13 genera [25]. Nevertheless, culture-dependent biodiversity studies on endophytic bacterial communities remain scarce [19]. Pyrosequencing could detect low-abundance bacteria in leaf salad vegetables that could not be identified by culture-dependent methods [26]. Additional, high-throughput sequencing also used in the analysis of soil microbial communities, and this method effectively revealed the changes in diversity of soil microbial communities in soils during the cultivation of *Panax* plants [21, 27, 28]. In the present study, high-throughput sequencing analysis of 16S ribosomal RNA (rRNA) genes was conducted to describe the diversity and composition of associations among different parts of *P. notoginseng*. The results clarified the tissue-wise diversity of bacterial endophytes in the samples collected from *P. notoginseng* as well as expanded the knowledge on plant–microbe relationships and the potential properties for plant growth promotion and biotransformation.

Methods
Processing of samples
Three-year-old *P. notoginseng* plants were collected from Wenshan, Yunnan Province, China, which is the main production area of *P. notoginseng*. These plant samples were used to analyze the bacterial endophytes in different parts of *P. notoginseng*. Six plants were randomly gathered from one plantation and served as one sample in our test sites of Wenshan Miaoxiang Notoginseng Technology, Co., Ltd. in August. There were three replicates from three plantations. The flowers (Fl), leaves (Le), stems (St), roots (Ro), and fibers (Fi) of all samples were separated, washed with running tap water, and rinsed thrice with distilled water. A single sample consisted of 1 g of each part from six plants as one sample. To sterilize the surface of the plant parts, the samples from each part were successively immersed in 70% ethanol for 5 min, 2.5% sodium hypochlorite for 1–2 min, and 70% ethanol for 1 min, and then rinsed five times with sterile Millipore water. The last portion of the washing water was inoculated in Luria–Bertani agar at 37 °C for 24 h to validate sterilization efficiency. A total of 15 samples were stored at − 80 °C until DNA extraction.

DNA extraction, polymerase chain reaction (PCR) amplification, and sequence processing
The total genomic DNA was extracted from all plant parts by using the MOBIO PowerSoil® Kit (MOBIO Laboratories, Inc., Carlsbad, CA, USA) in accordance with the manufacturer's instructions. The DNA quality of each sample was confirmed by utilizing a NanoDrop spectrophotometer (Thermo Fisher Scientific, Model 2000, MA, USA) and stored at − 20 °C for further PCR amplification. Bacterial 16S rRNA V1 hypervariable region genes were amplified by using the universal primers 27F/338R [29]. The forward and reverse primers contained an 8 bp barcode (Additional file 1: Table S1). PCRs were performed as described by Dong et al. with slight modifications [21]. The reaction systems were denatured at 94 °C for 3 min and then amplified for 25 cycles at 94 °C for 45 s, 55 °C for 30 s, and 72 °C for 60 s. A final extension of 10 min was added at the end of the program. Negative controls (no templates) were included to check DNA contamination of the primer or the sample. PCR products from each sample were separated with 1% agarose gel, purified with a MinElute Gel Extraction Kit (Qiagen, Valencia, CA, USA), and quantified with a Quant-iT PicoGreen dsDNA Assay Kit (Invitrogen, Carlsbad, CA, USA). The amplicons were pooled in equimolar ratios. The amplicon libraries were paired-end sequenced (2 × 250) by using an Illumina MiSeq platform in accordance with the manufacturer's protocol.

Data analysis

The data were processed by utilizing the QIIME pipeline [30]. Bacterial sequences were trimmed and assigned to each sample based on their barcodes. Sequences were binned into operational taxonomic units (OTUs) at 97% similarity level by using UPARSE (version 7.1 http://drive 5.com/uparse/). Chimeric sequences were identified and removed by using UCHIME. The phylogenetic affiliation of each 16S rRNA gene sequence was analyzed by using a RDP Classifier (http://rdp.cme.msu.edu/) against the Silva (SSU123) 16S rRNA database at a confidence threshold of 70% [31]. Rarefaction analysis based on Mothur v.1.21.1 was conducted to reveal the diversity indices, including Chao 1 and Shannon [32]. Principal coordinate analysis (PCoA) was performed to examine dissimilarities in the community composition among samples on the basis of Bray–Curtis distance metrics [33]. Statistical analyses were performed by using the R package [34].

Statistical analyses

SPSS version 16.0 was used for the statistical analyses (SPSS Inc., Chicago, IL, USA). The data were presented as mean $\pm$ SD of $n = 3$. No adjustments were implemented for multiple comparisons. The parameters were obtained for all treatment replicates and subjected one-way ANOVA.

The Minimum Standards of Reporting Checklist contains details of the details of the experimental design, and statistics, and resources used in this study (Additional file 2).

Results

Alpha diversity of bacterial endophytes among P. notoginseng parts

A total of 174,761 reads, with an average of 11,650 sequences per sample, were obtained from 15 samples through high-throughput sequencing analyses of 16S rRNA gene sequences (Table 1). A total of 10,351 OTUs, which ranged from 254 to 964, were found in all sequences. Alpha diversity indices (Chao 1 and Shannon) presented differences among the plant parts of P. notoginseng (Fig. 1). Chao 1 indicated a high number of species in the fibril samples and a low number of species in the leaf and root samples (Fig. 1A). H' revealed that the fibril samples had the highest diversity, whereas the root sample had the lowest diversity (Fig. 1B). The flower and stem displayed similar diversity levels.

Beta diversity of bacterial endophytes among P. notoginseng parts

The Bray–Curtis dissimilarity matrix was calculated to differentiate the bacterial communities among P.

Table 1 Bacterial numbers of sequences and OUTs in each sample

Samples	Sequences	OTUs
Flower-1	10,784	877
Flower-2	6818	657
Flower-3	23,711	908
Leaf-1	666	254
Leaf-2	7279	678
Leaf-3	806	256
Stem-1	22,538	849
Stem-2	2683	533
Stem-3	18,277	817
Root-1	4402	388
Root-2	12,424	726
Root-3	5944	676
Fibril-1	18,206	922
Fibril-2	12,035	846
Fibril-3	28,188	964

-1, -2, and -3 present three replicates of each P. notoginseng part

notoginseng parts (Fig. 2). PCoA ordination showed a strong clustering of the bacterial communities of underground (root and fibril) and aboveground parts (flower, leaf, and stem). The first and second principal components explained 50.79 and 19.3% of the total variation. PCoA indicated that the samples collected from the aboveground parts had similar profiles, whereas the samples from the underground parts were clustered together at opposite sides of the plots of the aboveground parts. Bacterial diversity in the aboveground parts differed from that in the underground parts.

Composition of bacterial endophytes among P. notoginseng parts

The reads from the 16S rRNA amplicon sequences that were generated from all samples mostly belonged to the 14 phyla (Fig. 3). The relative abundances of Proteobacteria, Actinobacteria, Verrucomicrobia, Bacteroidetes, Acidobacteria, Firmicutes, Gemmatimonadetes, and Chloroflexi reached 97.9, 97.2, 97.6, 98.2, and 97.7% in the samples from the flower, leaf, stem, root, and fibril, respectively (Fig. 3a). The relative abundance of Proteobacteria in the underground parts was significantly higher than in the aboveground parts. The abundance of Verrucomicrobia in the aboveground parts was markedly higher than in the underground parts. The relative abundances (< 1%) of Candidatus Saccharibacteria, Fusobacteria, Cyanobacteria, and Nitrospirae in the aboveground parts were higher than those in the underground parts

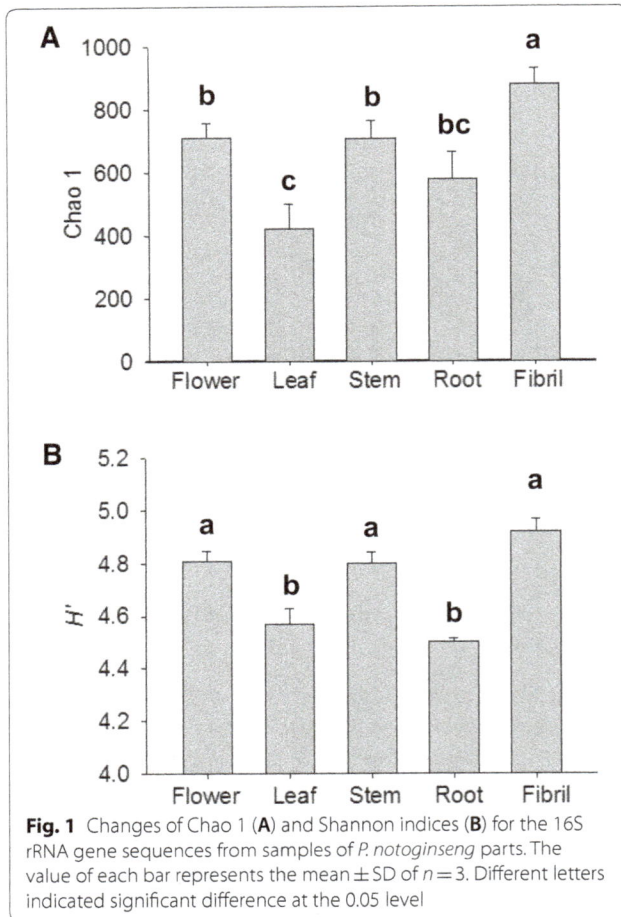

Fig. 1 Changes of Chao 1 (**A**) and Shannon indices (**B**) for the 16S rRNA gene sequences from samples of *P. notoginseng* parts. The value of each bar represents the mean ± SD of *n* = 3. Different letters indicated significant difference at the 0.05 level

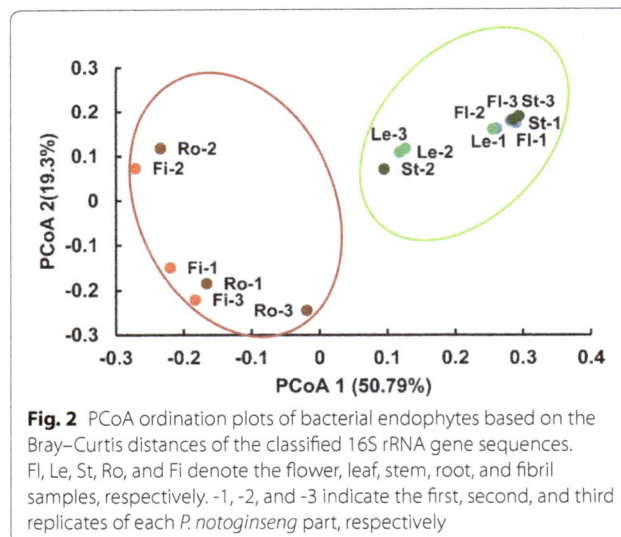

Fig. 2 PCoA ordination plots of bacterial endophytes based on the Bray–Curtis distances of the classified 16S rRNA gene sequences. Fl, Le, St, Ro, and Fi denote the flower, leaf, stem, root, and fibril samples, respectively. -1, -2, and -3 indicate the first, second, and third replicates of each *P. notoginseng* part, respectively

(Fig. 3b). The relative abundance of bacterial endophytes varied and depended on the *P. notoginseng* parts at the phylum level.

The relative abundances of the bacterial endophytes in the aboveground and underground parts showed considerable variation at the order level (Fig. 4 and Additional file 1: Table S2). The relative abundances of Bacillales, Chitinophagales, Gemmatimonadales, Solirubrobacterales, and Verrucomicrobiales in the aboveground parts were markedly higher than in the underground parts (*P* < 0.05). The abundances of Burkholderiales, Caulobacterales, Corynebacteriales, Myxococcales, and Sphingomonadales in the underground parts were significantly higher than those in the aboveground parts (*P* < 0.05). The bacterial endophytes in the samples from the aboveground parts with higher abundance at the order level were Chitinophagales, Rhizobiales, Solirubrobacterales, and Verrucomicrobiales. The bacterial endophytes in the samples from the underground parts with higher abundance at the order level were Burkholderiales, Rhizobiales, Sphingomonadales, and Verrucomicrobiales.

Heat map analysis of the relative abundances of bacterial endophytes at the genus level showed variations in the samples from the aboveground and underground parts (Fig. 5). The relative abundances of *Conexibacter, Gemmatimonas, Holophaga, Luteolibacter, Methylophilus, Prosthecobacter,* and *Solirubrobacter* in the aboveground parts were significantly higher than those in the underground parts (*P* < 0.05). The abundances of *Bradyrhizobium, Novosphingobium, Phenylobacterium, Sphingobium,* and *Steroidobacter* in the aboveground parts were markedly lower than those in the underground parts (*P* < 0.05). Among all samples, *Prosthecobacter* had the highest abundance at the genus level. The low abundance (< 1.0%) of bacterial endophytes was related to the samples from *P. notoginseng* parts at the genus level (Additional file 1: Table S3). The relative abundances of *Agrobacterium, Sphingobium* and *Shinella* in the root samples were significantly higher than in the fibril samples (*P* < 0.05). By contrast, the abundances of *Burkholderia* and *Steroidobacter* in the root samples were markedly lower than in the fibril samples (*P* < 0.05).

Discussion

In this study, the diversity of bacterial endophytes was associated with the different parts of *P. notoginseng*. Chao 1 and *H'* indices indicated that the fibril samples had the highest diversity among all of the samples from the different parts. Chao 1 revealed that *Stellera chamaejasme* L. displayed an increasing trend in species richness from the root samples to the stem and leaf samples [19]. The OTUs of the bacterial endophytes were randomly distributed among plant species and organs, and Chao 1 also revealed that the diversity of *Santiria apiculate* and *Rothmannia macrophylla* in the root samples was higher than that in the leaf samples [35]. PCoA showed that samples

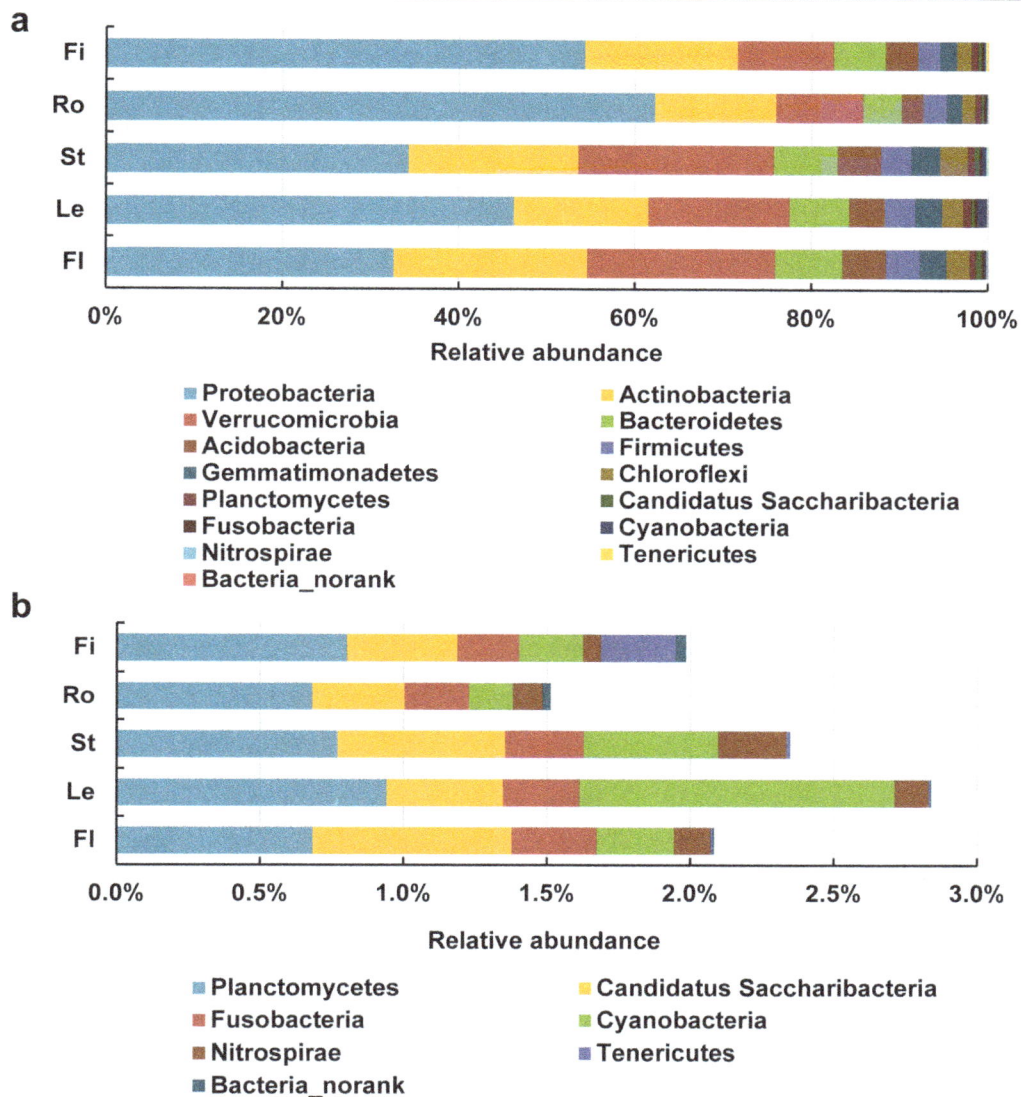

Fig. 3 Relative abundances of the bacterial community at the phylum level. **a** All bacterial endophytes at the phylum level. **b** Bacterial endophytes with low relative abundance (< 1%) at the phylum level. Fl, Le, St, Ro, and Fi refer to the flower, leaf, stem, root, and fibril samples, respectively. The value of each bar represents the mean of $n = 3$

from the aboveground parts were distinguishable from those from the underground parts. Principal component analysis (PCA) revealed that the leaf and stem samples of *S. chamaejasme* L. were clustered together and were different from the plots for the root [19], and that the stem and leaf samples of poplar trees were distinguishable from the root samples [10]. The bacterial endophytes from the fibril had the highest diversity.

In this study, Proteobacteria, Actinobacteria, Verrucomicrobia, Bacteroidetes, Acidobacteria, and Firmicutes were the main bacterial communities in *P. notoginseng* plants. A previous study detected Proteobacteria,

Actinobacteria, Bacteroidetes, and Acidobacteria in the *P. notoginseng* root [17]. Proteobacteria, Actinobacteria, Bacteroidetes, and Firmicutes were found in *P. ginseng* roots by using a culture-dependent method [16]. More than 300 endophytic actinobacteria and bacteria belonging to *Rhodococcus*, *Brevibacterium*, *Nocardioides*, *Streptomyces*, *Microbacterium*, *Nocardiopsis*, *Brachybacterium*, *Tsukamurella*, *Arthrobacter*, and *Pseudonocardia* were isolated from different tissues of *Dracaena cochinchinensis* L. [12]. The plant species influenced the selection of endophytes. The plant parts of *P.*

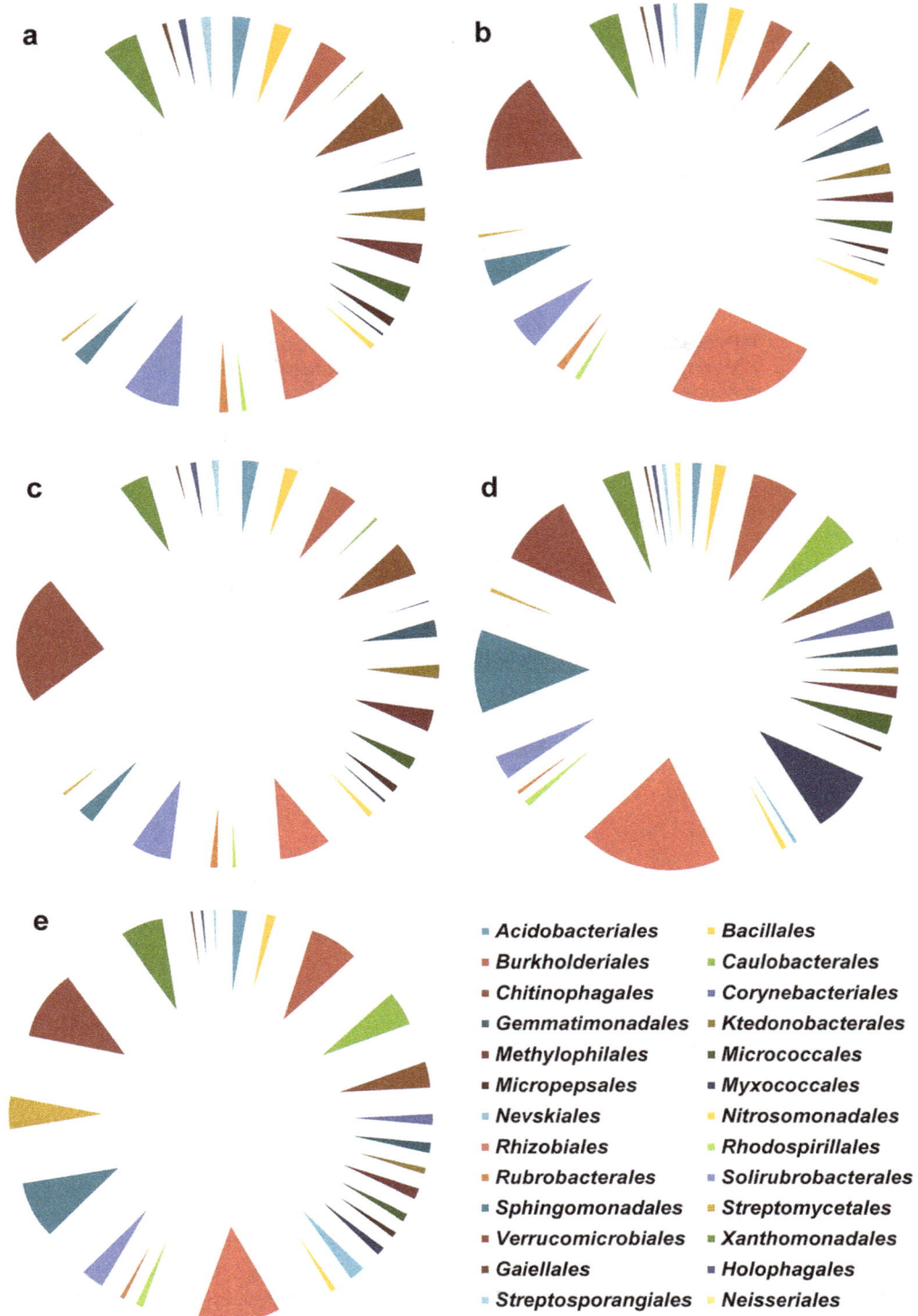

Fig. 4 Relative abundances of bacterial community (> 1%) at the order level. **a–e** Abundances of the bacterial endophytes from Fl, Le, St, Ro, and Fi. The value of each bar represents the mean of $n = 3$

Legend:
- *Acidobacteriales*
- *Bacillales*
- *Burkholderiales*
- *Caulobacterales*
- *Chitinophagales*
- *Corynebacteriales*
- *Gemmatimonadales*
- *Ktedonobacterales*
- *Methylophilales*
- *Micrococcales*
- *Micropepsales*
- *Myxococcales*
- *Nevskiales*
- *Nitrosomonadales*
- *Rhizobiales*
- *Rhodospirillales*
- *Rubrobacterales*
- *Solirubrobacterales*
- *Sphingomonadales*
- *Streptomycetales*
- *Verrucomicrobiales*
- *Xanthomonadales*
- *Gaiellales*
- *Holophagales*
- *Streptosporangiales*
- *Neisseriales*

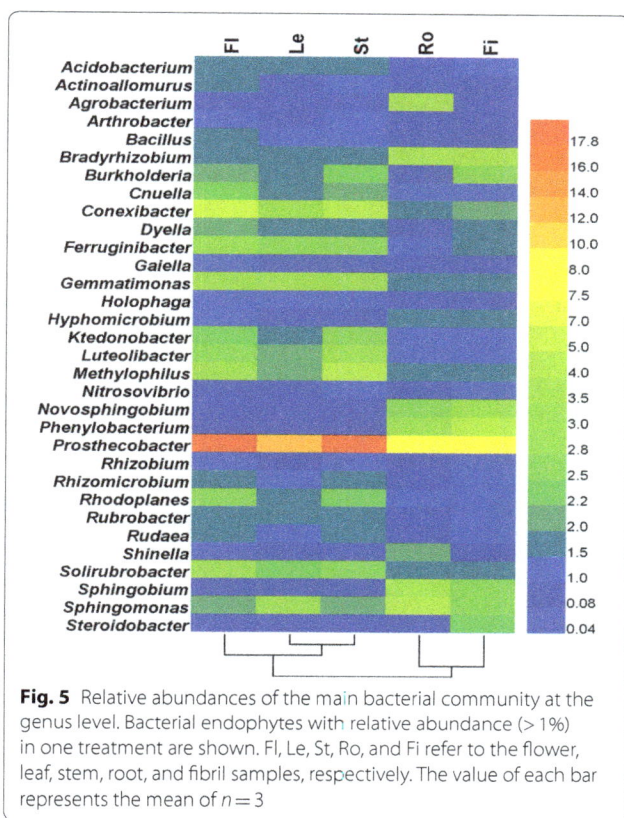

Fig. 5 Relative abundances of the main bacterial community at the genus level. Bacterial endophytes with relative abundance (> 1%) in one treatment are shown. Fl, Le, St, Ro, and Fi refer to the flower, leaf, stem, root, and fibril samples, respectively. The value of each bar represents the mean of $n = 3$

notoginseng represented the ecological niches for bacterial endophytes.

The composition of bacterial endophytes from the aboveground parts varied from that of the underground parts. The composition of bacterial endophytes was associated with the plant compartments [10]. The relative abundances of the bacterial endophytes in all samples showed considerable variations at the phylum and genus levels [19]. The relative abundances of the bacterial endophytes, including *Conexibacter, Gemmatimonas, Holophaga, Luteolibacter, Methylophilus, Prosthecobacter, Solirubrobacter, Bradyrhizobium, Novosphingobium, Phenylobacterium, Sphingobium,* and *Steroidobacter,* in the aboveground and underground parts differed significantly. Evident strains are *Gemmatimonas, Bradyrhizobium, Novosphingobium,* and *Sphingobium,* which can solubilize insoluble elements, induce plant stress resistance or produce antifungal antibiotics [36–39]. Endophytic *Bacillus altitudinis* served as elicitors of biomass and ginsenoside production [13]. Bacterial endophytes from *Zea* displayed anti-fungal activity against two fungal pathogens [40]. Li et al. have reported that the domain genera included *Rhizobium, Sulfurospirillum, Uliginosibacterium, Pseudomonas, Aeromonas* and *Bacteroides,* all of which could fix nitrogen and improve

plant growth [41]. The fungal endophytes communities in *Monarda citriodora* expressed anticancer and antimicrobial activities [42]. In view of the roles played by endophytes in plant growth and biotransformation, our findings contribute to the expansion of endophyte use in the production of *P. notoginseng* and its important metabolites. The information on the differences of endophytes in the aboveground and underground parts can serve as basis for the selection of functional bacteria. Importantly, higher saponins contents were detected in harvest 3-year-old *P. notoginseng* plants [43, 44]. Endophytes increased ginsenoside concentration and reduced morbidity [13, 14]. Thus, 3-year-old *P. notoginseng* plants served as the proper samples to analyze the endophytes. Additionally, the diversity of bacterial endophytes showed richness than fungal endophytes or exogenous bacteria in hour study (data not shown), and we focused on bacterial endophytes in different parts of *P. notoginseng.*

Conclusions
The diversity and composition of bacterial endophytes were associated with different plant parts of *P. notoginseng,* and bacterial endophytes from aboveground parts (flower, leaf, and stem) were distinguished from those from underground parts (root and fibril). Our results described the profiles of bacterial endophytes in *P. notoginseng* parts and provided insight into the exploitation of endophytes in the production of *P. notoginseng* and its important metabolites.

Abbreviations
Fl: flower; Le: leaf; St: stem; Ro: root; Fi: fibril; rRNA: ribosomal RNA; PCR: polymerase chain reaction; PCoA: principal coordinates analysis; RDP: ribosomal database project; OTUs: operational taxonomic units; H': Shannon index.

Authors' contributions
LD designed the work, analyzed the data, and wrote the manuscript. RC analyzed the data and collected samples. LX, GW and FW performed the experiment. JX and XG analyzed the data. YW and ZC performed the field experiment. SC designed the work and wrote this manuscript. All authors read and approved the final manuscript.

Author details
[1] Institute of Chinese Materia Medica, China Academy of Chinese Medical Sciences, Beijing 100700, China. [2] Wenshan Miaoxaing Notoginseng Technology, Co., Ltd., Wenshan 663000, China. [3] Institute of Sanqi Research, Wenshan University, Wenshan 663000, China. [4] College of Agriculture, Ludong University, Yantai 264025, China.

Acknowledgements
We thank Jun Qian for analysis of 16S rRNA gene sequences.

Competing interests
The authors declare that they have no competing interests.

Consent to publish
Not applicable.

Funding
This study was supported by the grants from the Fundamental Research Funds for the Central public welfare research institutes (No. ZXKT17049), Beijing Nova Program (No. Z181100006218020), the Major Science and Technology Programs in Yunnan Province (No. 2016ZF001-001), and the Science and Technology Project of Yantai (No. 2015ZH071).

References
1. Ng T. Pharmacological activity of sanchi ginseng (*Panax notoginseng*). J Pharm Pharmacol. 2006;58:1007–19.
2. Zhang H, Cheng Y. Solid-phase extraction and liquid chromatography-electrospray mass spectrometric analysis of saponins in a Chinese patent medicine of formulated *Salvia miltiorrhizae* and *Panax notoginseng*. J Pharmaceut Biomed. 2006;40:429–32.
3. Liu X, Wang L, Chen X, Deng X, Cao Y, Wang Q. Simultaneous quantification of both triterpenoid and steroidal saponins in various Yunnan Baiyao preparations using HPLC-UV and HPLC-MS. J Sep Sci. 2008;31:3834–46.
4. Du Q, Jerz G, Waibel R, Winterhalter P. Isolation of dammarane saponins from *Panax notoginseng* by high-speed countercurrent chromatography. J Chromatogr A. 2003;1008:173–80.
5. Sun H, Yang Z, Ye Y. Structure and biological activity of protopanaxatriol-type saponins from the roots of *Panax notoginseng*. Int Immunopharmac. 2006;6:14–25.
6. Hu Z, You C, Zhang T. Discussing the obstacles caused by continuous notoginseng cropping. J Wenshan Univ. 2011;24:6–11.
7. Liu L, Liu D, Jing H, Feng G, Zhang J, Wei M, et al. Overview on the mechanisms and control methods of sequential cropping obstacle of *Panax notoginseng* F. H. Chen. J Mountain Agri Biol. 2011;30:70–5.
8. Ma C, Li S, Gu Z, Chen Y. Measures of integrated control of root rot complex of continuous cropping *Panax notoginseng* and their control efficacy. Acta Agri Shanghai. 2006;22:63–8.
9. Larousse M, Rancurel C, Syska C, Palero F, Etienne C, Industri B, et al. Tomato root microbiota and *Phytophthora parasitica*-associated disease. Microbiome. 2017;5:56.
10. Beckers B, De Beek MO, Weyens N, Boerjan W, Vangronsveld J. Structural variability and niche differentiation in the rhizosphere and endosphere bacterial microbiome of field-grown poplar trees. Microbiome. 2017;5:25.
11. Hassan SED. Plant growth-promoting activities for bacterial and fungal endophytes isolated from medicinal plant of *Teucrium polium* L. J Adv Res. 2017;8:687–95.
12. Singh M, Kumar A, Singh R, Pandey K. Endophytic bacteria: a new source of bioactive compounds. Biotech. 2017;7:315.
13. Song X, Wu H, Yin Z, Lian M, Yin C. Endophytic bacteria isolated from *Panax ginseng* improved ginsenoside accumulation in adventitious ginseng root culture. Molecules. 2017;22:837.
14. Gao Y, Liu Q, Zang P, Li X, Ji Q, He Z, et al. An endophytic bacterium isolated from *Panax ginseng* C.A. Meyer enhances growth, reduces morbidity, and stimulates ginsenoside biosynthesis. Phytochem Lett. 2015;125:132–8.
15. Van Overbeek L, van Elsas J. Effects of plant genotype and growth stage on the structure of bacterial communities associated with potato (*Solanum tuberosum* L.). FEMS Microbiol Ecol. 2008;64:283–96.
16. Chowdhury E, Jeon J, Rim S, Park Y, Lee S, Bae H. Composition, diversity and bioactivity of culturable bacterial endophytes in mountain-cultivated ginseng in Korea. Sci Rep. 2017;7:10098.
17. Tan Y, Cui Y, Li H, Kuang A, Li X, Wei Y, et al. Diversity and composition of rhizospheric soil and root endogenous bacteria in *Panax notoginseng* during continuous cropping practices. J Basic Microb. 2016;9999:1–8.
18. Bodenhausen N, Horton M, Bergelson J. Bacterial communities associated with the leaves and the roots of Arabidopsis thaliana. PLoS ONE. 2013;8:e56329.

19. Jin H, Yang X, Yan Z, Liu Q, Li X, Chen J, et al. Characterization of rhizosphere and endophytic bacterial communities from leaves, stems and roots of medicinal *Stellera chamaejasme* L. Syst Appl Microbiol. 2014;37:376–85.
20. Dong L, Xu J, Feng G, Li X, Chen S. Soil bacterial and fungal community dynamics in relation to *Panax notoginseng* death rate in a continuous cropping system. Sci Rep. 2016;6:31802.
21. Dong L, Xu J, Zhang L, Yang J, Liao B, Li X, et al. High-throughput sequencing technology reveals that continuous cropping of American ginseng results in changes in the microbial community in arable soil. Chin Med. 2017;12:18.
22. Wani Z, Ashraf N, Mohiuddin T, Riyaz-Ul-Hassan S. Plant-endophyte symbiosis, an ecological perspective. Appl Microbiol Biotechnol. 2015;99:2955–65.
23. Kaul S, Sharma T, Dhar M. "Omics" tools for better understanding the plant-endophyte interactions. Front Plant Sci. 2016;7:955.
24. Checcucci A, Maida I, Bacci G, Ninno C, Bilia A, Biffi S, et al. Is the plant-associated microbiota of *Thymus* spp. adapted to plant essential oil? Res Microbiol. 2016;3:276–87.
25. Akinsanya M, Goh J, Lim S, Ting A. Diversity, antimicrobial and antioxidant activities of culturable bacterial endophyte communities in *Aloe vera*. FEMS Microbiol Lett. 2015;362:184.
26. Jackson C, Randolph K, Osborn S, Tyler H. Culture dependent and independent analysis of bacterial communities associated with commercial salad leaf vegetables. BMC Microbiol. 2013;13:274.
27. Dong L, Xu J, Zhang L, Cheng R, Wei G, Su H, Yang J, Qian J, Xu R, Chen S. Rhizospheric microbial communities are driven by *Panax ginseng* at different growth stages and biocontrol bacteria alleviates replanting mortality. Acta Pharm Sin B. 2018;8:272–82.
28. Dong L, Xu J, Li Y, Fang H, Niu W, Li X, et al. Manipulation of microbial community in the rhizosphere alleviates the replanting issues in *Panax ginseng*. Soil Biol Biochem. 2018;125:64–74.
29. Fierer N, Jackson J, Vilgalys R, Jackson R. Assessment of soil microbial community structure by use of taxon-specific quantitative PCR assays. Appl Environ Microbiol. 2005;71:4117–20.
30. Caporaso J, Bittinger K, Bushman F, DeSantis T, Andersen G, Knight R. PyNAST: a flexible tool for aligning sequences to a template alignment. Phylogenetics. 2010;26:266–7.
31. Katherine R, Carl J, Angela K, Nicoletta R, Franck C, Alejandro E, et al. Habitat degradation impacts black howler monkey (*Alouatta pigra*) gastrointestinal microbiomes. ISME J. 2013;7:1344–53.
32. Schloss P, Westcott S, Ryabin T, Hall J, Hartmann M, Hollister E, et al. Introducing mothur: open-source, platform-independent, community-supported software for describing and comparing microbial communities. Appl Environ Micro. 2009;75:7537–41.
33. Lozupone C, Lladser M, Dan K, Stombaugh J, Knight R. UniFrac: an effective distance metric for microbial community comparison. ISME J. 2010;5:169.
34. Oksanen J, Blanchet F, Kindt R, Simpson G. Vegan: community ecology package. Version 2.0-10. J Stat Softw. 2011;48:1–21.
35. Haruna E, Zin N, Kerfahi D, Adams J. Extensive overlap of tropical rainforest bacterial endophytes between soil, plant parts, and plant species. Microb Ecol. 2017. https://doi.org/10.1007/s00248-017-1002-2.
36. Mahanty T, Bhattacharjee S, Goswami M, Bhattacharyya P, Das B, Ghosh A, Tribedi P. Biofertilizers: a potential approach for sustainable agriculture development. Environ Sci Pollut Res Int. 2017;24:3315–35.
37. Berendsen RL, Pieterse CMJ, Bakker PHM. The rhizosphere microbiome and plant health. Trends Plant Sci. 2012;17:478–86.
38. Egamberdiyeva D. The effect of plant growth promoting bacteria on growth and nutrient uptake of maize in two different soils. Appl Soil Ecol. 2007;36:184–9.
39. Verma JP, Yadav J, Tiwari KN, Lavakush SV. Impact of plant growth promoting rhizobacteria on crop production. Int J Agri Res. 2010;5:954–83.
40. Shehata H, Lyons E, Jordan K, Raizada M. Relevance of in vitro agar based screens to characterize the anti-fungal activities of bacterial endophyte communities. BMC Microbiol. 2016;16:8.

41. Li Y, Liu Q, Liu Y, Zhu J, Zhang Q. Endophytic bacterial diversity in roots of *Typha angustifolia* L. in the constructed Beijing Cuihu Wetland (China). Res Microbiol. 2011;162:124–31.

42. Katoch M, Phull S, Vaid S, Singh S. Diversity, Phylogeny, anticancer and antimicrobial potential of fungal endophytes associated with *Monarda citriodora* L. BMC Microbiol. 2017;17:44.

43. Wei G, Dong L, Yang J, Zhang L, Xu J, Yang F, et al. Integrated metabolomic and transcriptomic analyses revealed the distribution of saponins in Panax notoginseng. Acta Pharm Sin B. 2018;8:458–65.

44. Yang J, Dong L, Wei G, Hu H, Zhu G, Zhang J, et al. Identification and quality of *Panax notoginseng* and *Panax vietnamensis* var. *fuscidicus* through integrated DNA barcoding and HPLC. Chin Herbal Med. 2018;10:177–83.

3

Approaches in studying the pharmacology of Chinese Medicine formulas: bottom-up, top-down—and meeting in the middle

Tao Huang[1], Linda L. D. Zhong[1,2], Chen-Yuan Lin[1,3], Ling Zhao[1], Zi-Wan Ning[1], Dong-Dong Hu[1], Man Zhang[1,4], Ke Tian[1], Chung-Wah Cheng[2], Zhao-Xiang Bian[1,2]* and for MZRW Research Group

Abstract

Investigating the pharmacology is key to the modernization of Chinese Medicine (CM) formulas. However, identifying which are the active compound(s) of CM formulas, which biological entities they target, and through which signaling pathway(s) they act to modify disease symptoms, are still difficult tasks for researchers, even when equipped with an arsenal of advanced modern technologies. Multiple approaches, including network pharmacology, pharmaco-genomics, -proteomics, and -metabolomics, have been developed to study the pharmacology of CM formulas. They fall into two general categories in terms of how they tackle a problem: bottom-up and top-down. In this article, we compared these two different approaches in several dimensions by using the case of MaZiRenWan (MZRW, also known as Hemp Seed Pill), a CM herbal formula for functional constipation. Multiple hypotheses are easy to be proposed in the bottom-up approach (e.g. network pharmacology); but these hypotheses are usually false positives and hard to be tested. In contrast, it is hard to suggest hypotheses in the top-down approach (e.g. pharmacometabolomics); however, once a hypothesis is proposed, it is much easier to be tested. Merging of these two approaches could results in a powerful approach, which could be the new paradigm for the pharmacological study of CM formulas.

Keywords: Bottom-up, Chinese medicine formula, Focused network pharmacology, Pharmacometabolomics, Top-down

Background

Unknown active constituents and unclear mechanism-of-actions have sparked criticism when Chinese medicine (CM) formula is getting more popular today [1, 2]. Thus, investigating the pharmacology is important to the modernization of CM formula. However, the pharmacological study of a CM formula is much more complicated than that of a single compound. With a single compound study, researchers need only determine which biological

target(s) it acts on, and which disease pathway(s) it alters (Fig. 1a). With a formula study, there is much more to be done and many more factors to be considered. Firstly, the CM formula is comprised of several herbs, each of which contains hundreds, possibly thousands, of compounds, many of which could be unique to that herb. Secondly, not all the compounds from herb are involved in the pharmacological activity—some of them are removed during preparation, while some of them are just passed by. Thirdly, most compounds from herbs are weak modulators of biological targets, thus the effect of an individual compound is hard to determine. Fourthly, the herbal compounds may have multiple pharmacological actions, some of which are not directly correlated with symptom

*Correspondence: bianzxiang@gmail.com
[2] Hong Kong Chinese Medicine Clinical Study Centre, Hong Kong Baptist University, Room 307, Jockey Club School of Chinese Medicine, 7 Baptist University Road, Kowloon, Hong Kong, Hong Kong SAR, China

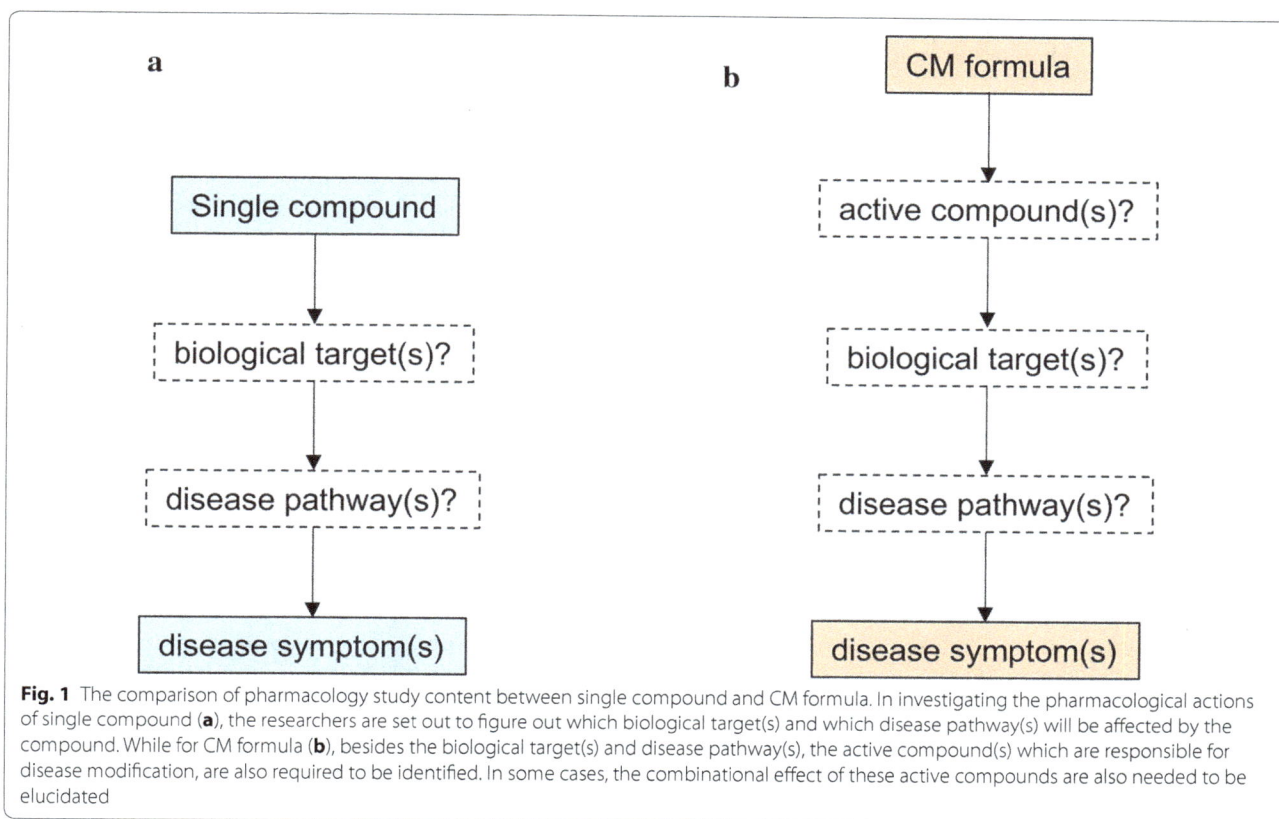

Fig. 1 The comparison of pharmacology study content between single compound and CM formula. In investigating the pharmacological actions of single compound (**a**), the researchers are set out to figure out which biological target(s) and which disease pathway(s) will be affected by the compound. While for CM formula (**b**), besides the biological target(s) and disease pathway(s), the active compound(s) which are responsible for disease modification, are also required to be identified. In some cases, the combinational effect of these active compounds are also needed to be elucidated

improvement; to identify the targets and pathways that are truly involved is not easy. Lastly, the complex interactions (synergistic or antagonistic) between herb compounds are hard to determine.

Multiple approaches have been utilized and developed for investigating the pharmacology of CM formula, including network pharmacology, pharmaco-genomics, -proteomics, and -metabolomics. These approaches have been successfully applied in studying the pharmacology of the Liu-Wei-Di-Huang pill, Qing-Luo-Yin, and other CM formulas [3–11]. In particular, there are reviews discussing the theory, methodology and applications of CM network pharmacology [12–19]. We used several of these methodologies to investigate the pharmacology of a CM formula MaZiRenWan (MZRW, also known as Hemp Seed Pill) [20, 21]. Based on the nature, we observe that most of these approaches fall into one of two categories in terms of how they tackle the problem: bottom-up, or top-down (Fig. 2).

In the context of medicinal herb research, by bottom-up, we mean starting with the many smaller units, i.e. isolated constituents, and determining their larger role in a disease pathway (Fig. 2a). By top-down, we mean starting with the disease pathway, and determining which constituents are involved in regulating it (Fig. 2b). These two contrasting approaches are equally effective—and are

seen in other contexts such as nanotechnology, neuroscience, psychology, public health, ecology, management, and organization [22]. For example, in cognitive process, bottom-up cognition is focusing on details primarily, then the whole landscape. While a top-down approach is used by the person who focus on the big picture first and from that figure out details to support it [23]. In this article, we will compare these two distinct approaches in the investigation of pharmacology of one CM formula, MZRW for functional constipation (FC).

MZRW is an herbal formula for constipation from traditional chinese medicine (TCM). About 2000 years ago, MZRW was firstly recorded in *Discussion of Cold-Induced Disorders* (*Shang Han Lun*) [24, 25]. It is comprised of six herbs, namely *Fructus cannabis* (*Huo Ma Ren*), *Radix et rhizoma rhei* (*Da Huang*), *Semen Armeniacae Amarum* (*Ku Xing Ren*), *Radix paeoniae Albo* (*Bai Shao*), *Cortex magnolia officinalis* (*Hou Pu*), and *Fructus aurantii immaturus* (*Zhi Shi*) [26]. In TCM theory, MZRW can drain heat, unblock the bowel, promote the movement of Qi, and moisten the intestines [26].

We chose MZRW because a systematic review of the published literature showed that MZRW is the most frequently used TCM formula for constipation [27] yet there is little if any strict clinical evidence of its efficacy. To that end, we demonstrated that MZRW is significantly

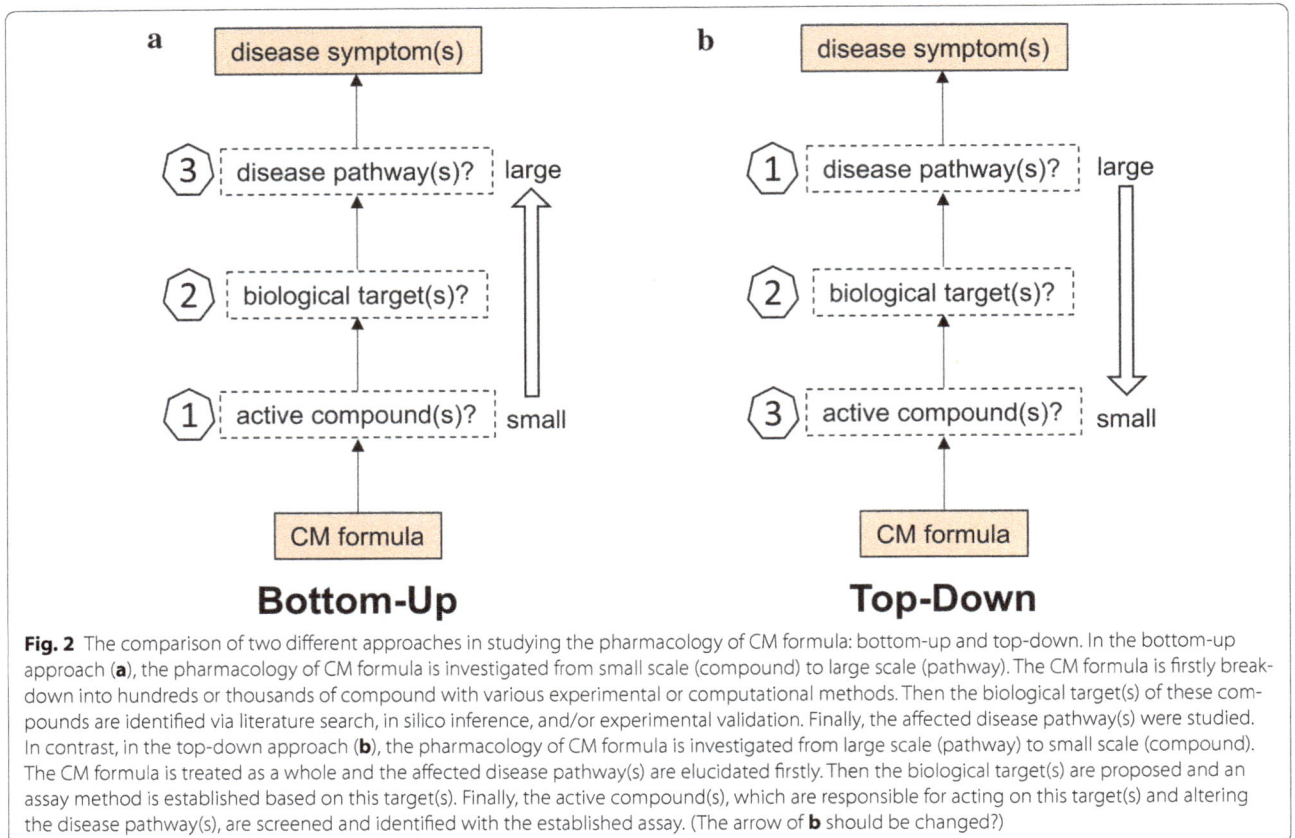

Fig. 2 The comparison of two different approaches in studying the pharmacology of CM formula: bottom-up and top-down. In the bottom-up approach (**a**), the pharmacology of CM formula is investigated from small scale (compound) to large scale (pathway). The CM formula is firstly break-down into hundreds or thousands of compound with various experimental or computational methods. Then the biological target(s) of these compounds are identified via literature search, in silico inference, and/or experimental validation. Finally, the affected disease pathway(s) were studied. In contrast, in the top-down approach (**b**), the pharmacology of CM formula is investigated from large scale (pathway) to small scale (compound). The CM formula is treated as a whole and the affected disease pathway(s) are elucidated firstly. Then the biological target(s) are proposed and an assay method is established based on this target(s). Finally, the active compound(s), which are responsible for acting on this target(s) and altering the disease pathway(s), are screened and identified with the established assay. (The arrow of **b** should be changed?)

better than placebo in improvement of bowel movement during drug treatment, while such effect is more sustainable than placebo during 8 weeks follow-up, in the randomized, placebo-controlled clinical study with 120 FC patients [26]. Recently, we have finished a larger clinical study including 291 FC patients to compare the efficacy of MZRW with that of Senna (commonly used laxative in Hong Kong) and placebo [28]. The results showed that, both MZRW and Senna are better than placebo during the treatment period; while the efficacy of MZRW is more sustainable than that of Senna and placebo in the follow-up period. We also identified ten major compounds from MZRW in rat plasma by UPLC–MS/MS [29] to facilitate the pharmacokinetic study of MZRW in healthy volunteers [30].

On top of this solid clinical evidence and pharmacokinetic data, we set out to elucidate the pharmacology of MZRW for FC. We tried different methodologies to determine (1) which active compound(s) are in MZRW, and how they act (2) on which biological target(s), (3) through which signaling pathway(s) to alter the bowel movement, as slow bowel movement is the major symptom of FC patients. Doing this work eventually we realized that every methodology has its own advantages and

disadvantages, but they can be compared in an efficient way: bottom-up versus top-down (Table 1). In the following sections we will first describe these two different approaches; then describe their application in the analysis of MZRW; and conclude with the take-home lessons for doing similar research on other CM formulas.

Bottom-up approaches

In the bottom-up approach, researchers start with compounds, look for biological targets, and work toward understanding the biochemistry of the disease pathway(s) (Fig. 2a).

Network pharmacology is the representative methodology of the bottom-up approach. Firstly, the compounds have been identified as constituents of these herbs of CM formula via literature/database search, and/or LC–MS identification, etc. Secondly, the known biological targets of these compounds are collected by literature/database search and/or predicted by various computational tools, such as inverse docking, bioactivity spectra analysis, and chemical similarity searching. Thirdly, the biological targets are used to build a network based on a molecular interaction database, and the relevant signaling pathways can be focused on with enrichment analysis

Table 1 Bottom-up and top-down approaches in pharmacological research of CM formula

Approach	Bottom-up	Top-down
Representative methodology	Network pharmacology	Pharmacogenomics, Pharmacoproteomics, Pharmcometabolomics
Question solving order	From small (compounds) to large (disease pathways)	From large (biological pathways) to small (compound)
Hypothesis forming	Easy	Hard
Multiple hypotheses producing	Yes	No, usually single
Hypothesis testing	Hard	Easy

tools. Finally, by using this network, the hypotheses, that which compound(s) could modify the disease symptoms through which target(s)/pathway(s), are generated. Then each potentially active compound is tested to determine whether it, in fact, affects the pathways involved in the disease. In general, it is easy to generate multiple hypotheses with network pharmacology. However, inevitably, a number of these hypotheses are just false positives, and testing so many hypotheses is mission impossible (Table 1), as can be seen with our work on MZRW [21].

The first problem is the huge number of compounds in any herbal formula. There are only six herbs in MZRW; however, the number of unique compounds in these six herbs, based on a database constructed from a literature search, is greater than one thousand. Due to one compound could act on multiple targets, one thousand compounds would result in ten thousand hypotheses; it would be impractical if not impossible to test them all. Thus, we used several ways to reduce the number of candidate compounds. Firstly, the compounds that were detected in extracts and biological samples with LC-MS were kept, while the remaining were discarded. This method resulted in 97 candidate compounds, a feasible number for testing. Secondly, to reduce redundancy, we used chemical structure clustering analysis to classify the 97 compounds into small component groups. Within each component group, the candidate compounds are similar to each other. Based on the well-known observation that "similar compounds have similar bioactivities" [31], a compound was selected from each component group and its pharmacological action was considered representative of that group (Fig. 3). Thirdly, we used rat colonic segments in an organ bath to determine which, if any, of these representative compounds enhanced colonic motility, in the phenotypic symptom we had chosen to model FC. Finally, we had 5 representative compounds that were active in reducing FC: emodin, amygdalin, albiflorin, honokiol, and naringin.

The second problem with network pharmacology in particular and the bottom-up approach in general is similar to the first: there are a huge number of hitting biological targets. Within a literature/database search and chemical similarity search [32], we found 10 + targets for each of the 5 representative compounds. Although there might be some novel targets related to disease modification, we still thought that the number of biological targets that could explain the pharmacological actions of MZRW was overestimated. To solve this problem, we checked the target-disease link with a literature search. Finally,

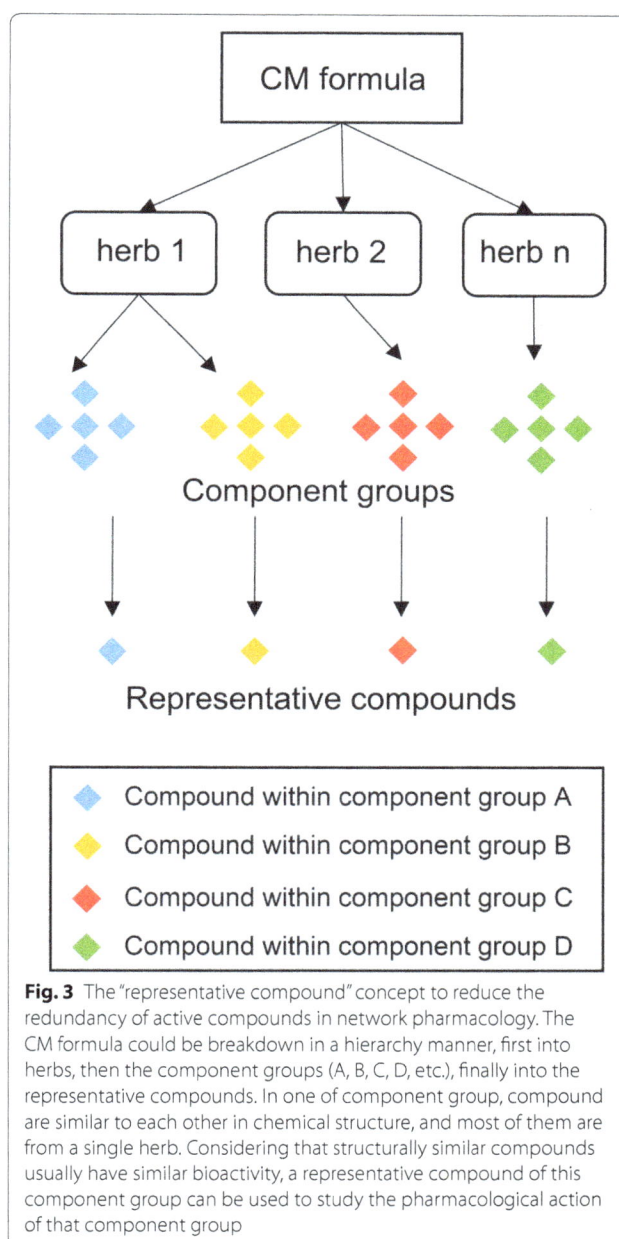

Fig. 3 The "representative compound" concept to reduce the redundancy of active compounds in network pharmacology. The CM formula could be breakdown in a hierarchy manner, first into herbs, then the component groups (A, B, C, D, etc.), finally into the representative compounds. In one of component group, compound are similar to each other in chemical structure, and most of them are from a single herb. Considering that structurally similar compounds usually have similar bioactivity, a representative compound of this component group can be used to study the pharmacological action of that component group

7 targets (ACHE, ESR2, CYP19A1, PTGS1, PTGS2, ADORA1, CNR1), either referenced in the literature or predicted by computational tool, were found have direct link with constipation.

The third problem is the large number of predicted pathways. Previous reported network pharmacology studies suggest huge networks involving dozens or hundreds signaling pathways. However, most of these pathways are not directly related with disease modifications, and testing such pathways would cause time and funding waste in experimental validation. For our purposes, only the disease pathways matters. With all the efforts described above, we were able to minimize the number of predicted pathways into five disease pathways: acetylcholine-, estrogen-, prostaglandin-, cannabinoid-, and purine. All of them have been shown to be related with bowel movement evidenced by human and animal studies.

In summary, in the traditional network pharmacology, a huge number of compounds, targets, and pathways generates too many hypotheses to be tested in real time. With MZRW, only by selecting representative compounds, targets and pathways were we able to generate a feasible number of hypotheses for testing. This new approach was named after "focused network pharmacology" [21].

Top-down approaches

In the top-down approach, the researchers solve the key questions in the large-to-small manner: from disease pathway(s), to biological target(s), to compound(s) (Fig. 2b). Compared with the bottom-up approach (network pharmacology), the top-down approach is relatively less used in studying the pharmacology of CM formulas [33, 34].

Representative methodologies of top-down approach are pharmaco-omics, including pharmacogenomics, pharmacoproteomics, and pharmacometabolomics. Pharmaco-omics has two meaning. The first would be to study the effects of a CM formula on specific biomarkers (genes, proteins, metabolites, etc.) during drug treatment. The second would be study of the effects of a specific genotype (or protein/metabolite level) on the efficacy of treatment CM formula. Here we use the first definition. Firstly, change of biomarker levels in samples (biofluids or tissues) before and after drug treatment are measured with genomics, proteomics or metabolomics technologies. Significant altered biomarkers are attributed to the drug treatment effect. To select specific biomarkers for further study, the biomarker alteration profile of the drug treatment group is compared with that of placebo group, or positive drug group. The effect of a CM formula on such specific biomarkers and associated

disease pathway is validated through animal study. Secondly, within the focused disease pathway, one protein is proposed as a candidate target on which the CM formula acts. Thirdly, by using this target, an easy-to-handle screening assay is established and used to identify active compounds from the CM formula. Although it is quite hard, after a few hypotheses are suggested, they are readily validated through animal study (Table 1). We will explain the process in detail with our pharmacometabolomic (top-down) study of MZRW [20].

In the first step, we used samples and data from our previous clinical study comparing the efficacy of MZRW with that of Senna and placebo in 291 FC patients [28]. During this study, we randomly collected serum samples before and after treatment. The serum samples were subjected to untargeted metabolomics analysis, and about 2700 fragments were found in positive and negative modes. The degree of change in these fragments before and after treatment in each patient was calculated, and these alterations were correlated with the improvement of complete spontaneous bowel movement (CSBM), the major endpoint of this clinical study. By comparing the correlation profile in three groups, we found several fragments were significantly correlated with the CSBM improvement in MZRW group, but not in Senna or placebo groups. After analysis with Metabolite and Tandem MS Database (https://metlin.scripps.edu), 15 of these fragments were identified, and 4 of them were found to be structurally closely related to the fatty acid amide (FAA). The one with the most significant correlation of MZRW efficacy was oleamide, an endogenous FAA which is well-known for intestinal motility regulation [35]. Based on this complex analysis, we were able to link MZRW with the oleamide signaling pathway (the disease pathway).

In the second step, we tested which proteins in the oleamide signaling pathways are affected by MZRW. In the mouse models, we found that, the colonic fatty acid amide hydrolase (FAAH) was significantly up-regulated in colon tissue after MZRW treatment. Thus, we identified FAAH as the major target of MZRW for FC.

To complete the third step, we are establishing a cell-based assay to test which compounds from MZRW may regulate FAAH to control the level of oleamide in the colon. At this rate, we predict it will take several years to finish the compound screening; however, we have confidence we will ultimately succeed.

In summary, the most difficult part of the top-down approach is identifying which disease pathway is affected by the CM formula. Sample collection can take years and the data analysis is complex; however, once the hypothesis is generated, it is easy to be tested. We believe that advances in technology/computation will speed things up and make the top-down approaches are more feasible.

Conclusions

In this article, we compared the bottom-up and top-down approaches in the study of CM herbal formula, particular with the example of MZRW for FC. The bottom-up approach starts with compounds and ends with biological pathways or networks; while the top-down approach begins with pathways and ends with individual compounds. Multiple hypotheses are readily proposed in the bottom-up approach (e.g. network pharmacology); but these hypotheses are hard to test due to the huge numbers of compounds/targets/pathways and high false positive predictions. In contrast, long-term sample collection and complex data analysis makes it hard to suggest hypotheses in the top-down approach; however, once a hypothesis is found, it is much easier to be tested. In the past decade, the bottom-up approach has been frequently applied to CM formulas, but the impact was restricted because it is relatively less testable. In the future, the top-down approach would be more favorably adopted by the researchers, because it is much more testable and will deliver more accurate and concentrated results.

We also image a hybrid model where the bottom-up and top-down approaches meet in the middle. This new approach, utilizing the predicted and validated compound-target link in the bottom-up approach, in the compound screening process of the top-down approach, could reduce the time and cost of identifying the active compounds. The merging of two distinct approaches, bottom-up and top-down, will generate a powerful new approach in the study of the pharmacology of CM formula in the near future.

Abbreviations
CM: Chinese medicine; CSBM: complete spontaneous bowel movement; FAA: fatty acid amide; FAAH: fatty acid amide hydrolase; FC: functional constipation; MZRW: MaZiRenWan; TCM: traditional Chinese medicine.

Authors' contributions
ZXB and TH designed this article. TH carried out the data collection and analysis. TH and ZXB wrote the manuscript. LLDZ, CWC, CYL, LZ, ZWN, DDH, KT and MZ made contributions to the manuscript preparation. All authors read and approved the final manuscript.

Author details
[1] Institute of Brain and Gut Research, School of Chinese Medicine, Hong Kong Baptist University, Room 307, Jockey Club School of Chinese Medicine, 7 Baptist University Road, Kowloon, Hong Kong, Hong Kong SAR, China. [2] Hong Kong Chinese Medicine Clinical Study Centre, Hong Kong Baptist University, Room 307, Jockey Club School of Chinese Medicine, 7 Baptist University Road, Kowloon, Hong Kong, Hong Kong SAR, China. [3] YMU-HKBU Joint Laboratory of Traditional Natural Medicine, Yunnan Minzu University, Kunming 650500, China. [4] Guangzhou Research Institute of Snake Venom, Guangzhou Medical University, Guangzhou 510000, China.

Acknowledgements
The authors thank all the members of the MZRW research group, including Shu-hai Lin and Yan-hong Li for their great help and support.

Competing interests
The authors declare that they have no competing interests.

Consent to publish
Not applicable.

Funding
This study was supported by Health and Health Services Fund, Hong Kong SAR, P. R. China (Project No. 09101501) and Shenzhen Science and Technology Innovations Committee (No. JCYJ20140419130444178).

References
1. Coghlan ML, Haile J, Houston J, Murray DC, White NE, Moolhuijzen P, Bellgard MI, Bunce M. Deep sequencing of plant and animal DNA contained within traditional Chinese medicines reveals legality issues and health safety concerns. PLoS Genet. 2012;8(4):e1002657.
2. Chen CH, Dickman KG, Moriya M, Zavadil J, Sidorenko VS, Edwards KL, Gnatenko DV, Wu L, Turesky RJ, Wu XR, et al. Aristolochic acid-associated urothelial cancer in Taiwan. Proc Natl Acad Sci USA. 2012;109(21):8241–6.
3. Wu L, Gao X, Cheng Y, Wang Y, Zhang B, Fan X. Symptom-based traditional Chinese medicine slices relationship network and its network pharmacology study. Zhongguo Zhong yao za zhi = Zhongguo zhongyao zazhi = China Journal of Chinese Materia Medica. 2011;36(21):2916–9.
4. Liu Q, Zhang Z, Fang L, Jiang Y, Yin X. Application of network pharmacology and high through-put technology on active compounds screening from traditional Chinese medicine. Zhongguo Zhong yao za zhi = Zhongguo zhongyao zazhi = China Journal of Chinese Materia Medica. 2012;37(2):134–7.
5. Xu H, Huang L, Lu P, Yang H. Application of ADME process in vivo in combination with network pharmacology in study of traditional Chinese medicine. Zhongguo Zhong yao za zhi = Zhongguo zhongyao zazhi = China Journal of Chinese Materia Medica. 2012;37(2):142–5.
6. Zhang X, Gu J, Cao L, Li N, Ma Y, Su Z, Ding G, Chen L, Xu X, Xiao W. Network pharmacology study on the mechanism of traditional Chinese medicine for upper respiratory tract infection. Mol BioSyst. 2014;10(10):2517–25.
7. Lu M, Wang TY, Tian XX, Shi XH, Fan GW, Zhang Y, Zhu Y. Interaction of anti-thrombotic and anti-inflammatory activities of commonly used traditional Chinese medicine for promoting blood circulation and removing blood stasis revealed by network pharmacology analysis. Yao xue xue bao =Acta Pharmaceutica Sinica. 2015;50(9):1135–41.
8. Hu RF, Sun XB. Design of new traditional Chinese medicine herbal formulae for treatment of type 2 diabetes mellitus based on network pharmacology. Chin J Nat Med. 2017;15(6):436–41.
9. Suo T, Liu J, Chen X, Yu H, Wang T, Li C, Wang Y, Wang C, Li Z. Combining chemical profiling and network analysis to investigate the pharmacology of complex prescriptions in traditional Chinese medicine. Sci Rep. 2017;7:40529.
10. Tang HC, Huang HJ, Lee CC, Chen CYC. Network pharmacology-based approach of novel traditional Chinese medicine formula for treatment of acute skin inflammation in silico. Comput Biol Chem. 2017;71:70–81.
11. Zhang B, Wang X, Li S. An integrative platform of TCM network pharmacology and its application on a herbal formula, Qing-Luo-Yin. Evid-Based Complement Altern Med eCAM. 2013;2013:456747.
12. Li S. Network target: a starting point for traditional Chinese medicine network pharmacology. Zhongguo Zhong yao za zhi = Zhongguo zhongyao zazhi = China Journal of Chinese Materia Medica. 2011;36(15):2017–20.
13. Li J, Lu C, Jiang M, Niu X, Guo H, Li L, Bian Z, Lin N, Lu A. Traditional chinese medicine-based network pharmacology could lead to new multicompound drug discovery. Evid-based Complement Altern Med eCAM. 2012;2012:149762.

14. Liu ZH, Sun XB. Network pharmacology: new opportunity for the modernization of traditional Chinese medicine. Yao xue xue bao = Acta Pharmaceutica Sinica. 2012;47(6):696–703.

15. Li S, Zhang B. Traditional Chinese medicine network pharmacology: theory, methodology and application. Chin J Nat Med. 2013;11(2):110–20.

16. Yang M, Chen JL, Xu LW, Ji G. Navigating traditional chinese medicine network pharmacology and computational tools. Evid-Based Complement Altern Med eCAM. 2013;2013:731969.

17. da Hao C, Xiao PG. Network pharmacology: a Rosetta Stone for traditional Chinese medicine. Drug Dev Res. 2014;75(5):299–312.

18. Li S, Fan TP, Jia W, Lu A, Zhang W. Network pharmacology in traditional chinese medicine. Evid-Based Complement Altern Med eCAM. 2014;2014:138460.

19. Wu XM, Wu CF. Network pharmacology: a new approach to unveiling traditional Chinese medicine. Chin J Nat Med. 2015;13(1):1–2.

20. Huang T, Zhao L, Lin C-y, Lu L, Ning Z-w, Zhong LDD, Yang ZJ, Bian ZX. Chinese herbal medicine (MaZiRenWan) improves bowel movement in functional constipation through down-regulating oleamide. 2018 (unpublished data).

21. Huang T, Ning ZW, Hu DD, Zhang M, Zhao L, Lin CY, Zhong LLD, Yang ZJ, Xu HX, Bian ZX. Uncovering the mechanisms of Chinese herbal medicine (MaZiRenWan) for functional constipation by focused network pharmacology approach. Front Pharmacol. 2018;9:270. https://doi.org/10.3389/fphar.2018.00270.

22. Top-down and bottom-up design. https://en.wikipedia.org/wiki/Top-down_and_bottom-up_design. Accessed 20 Feb 2018.

23. Biederman I, Glass AL, Stacy EW. Searching for objects in real-world scenes. J Exp Psychol. 1973;97(1):22.

24. Mitchell C, Chang C-C, Ye F, Wiseman N, Zhang Z. Shang Han Lun: on cold damage, translation and commentaries. Brookline: Paradigm Publications; 1998.

25. Zhang Z, Ye F, Wiseman N, Mitchell C, Feng Y. Shang Han Lun: on cold damage, translation and commentaries. Brookline: Paradigm Publications; 1999.

26. Cheng CW, Bian ZX, Zhu LX, Wu JC, Sung JJ. Efficacy of a Chinese herbal proprietary medicine (Hemp Seed Pill) for functional constipation. Am J Gastroenterol. 2011;106(1):120–9.

27. Zhong LL, Zheng G, Da Ge L, Lin CY, Huang T, Zhao L, Lu C, Lu AP, Bian ZX. Chinese herbal medicine for constipation: zheng-based associations among herbs, formulae, proprietary medicines, and herb-drug interactions. Chin Med. 2016;11:28.

28. Zhong LL, Cheng CW, Kun W, Dai L, Hu DD, Ning ZW, Xiao HT, Lin CY, Zhao L, Huang T, Tian K, Chan KH, Lam TW, Chen XR, Wong CT, Li M, Lu AP, Wu CY, Bian ZX. Chinese herbal medicine (MaZiRenWan) improves functional constipation with excessive pattern versus Senna and placebo. 2018 (provisionally accepted).

29. Hu D-D, Han Q-B, Zhong LL-D, Li Y-H, Lin C-Y, Ho H-M, Zhang M, Lin S-H, Zhao L, Huang T. Simultaneous determination of ten compounds in rat plasma by UPLC-MS/MS: application in the pharmacokinetic study of Ma-Zi-Ren-Wan. J Chromatogr B. 2015;1000:136–46.

30. Hu DD, Zhong LLD, Kun W, Mu HX, Lin CY, Zhao L, Dai L, Huang T, Bian ZX. Evaluation of the pharmacokinetics and renal excretion of Ma-Zi-Ren-Wan in health subjects. World J Tradit Chin Med. 2017;3(2):8–15.

31. Bender A, Glen RC. Molecular similarity: a key technique in molecular informatics. Org Biomol Chem. 2004;2(22):3204–18.

32. Huang T, Mi H, Lin CY, Zhao L, Zhong LL, Liu FB, Zhang G, Lu AP, Bian ZX, for MG. MOST: most-similar ligand based approach to target prediction. BMC Bioinform. 2017;18(1):165.

33. Sun H, Zhang A, Yan G, Han Y, Sun W, Ye Y, Wang X. Proteomics study on the hepatoprotective effects of traditional Chinese medicine formulae Yin-Chen-Hao-Tang by a combination of two-dimensional polyacrylamide gel electrophoresis and matrix-assisted laser desorption/ionization-time of flight mass spectrometry. J Pharm Biomed Anal. 2013;75:173–9.

34. Wang X, Wang Q, Zhang A, Zhang F, Zhang H, Sun H, Cao H, Zhang H. Metabolomics study of intervention effects of Wen-Xin-Formula using ultra high-performance liquid chromatography/mass spectrometry coupled with pattern recognition approach. J Pharm Biomed Anal. 2013;74:22–30.

35. Capasso R, Matias I, Lutz B, Borrelli F, Capasso F, Marsicano G, Mascolo N, Petrosino S, Monory K, Valenti M, et al. Fatty acid amide hydrolase controls mouse intestinal motility in vivo. Gastroenterology. 2005;129(3):941–51.

4

Cost-consequence analysis of salvianolate injection for the treatment of coronary heart disease

Pengxin Dong[1,2†], Hao Hu[3†] ⓘ, Xiaodong Guan[4], Carolina Oi Lam Ung[3], Luwen Shi[2,4], Sheng Han[2*] and Shuwen Yu[1,5*]

Abstract

Background: Complicated with the impact of aging population and urbanization, coronary heart disease (CHD) incurs more and more disease burdens in China. Salvianolate injection is a Chinese patent drug widely used for treating CHD in China. A series of studies have verified the efficacy of salvianolate injection, but the high drug cost has raised concerns. It is, therefore, important to conduct cost-consequence analysis to demonstrate whether salvianolate injection is associated with outcome improvement and cost containment. The aim of this study was to retrospectively evaluate the cost-consequence of salvianolate injection for the treatment of coronary heart disease by combining salvianolate injection with conventional treatment from a societal perspective.

Methods: We retrospectively studied hospitalized patients with CHD from August 2011 to December 2015 by using electronic medical record database. Patients who received salvianolate injection combined with conventional treatment were selected as exposed group, while those who received conventional treatment alone were selected as unexposed group. Propensity score matching (PSM) analysis was used to balance the characteristics of patients. After PSM, we evaluated hospital stay, total nitrates dosage, total medical costs, and subcategories costs. Patients with chronic ischemic heart disease were analyzed as a highly selected subcohort.

Results: For the overall group, hospital stay was significantly decreased by 2.9 days ($P < 0.05$) and total nitrates dosage was significantly decreased by 172.4 mg ($P < 0.05$) in exposed group; cost savings of pharmacy cost, examination cost, laboratory cost, operation cost and treatment was observed as significant (at $P < 0.05$); and the additional expenditure of Chinese patent drug (1174.9 CNY) was less than the saving of total medical costs (2636.4 CNY). For chronic ischemic heart disease subcohort, compared with unexposed group, significant decreases were also found in hospital stay and total nitrates dosage ($P < 0.05$); cost savings were significant ($P < 0.05$) for exposed group in terms of total medical costs (4339.5 CNY) and subcategories costs (including pharmacy cost, examination cost, operation cost and treatment cost); and the additional expenditure of Chinese patent drug (1189.3 CNY) was less than the saving of total medical costs.

Conclusion: Compared with conventional treatment for the treatment of CHD, combination of salvianolate injection and conventional treatment was associated with a reduction in hospital stay and total nitrates dosage. The acquisition cost of Chinese patent drug (including salvianolate injection) was offset by a higher reduction in total medical costs, especially for chronic ischemic heart disease.

*Correspondence: hansheng@bjmu.edu.cn; jnquans@sina.com
†Pengxin Dong and Hao Hu share co-first authorship
[1] School of Pharmaceutical Sciences, Shandong University, Jinan, Shandong, China
[2] International Research Center of Medical Administration, Peking University, Beijing, China

Keywords: Cost-consequence analysis, Salvianolate injection, Coronary heart disease, Chronic ischemic heart disease, Traditional Chinese medicine, Pharmacoeconomics

Background

Coronary heart disease (CHD) incurs great costs and heavy economic burdens worldwide [1, 2]. According to the findings from the Global Burden of Disease Study 2013, 92.94 million people were suffering from this disease [3]. As for China, complicated with the impact of aging population and urbanization, CHD prevalence and mortality increased sharply during the past few decades [4, 5]. In 2014, a total of 500,946 Chinese patients received percutaneous coronary intervention due to CHD, causing high medical expenditure for CHD patients in China [6].

Based on the guidelines introduced by the National Health and Family Planning Commission of the People's Republic of China, traditional Chinese medicine (TCM) is considered one of the general treatment for CHD [7]. TCM regards CHD as "thoracic obstruction". The primary TCM syndrome of CHD is blood stasis. Therefore, the major objectives of TCM therapy is to promote blood circulation, remove blood stasis and dredge collaterals [8, 9]. Comparing with western medicine, TCM functions through multiple paths and multiple target spots, so that it is always expected to improve patients' overall health status [10].

Salvianolate injection is a TCM injection made from the root of a Chinese herb called red-rooted salvia. The indication of salvianolate injection is CHD with stable angina pectoris. The syndrome differentiation in TCM of salvianolate injection is blood stasis syndrome, usually occurring in CHD, arrhythmia and congestive heart failure. Pharmacological studies indicated that salvianolate injection could protect cardiomyocytes via reducing the levels of proinflammatory cytokines and inhibiting reactive oxygen species production [11, 12]. A systematic review made by Zhang [13] in 2016 showed that the combined use of salvianolate injection and western medicine improved both the total effective rate and the electrocardiogram effective rate. Safety of salvianolate injection was confirmed in an overview of systematic reviews made by Liu [14]. In that study, adverse reaction rate of salvianolate injection was considered equivalent to conventional treatment and lower than other TCM injections. Given its favorable efficacy and safety, doctors in China usually supplement conventional treatment with salvianolate injection for CHD patients [15, 16]. According to a ranking list of TCM for cardiovascular and cerebrovascular diseases in March 2016, salvianolate injection had the highest market share in five of the seven Chinese biggest cities [17].

However, the high costs of salvianolate injection has raised concerns. It is, therefore, important to conduct cost-consequence analysis to demonstrate whether salvianolate injection is associated with outcome improvement and cost containment. As shown in the current literature, some studies had tried to conduct economic evaluation of salvianolate injection for CHD. A prospective study to compare cost-consequence of salvia injection, tanshinone II A injection, salvianolate injection, and salvia Kawashima injection for coronary heart disease angina, found salvianolate injection had better cost-consequence [18]. Another study also compared the cost-consequence of these four types of injections and found salvianolate injection showed comparative advantages in term of cost-consequence [19]. However, the above studies only included drug cost and infusion cost without comprehensive assessment of direct medical cost of salvianolate injection for CHD. In addition, they did not consider the impact of salvianolate injection use on possible cost saving on western medicine cost and surgery cost, etc.

The aim of this study was to retrospectively evaluate the cost-consequence of salvianolate injection for the treatment of CHD by combining salvianolate injection with conventional treatment from a societal perspective. Using the medical record database from real world, it is expected to provide references for doctors and policymakers when they need to make clinical or policy decisions about salvianolate injection. Moreover, this study is expected to contribute to the field of pharmacoeconomics of TCM products which is still at the very early development stage in need of further exploratory investigations.

Methods
Study population

To realize the research objective, a retrospective cohort study was applied. The minimum standards of reporting checklist of detailed information about experimental design, and statistics, and resources was used in this study (see Additional file 1).

The study cohort was drawn from the electronic medical record database of the Anyang People's Hospital. The hospital is a 1500-bed, university affiliated tertiary hospital, which is a regional medical center in Henan Province. This study was conducted in 2016 using data from the electronic medical record database since its implementation in August 2011. To collect as many samples as possible, we retrospectively reviewed the inpatients who were admitted to hospital between August 2011 and December 2015. For each sample, the data was retrieved from the day of hospital admission until the day of hospital discharge or hospital death.

In order to extract the study population comprehensively, samples were recruited based on a wide range of diagnosis. Eligible patients included those with ICD-10 code I20 for angina pectoris, or I25 for chronic ischemic heart disease, or description of "angina", "coronary heart disease", "coronary artery", "myocardial infarction", "heart failure", "myocardium", "atrial fibrillation" or "palpitation" in their admitting diagnosis. After preliminary extraction, we performed a manual check to ensure all of study samples were patients with CHD. Patients who received other TCM except salvianolate injection during their hospital stay were excluded from the study.

Among all types of CHD, chronic ischemic heart disease is the most widespread subcategory of CHD. Therefore, we also selected patients with chronic ischemic heart disease in both exposed group and unexposed group as a highly selected subcohort. This subcohort included patients with ICD-10 code I25 or description "coronary heart disease" or "coronary artery".

Exposure and outcomes

In the study cohort, patients who received salvianolate injection combined with conventional treatment were selected as exposed group, while those who received conventional treatment alone were selected as unexposed group. According to the medication guide of CHD, conventional treatment included β-blockers, nitrates, calcium channel blockers, lipid regulating agents, anticoagulants and antiplatelet agents, ACE inhibitors and angiotensin receptor blockers. In this study, conventional treatment referred to the treatment included neither salvianolate injection nor other TCM products.

The study outcomes were hospital stay, total nitrates dosage, total medical costs and subcategories costs. At the beginning, we divided total medical costs into 13 subcategories costs: supplies cost, pharmacy cost, examination cost, laboratory cost, operation cost, treatment cost, Chinese patent drug cost, bed cost, nursing cost, blood cost, Chinese herb cost, diet cost, and others cost. Costs composition analysis indicated that among 13 subcategories costs, the accumulative constituent ratio of supplies cost, pharmacy cost, examination cost, laboratory cost, operation cost, treatment cost and Chinese patent drug cost was over 90%. Therefore, we incorporated these seven subcategories costs into final analysis.

Except the outcome measurement above, we also collected the following characteristics of patients: age, sex, diastolic blood pressure, systolic blood pressure, whether or not the patient had joined a medical reimbursement program, nitrates dosage, and administration of nitrates used prior to salvianolate injection.

Propensity score matching for bias

The major bias in the present study was "selection bias". In particular, if physicians tended to prescribe salvianolate injection for patients in worse conditions, the cost-consequence would be underestimated. On the contrary, if physicians tended to prescribe salvianolate injection for patients in milder conditions, the cost-consequence would be overestimated. We performed a 1:1 propensity score matching (PSM) analysis to reduce bias [20, 21].

Considering medication background of CHD and data accessibility, we selected age, sex, blood pressure, whether or not the patient had joined a medical reimbursement program as covariates for elementary matching, caliper set at 0.05.

Then, in order to evaluate total nitrates dosage impartially, nitrates dosage and administration of nitrates used prior to salvianolate injection were selected as covariates for further matching, caliper set at 0.01. We selected nitrates dosage and administration of nitrates used prior to salvianolate injection as covariates because nitrates use was an important indicator of the severity of CHD.

In this study, we regarded nitrates use as not only a baseline characteristic but also a clinical outcome. For exposed group, with the first exposure point of salvianolate injection used, the previous line of nitrates exposure was used as a baseline, followed by the use of nitrates as an outcome. For unexposed group, because the first exposure time point of salvianolate injection could not be determined, so we calculated the time for each patient in the exposure group from admission to the first use of salvianolate injection as time interval. Then, for patients in unexposed group, nitrates use during the corresponding time interval was set as a baseline; and nitrates use post time interval was set as an outcome.

The whole flow chart of PSM was summarized as Fig. 1.

Statistical analysis

All analyses were performed using R3.3.3 software. First, descriptive analysis was conducted. Numerical variables were expressed as mean ($\pm$standard deviation [SD]). Categorical variables were expressed as percentage.

To test the exposure effects, we performed paired t test to assess differences between exposed group and unexposed group. Due to existence of null value, subcategories costs were analyzed with t test. A 2-tailed P value < 0.05 was considered as significant.

Because this study used PSM to select data, sensitivity analysis was performed for data selection and matching methods. In addition, different statistical test methods were used in this study to verify the sensitivity of the statistical test results to the statistics method.

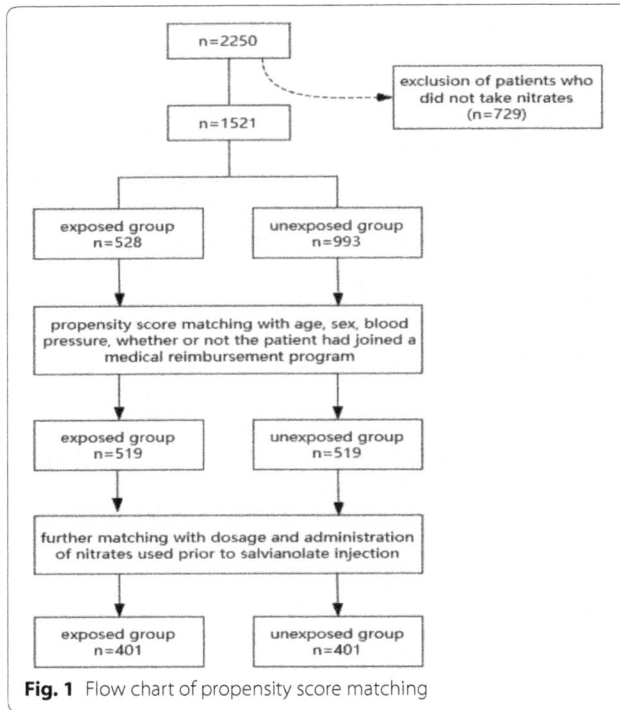

Fig. 1 Flow chart of propensity score matching

Results
Propensity score matching
First, 2250 patients were collected from the hospital.

Second, 729 patients who did not take nitrates were excluded. Third, a total of 802 patients were successfully matched after PSM.

The baseline characteristics of patients before PSM was summarized in Table 1. There were significant ($P < 0.05$) differences in age, diastolic blood pressure, systolic blood pressure, and medical reimbursement between exposed (conventional treatment + salvianolate injection) group and unexposed (conventional treatment + salvianolate injection) group.

After PSM, as shown in Table 2, there were no significant differences in baseline characteristics between exposed (conventional treatment + salvianolate injection) group and unexposed (conventional treatment + salvianolate injection) group.

Cost-consequence analysis of overall cohort
For the overall cohort, as shown in Table 3, hospital stay in exposed group was significantly decreased by 2.9 days compared with unexposed group (11.7 [±7.5] vs 14.6 [±1.5] days; $P < 0.05$). Total nitrates dosage was significantly decreased by 172.4 mg in exposed group compared with unexposed group (457.7 [±511.4] vs 630.1 [±650.4] mg; $P < 0.05$). A decrease of 2636.4 CNY in total medical costs was found in patients who received combination of conventional treatment and salvianolate injection (14,726.3 [±18,165.8] vs 17,362.7 [±22,161.8] CNY; $P = 0.054$), although there was no significant difference

Table 1 Baseline characteristics before propensity score matching

Characteristic	Conventional treatment + salvianolate injection (n = 635)	Conventional treatment (n = 1615)	P
Age (years)	63.3 (±13.01)	60.4 (±18.01)	< 0.05
Male sex (%)	50	50	0.414
Diastolic blood pressure (mmHg)	71.1 (±6.55)	73 (±7.84)	< 0.05
Systolic blood pressure (mmHg)	122.2 (±10.87)	123.7 (±13.72)	< 0.05
Medical reimbursement (%)	80	90	< 0.05

Table 2 Baseline characteristics after propensity score matching

Characteristic	Conventional treatment + salvianolate injection (n = 401)	Conventional treatment (n = 401)	P
Age (years)	64.2 (±12.2)	65.8 (±12.2)	0.069
Male sex (%)	60	60	1
Diastolic blood pressure (mmHg)	71.3 (±6.5)	71.1 (±6.3)	0.724
Systolic blood pressure (mmHg)	122.7 (±10.9)	122.6 (±11.8)	0.825
Medical reimbursement (%)	90	90	1
Dosage of nitrates (mg)	19.3 (±123.5)	19.3 (±123.5)	1
Administration of nitrates[a]	0.2	0.2	1

[a] Using only oral nitrates was set as 0; using only nitrates injections was set as 1; using both dosage forms was set at 2

Table 3 Comparison of clinical and economic outcomes in overall cohort

Outcome	Conventional treatment + salvianolate injection (n = 401)	Conventional treatment (n = 401)	Difference	P
Hospital stay (days)	11.7 (±7.5)	14.6 (±11.5)	−2.9	<0.05
Total nitrates dosage (mg)	457.7 (±511.4)	630.1 (±650.4)	−172.4	<0.05
Total medical costs (CNY)	14,726.3 (±18,165.8)	17,362.7 (±22,161.8)	−2636.4	0.054
Subcategories costs (CNY)				
Supplies cost	5538.6 (±13,486.6)	5770.9 (12,458.5)	−232.3	0.801
Pharmacy cost	3122.5 (±3124.2)	4890.1 (±5218.0)	−1767.6	<0.05
Examination cost	1410.6 (±1277.5)	1954.9 (±2427.2)	−544.3	<0.05
Laboratory cost	1351.7 (±818.3)	1564.2 (±1330.3)	−212.5	<0.05
Operation cost	2626.2 (±1884.2)	4223.2 (±3211.2)	−1597.0	<0.05
Treatment cost	447.4 (±831.6)	1005.7 (±1687.1)	−558.3	<0.05
Chinese patent drug cost	1316.6 (±581.0)	141.7 (±474.6)	1174.9	<0.05

between exposed group and unexposed group at $P < 0.05$ level.

As for subcategories costs, in exposed group, pharmacy cost, examination cost, laboratory cost, operation cost, and treatment cost were significantly ($P < 0.05$) lower, while Chinese patent drug cost was significantly (1316.6 [±581.0] vs 141.7 [±474.6] CNY; $P < 0.05$)

higher. Supplies cost did not significantly ($P = 0.801$) differ between exposed group and unexposed group.

As presented in Fig. 2, compared with unexposed group, exposed group had cost-saving in total medical costs and subcategories costs except Chinese patent drug cost. However, even with additional expenditure of 1174 CNY for Chinese patent drug, there was still 2636.4 CNY cost saving in total medical costs for exposed group.

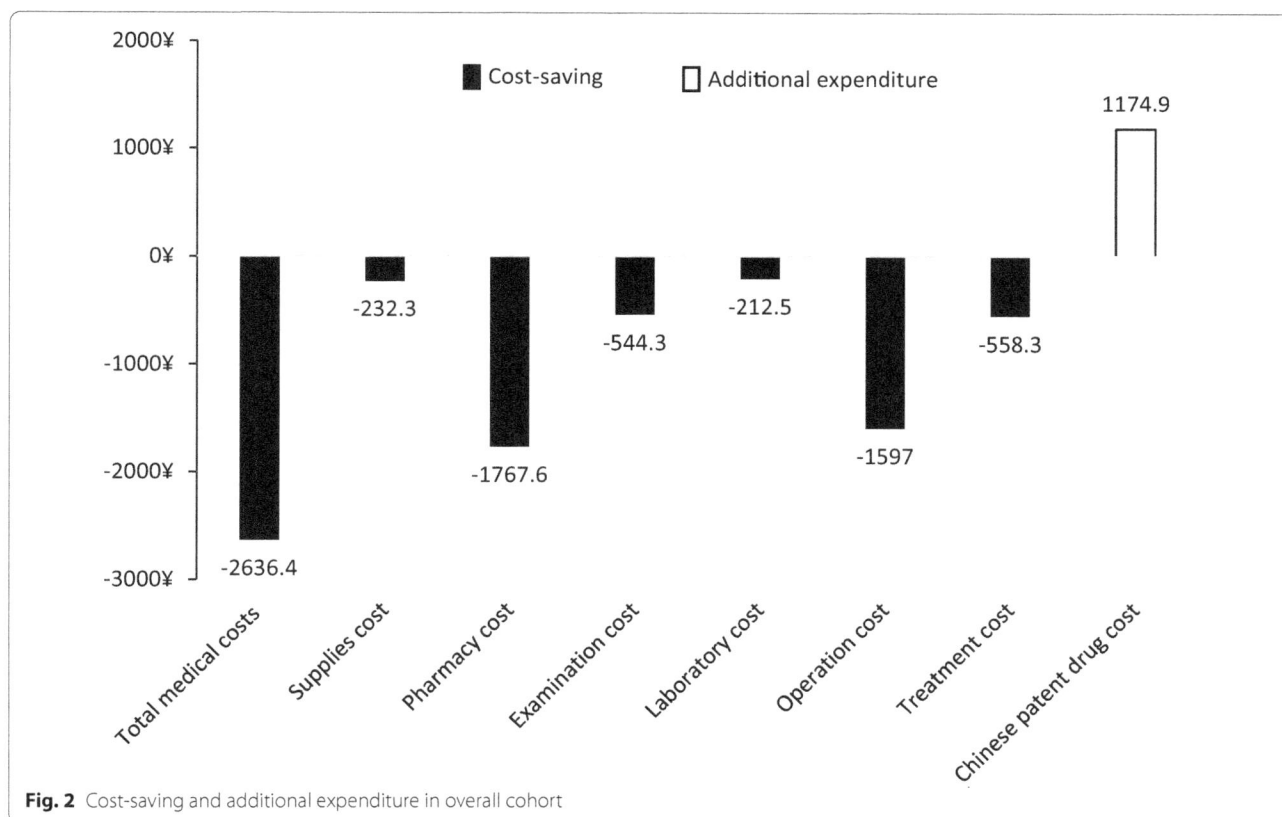

Fig. 2 Cost-saving and additional expenditure in overall cohort

Table 4 Comparison of clinical and economic outcomes in subcohort of chronic ischemic heart disease

Outcome	Conventional treatment + salvianolate injection (n = 129)	Conventional treatment (n = 129)	Difference	P
Hospital stay (d)	11.9 (±7.7)	15.5 (±13.0)	−3.6	<0.05
Total nitrates dosage (mg)	452.7 (±490.1)	703.4 (±845.2)	−250.7	<0.05
Total medical costs (CNY)	12,694.9 (±20,609.5)	17,034.4 (±21,251.3)	−4339.5	<0.05
Subcategories costs (CNY)				
Supplies cost	3760.4 (±15,171.77)	5158.4 (±9740.56)	−1398	0.382
Pharmacy cost	3308.2 (±3660.5)	4925.7 (±5065.2)	−1617.5	<0.05
Examination cost	1551.1 (±1403.78)	1957.2 (±1742.96)	−406.1	<0.05
Laboratory cost	1365.6 (±823.26)	1627.4 (±1384.94)	−261.8	0.07
Operation cost	2592.7 (±2243.94)	4705.1 (±3228.53)	−2112.4	<0.05
Treatment cost	462 (±895.68)	1042 (±1678.62)	−580	<0.05
Chinese patent drug cost	1334.9 (±637.9)	145.6 (±378.8)	1189.3	<0.05

Cost-consequence analysis of chronic ischemic heart disease subcohort

For the chronic ischemic heart disease subcohort, the results of cost-consequence analysis is reported in Table 4. Hospital stay in exposed group was 11.9 (±7.7) days, which was significantly 3.6 days less than 15.5 (±13.0) days of unexposed group ($P < 0.05$). Total nitrates dosage of patients in exposed group was significantly 250.7 mg lower than that of unexposed group

(457.7 [±511.4] vs 703.4 [±845.2] mg; $P < 0.05$). Comparison of total medical costs indicated a significant cost saving of 4339.5 CNY in exposed group (12,694.9 [±20,609.5] vs 17,034.4 [±21,251.3] CNY; $P < 0.05$).

Among the subcategories costs, pharmacy cost, examination cost, operation cost, and treatment cost were significantly ($P < 0.05$) lower in exposed group, while patients in exposed group incurred significantly ($P < 0.05$) more Chinese patent drug cost. Supplies cost ($P = 0.382$)

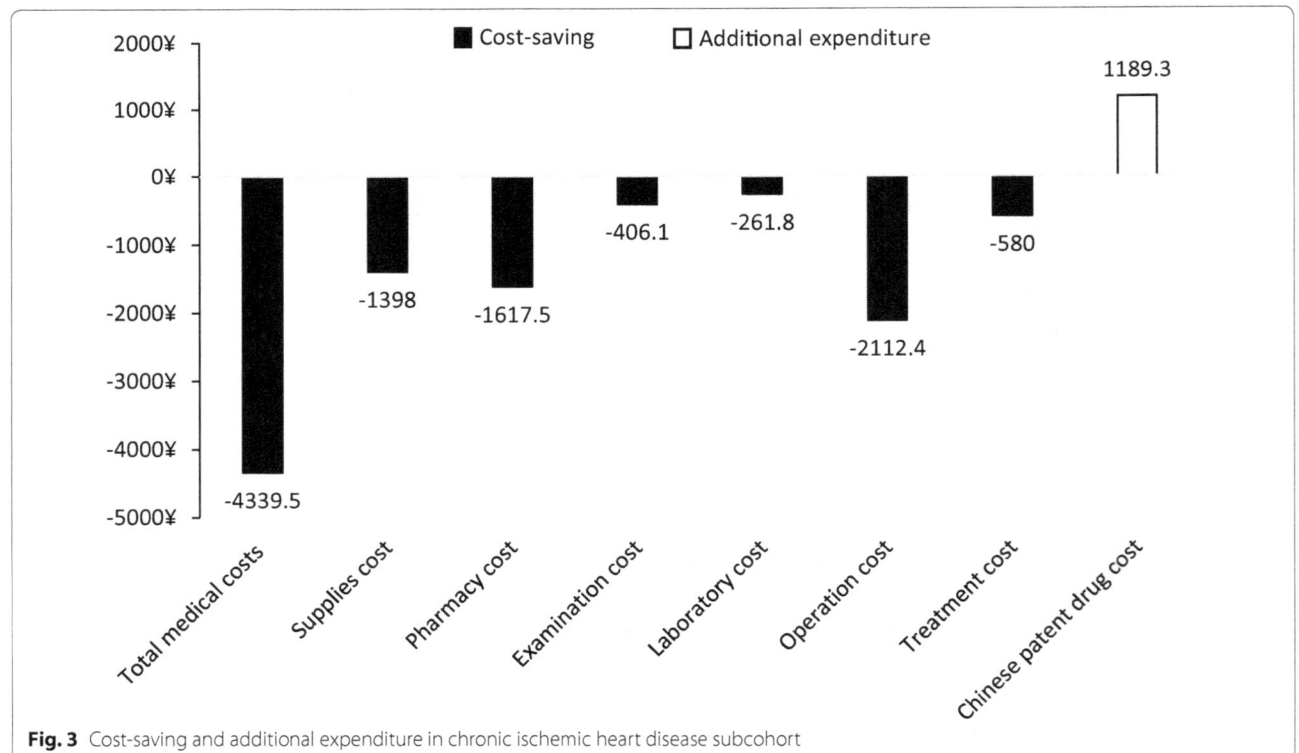

Fig. 3 Cost-saving and additional expenditure in chronic ischemic heart disease subcohort

and laboratory cost ($P = 0.007$) were not significantly different between exposed group and unexposed group.

As shown in Fig. 3, there was obvious cost saving for exposed group in supplies cost (1398 CNY), pharmacy cost (1617.5 CNY) and operation cost (2112.4 CNY). Although the combination use of conventional treatment and salvianolate injection caused additional expenditure of Chinese patent drug (1189.3 CNY), it still resulted in 4339.5 CNY saving of total medical costs compared with unexposed group.

Sensitivity analysis

The results of the sensitivity analysis for PSM showed that, within either the overall cohort or subcohort, the study results were insensitive to whether patients receiving nitrate medications, nitrate base usage, and what caliper values were used for PSM. The results were thus approved to be robust.

For sensitivity analysis for statistics methods, the results showed that the test results of the total medical costs difference were sensitive to the choice of statistical methods: the results obtained by using t test were not significant, while the results obtained using Wilcoxon rank-sum test were mostly significant at the 95% level. Since the data of total medical costs did not follow a normal distribution, it tended to accept non-parametric test results.

Discussion

Economic value is an essential component in the assessment for a drug applied in clinic [22, 23]. Especially for TCM products, economic evaluation is becoming more and more important for their use and imbursement and may even influence their international market access [24]. This study compared the cost-consequence of salvianolate injection combined with conventional treatment and conventional treatment alone. The result provides a reference for doctors who used salvianolate injection to achieve the best balance between the effectiveness and economic value of salvianolate injection for CHD. At the same time, it also provides a reference for policy marker to make decisions about including salvianolate injection into drug formulary to promote rational use of drugs in the clinical practice for CHD.

For the purpose of pharmacoeconomic evaluation, data obtained in real world is considered more instructive than data extracted from clinical trials [25]. In this study, we retrospectively analyzed the CHD treatment in electronic medical record database. This study setting was similar to real world. It is indicated that real world study design could bring about many external confounding factors [26]. To control confounding factors and reduce bias, a PSM analysis was performed in this study to balance

baseline characteristics between exposed group and unexposed group. Therefore, the study results provided reliable information of cost-consequence about salvianolate injection for CHD treatment.

Our findings showed a shorter hospital stay and a lower nitrates dosage observed in exposed group relative to unexposed group, for both overall CHD cohort and subcohort of chronic ischemic heart disease. Hospital stay and nitrates dosage were generally regarded as two representative indicators for CHD treatment [27–29]. Therefore, the shorter hospital stay and lower nitrate dosage could be regarded as indirect reflections of a better clinic effectiveness of the combined use of salvianolate injection and conventional treatment.

In addition to clinical consequence of shorter hospital stay and lower nitrates dosage, cost savings of total medical costs and subcategories costs (except Chinese patent drug cost) were observed in exposed group. The increase of Chinese patent drug cost was partially due to use of salvianolate injection. However, such increase in costs was offset by cost savings associated with the improvement of health status with the use of salvianolate injection. For overall cohort, salvianolate injection saved 2636.4 CNY total medical costs per patient admission. The result had an obvious economic value, but it was not statistically significant at $P < 0.05$. Accordingly, a further research with larger sample size will be need to reconfirm the conclusion. For chronic ischemic heart disease subcohort, the cost savings were more notable (4339.5 CNY). It indicated that salvianolate injection had a better cost consequence in this subcohort of chronic ischemic heart disease.

Nevertheless, some limitations of this study deserve to be mentioned for future research. First, we analyzed the patients who were admitted to hospital between 2011 and 2015. The long-time span might give rise to a time-dependent bias. Second, we extracted the data from a single hospital, so the generalizability of the results might be limited. Hence, a further study based on a bigger medical record data from more hospitals is warranted. Third, because of the limited data in the original medical record, this study did not include CHD severity and complications into analysis. While PSM used in this study can increase the comparison reliability to a great extent, future study using more comprehensive data about CHD will provide further information about cost-consequence of salvianolate injection for treatment of subcategory of CHD.

Conclusions

Compared with conventional treatment for CHD, combination of salvianolate injection and conventional treatment was associated with a reduction in hospital stay and total nitrates dosage. The acquisition cost of Chinese patent drug (including salvianolate injection) was offset by a higher reduction in total medical costs, especially for patients with chronic ischemic heart disease.

Abbreviations
CHD: coronary heart disease; PSM: propensity score matching; TCM: traditional Chinese medicine.

Authors' contributions
SH, SY and LS conceptualized the study and acquired the data. PD, HH, XG, COLU, and SH carried out data analysis and drafted the manuscript. All authors reviewed the final manuscript. All authors read and approved the final manuscript

Author details
[1] School of Pharmaceutical Sciences, Shandong University, Jinan, Shandong, China. [2] International Research Center of Medical Administration, Peking University, Beijing, China. [3] State Key Laboratory of Quality Research in Chinese Medicine, Institute of Chinese Medical Sciences, University of Macau, Taipa, Macao. [4] School of Pharmaceutical Science, Peking University Health Science Center, Beijing, China. [5] Shandong University Affiliated Jinan Central Hospital, Jinan, Shandong, China.

Acknowledgements
We acknowledge the constructive comments on early vision from the colleagues of the International Research Center of Medicinal Administration at Peking University and the Institute of Chinese Medical Sciences at University of Macau. We also appreciate the professional comments from three anonymous reviewers.

Competing interests
The authors declare that they have no competing interests.

Consent for publication
Not applicable.

Funding
This study was funded by Shanghai Green Valley Pharmaceutical Co., Ltd. However, the funding body played no role in the design of the study and collection, analysis, and interpretation of data and in writing the manuscript.

References
1. Sanchis-Gomar F, Perez-Quilis C, Leischik R, et al. Epidemiology of coronary heart disease and acute coronary syndrome. Ann Transl Med. 2016;4(13):256.
2. Kalra A, Bhatt DL, Rajagopalan S, et al. Overview of coronary heart disease risk initiatives in South Asia. Curr Atheroscler Rep. 2017;19(6):25.
3. Murray CJL, Barber RM, Foreman KJ, et al. Global, regional, and national disability-adjusted life years (DALYs) for 306 diseases and injuries and healthy life expectancy (HALE) for 188 countries, 1990–2013: quantifying the epidemiological transition. Lancet. 2015;386(10009):2145–91.
4. He Y, Lam TH, Jiang B, et al. Changes in BMI before and during economic development and subsequent risk of cardiovascular disease and total mortality: a 35-year follow-up study in China. Diabetes Care. 2014;37(9):2540–7.
5. Zhao D, Liu J. Cardiovascular disease in China: increasing burden ahead for prevention. Chin J Cardiol. 2012;40(3):177.
6. Chen WW, Gao RL, Liu LS, et al. Summary of the China cardiovascular disease report 2015. Chin Circ J. 2016;31(6):521–8.
7. Committee on Rational Drug Use of the National Health and Family Planning Commission, China Pharmacist Association. Rational drug use guidelines in coronary heart disease. Chin J Front Med Sci (Elect Ver). 2016;8(6):19–108.
8. Li GH, Jiang HY, Xie YM, et al. Analysis of traditional Chinese medicine syndrome, traditional Chinese medicine and western medicine in 84697 patients with coronary heart disease based on big data. Chin J Chin Mater Med. 2014;39(18):3462–8.
9. Jiang WB, Gu N. The development of the research on the treatment of blood stasis of coronary heart disease by Chinese traditional medicine injection. J Pract Tradit Chin Med. 2014;30(4):367.
10. Wu Y, Wang YL. The clinical status and research progress of TCM treatment for blood stasis of coronary heart disease. Mod J Integr Tradit Chin West Med. 2016;25(25):2844–7.
11. Meng C, Zhuo XQ, Xu GH, et al. Protection of salvianolate against atherosclerosis via regulating the inflammation in rats. J Huazhong Univ Sci Technol Med Sci. 2014;34(5):646–51.
12. Fei A, Cao Q, Chen S, et al. Salvianolate inhibits reactive oxygen species production in H_2O_2-treated mouse cardiomyocytes in vitro via the TGFβ pathway. Acta Pharmacol Sin. 2013;34(4):496–500.
13. Zhang D, Wu J, Liu S, et al. Salvianolate injection in the treatment of unstable angina pectoris: a systematic review and meta-analysis. Medicine. 2016;95(51):e5692.
14. Liu Y, Yan YY, Zhai SD. Salvianolate for treatment of angina: an overview of systematic reviews. Chin J Clin Pharmacol. 2016;32(6):560–2.
15. Song YQ, Xu XY, Sun RD. An overview of the clinical application of the salvianolate injection. Chin J Pharmacoepidemiol. 2012;21(8):404–7.
16. Chang YP, Zhang H, Xie YM, et al. Analysis of salvianolate injection combined with usual drugs in treatment of coronary heart disease in real world. Chin J Chin Mater Med. 2013;38(18):3186–9.
17. Menet. Ranking list of Chinese patent drug in hospital. [DB/OL]. 2016. http://shuju.menet.com.cn/homePage.jsp#. Accessed 15 Mar 2018.
18. Zhang YF, Qin ZL, Liu J, et al. Pharmacoeconomics research of 4 kinds of salvia miltiorrhiza preparations for the treatment of coronary heart disease angina pectoris. Chongqing Med. 2016;45(8):1081–3.
19. Liu CD, Li HM. Pharmacoeconomic analysis of radix salvia miltiorrhiza injection in treatment of coronary heart disease. Tianjin Pharm. 2011;23(2):55–76.
20. Gillespie IA, Floege J, Gioni I, Drüeke TB, Francisco AL, Anker SD, Kubo Y, Wheeler DC, Froissart M. Propensity score matching and persistence correction to reduce bias in comparative effectiveness: the effect of cinacalcet use on all-cause mortality. Pharmacoepidemiol Drug Saf. 2015;24(7):738–47.
21. Kosuke I, Marc R. Covariate balancing propensity score. J R Stat Soc. 2015;76(1):243–63.
22. Ikeda S, Murata T, Kobayashi M. Role of pharmacoeconomic analysis in pricing decision in Japan. Value Health. 2015;18(7):A533.
23. Franken M, Nilsson F, Sandmann F, de Boer A, Koopmanschap M. Unravelling drug reimbursement outcomes: a comparative study of the role of pharmacoeconomic evidence in Dutch and Swedish reimbursement decision making. Pharmacoeconomics. 2013;31(9):781–97.
24. Lin AX, Chan G, Hu Y, Ouyang D, Ung CO, Shi L, Hu H. Internationalization of traditional Chinese medicine: current international market, internationalization challenges and prospective suggestions. Chin Med. 2018;13(1):9.
25. Makady A, Ham RT, De BA, et al. Policies for use of real-world data in health technology assessment (HTA): a comparative study of six HTA agencies. Value Health. 2017;20(4):520–32.
26. Dimick JB, Livingston EH. Comparing treatments using observational study designs: what can we do about selection bias. Arch Surg. 2010;145(10):927.

27. Miao Y, Gao Z, Xu F, Wand X, Chen K, Zhang D. Clinical observation on salvianolate for the treatment of angina pectoris in coronary heart disease with heart-blood stagnation syndrome. Tradit Chin Drug Res Clin Pharmacol. 2006;2:140–4.

28. Qiu YH, Xue L, Gao XQ. Effect of salvianolate injection on cardiac function and inflammation factors in patients with chronic heart failure. Chin J Exp Tradit Med Formulae. 2013;7:85.

29. Feng Z, Deng Y, Chen X. The phase IV clinical observation study of salvianolate injection on recovery stage of cerebral infarction (blood stasis type). Pract Clin J Integr Tradit Chin West Med. 2013;8:6.

5

Combination of *Salvia miltiorrhiza* and ligustrazine attenuates bleomycin-induced pulmonary fibrosis in rats via modulating TNF-α and TGF-β

Chengliang Huang[1], Xu Wu[2], Shengpeng Wang[3], Wenjun Wang[1], Fang Guo[1], Yuanyuan Chen[1], Bi Pan[1], Ming Zhang[1] and Xianming Fan[1*]

Abstract

Background: Idiopathic pulmonary fibrosis (IPF), a chronic, progressive, fibrosing interstitial lung disease, is associated with extremely poor prognosis, and lacks effective treatment. The frequently used immunosuppressive therapies such as dexamethasone (DEX) are often associated with side effects. Recently, combination of two Chinese herbal medicine preparations, *Salvia miltiorrhiza* and ligustrazine (SML), serves as an alternative medicine for treatment of IPF in clinical practices in China. The aim of this study is to compare the anti-fibrotic effect of SML with that of DEX and to investigate the underlying mechanisms.

Methods: A rat model of bleomycin (BLM) induced pulmonary fibrosis was used in this study. Ninety rats were assigned to six groups: control group; BLM-group; BLM and dexamethasone group (BLM + DEX); BLM + low-dose SML; BLM + medium-dose SML and BLM + high-dose SML. Rats were sacrificed on day 7, 14 and 28 after treatment. The extent of alveolitis and fibrosis was observed by H&E and Masson's trichrome staining. The expressions of TNF-α, TGF-β1 and SMAD4 were determined and quantified by immunohistochemical analysis. The serum levels of TNF-α and TGF-β1 were further quantified by ELISA kits.

Results: Both DEX and SML treatment attenuated BLM-induced lung injury and pathological collagen deposition in rats, showing improved alveolitis and fibrosis scores on day 7, 14, 28, compared to the BLM group ($p < 0.05$). The anti-fibrotic effect of SML was in a dose-dependent manner, and the medium- and high-dose SML showed comparable effect with DEX on day 14 and 28. Expressions of TNF-α, TGF-β1 and SMAD4 were significantly decreased in the DEX- and SML-treated groups compared with BLM groups ($p < 0.05$). Medium- and high-dose SML showed better repression of TNF-α, TGF-β1 and SMAD4 expression compared to DEX at all time points ($p < 0.05$). Notably, SML at different dosages did not affect serum levels of alanine aminotransferase, aspartate aminotransferase and creatinine.

Conclusions: SML is safe and effective in repressing BLM-induced pulmonary fibrosis, which might be through modulating the expression of TNF-α and TGF-β1. Our findings advocate the use of SML for IPF, which might serve as a better treatment option over DEX.

Keywords: Ligustrazine, Pulmonary fibrosis, *Salvia miltiorrhiza*, SMAD4, TNF-α

*Correspondence: fxm129120@sina.com
[1] Department of Respiratory Medicine II, The Affiliated Hospital
of Southwest Medical University, Luzhou, Sichuan, China

Background

Idiopathic pulmonary fibrosis (IPF) is a chronic, progressive, fibrosing interstitial lung disease characterized by alveolar epithelial cell injury, aberrant proliferation of fibroblasts and excessive extracellular matrix (ECM) deposition leading to progressive fibrosis and loss of lung function, which accounts for about 20% of all cases of interstitial lung disease [1]. IPF is the most common and severe among the idiopathic interstitial pneumonias [2] and is associated with extremely poor prognosis with median survival time of 2–3 years [3]. Several risk and predisposing factors, including cigarette smoking, viral infections, gastro-oesophageal reflux and surfactant protein polymorphisms, have been reported to contribute to the pathogenesis of IPF [4, 5]. Although the pathological mechanisms remain unclear, increasing evidences demonstrate that repetitive injury to the alveolar epithelial cells drives aberrant wound healing responses, resulting in fibrosis [1, 6]. Several cytokines and chemokines have been reported to involved in this process [5, 6]. Among them, TGF-β, the major profibrotic mediator, plays central role in the development of fibrosis by inducing differentiation of lung fibroblasts into myofibroblasts, stimulating ECM accumulation and epithelial mesenchymal transition (EMT) [7, 8]; TNF-α, the cytokine with inflammatory and fibrotic properties, stimulates collagen synthesis, induces TGF-β and promotes proliferation of fibroblasts [8, 9]. Elevated levels of TGF-β and TNF-α have been found in the lungs of animals in experimental models of pulmonary fibrosis and in patients with IPF [10, 11]. Blocking of TNF-α and TGF-β signalling resulted in attenuation of fibrosis in rodents [12, 13], which served as a promising therapeutic strategy for IPF.

Currently, lung transplantation is the only effective treatment for IPF. The frequently used immunosuppressive therapies such as dexamethasone are often associated with side effects and have not been proven to improve the survival and quality of life of the patients [14]. Notably, the combination of two Chinese herbal medicine preparations, Salvia miltiorrhiza (Danshen) injection and ligustrazine injection, has been widely used for treatment of IPF in clinical practices, showing good efficacy and few side effects [15, 16]. Danshen, the root and rhizome of Salvia miltiorrhiza Bge., is widely used in traditional Chinese medicine for the treatment of various ailments such as those affecting the circulatory, hepatic and respiratory systems [17]. Recent studies has shown that Salvia miltiorrhiza and its main constituents dramatically attenuated pulmonary fibrosis in mice models through reducing inflammation [18, 19]. Furthermore, ligustrazine, the main active ingredient of Ligusticum chuanxiong hort (Chuanxiong), has been proved to have protective effects against lung fibrosis induced

by hyperoxia and bleomycin [20, 21]. The pair of Salvia miltiorrhiza and ligustrazine has been commercially available in China as a compound preparation, namely Danshen–ligustrazine injection. Despite the potential in treating IPF, the mechanisms underlying the actions of combination of Salvia miltiorrhiza and ligustrazine (SML) in pulmonary fibrosis are not fully elucidated. In the present study, we aimed to compare the anti-pulmonary fibrosis effects of SML with that of DEX in a rat model of bleomycin-induced pulmonary fibrosis and to investigate the underlying mechanisms.

Methods

The minimum standards of reporting checklist (Additional file 1) contains details of the experimental design, and statistics, and resources used in this study.

Chemicals and reagents

Bleomycin (BLM-A5) was purchased from Tianjin Taihe Pharmaceuticals Ltd (Tianjin, China). Salvia miltiorrhiza injection, the standard aqueous extract of Salvia miltiorrhiza, was purchased from Sichuan Sanjing Shenghe Pharmaceuticals Ltd. (Sichuan, China). Ligustrazine injection was purchased from Henan Furen Pharmaceuticals Ltd. (Henan, China). The immunohistochemistry kits used for the detection of TNF-α, TGF-β1 and SMAD4 were purchased from Dako (cat. no. K500711). ELISA kits for detection of serum TNF-α and TGF-β1 were obtained from MultiSciences (China). All other chemicals and reagents used were of analytical grade or of the highest grade available.

Animals

Ninety male Sprague–Dawley rats weighing about 180–220 g (6–7 weeks) were obtained from the animal center of Southwest Medical University (Luzhou, China). Animals were housed 2–3 per cage in a controlled environment (temperature, 25 ± 2 °C; humidity, 30–70%) with an alternating 12 h light/dark photoperiod. The rats were acclimatized for a week before the start of the experiment and fed with standard rodent chow and water ad libitum. The study was approved by Southwest Medical University Animal Ethics Committee and conducted in accordance with the Guide for the Care and Use of Laboratory Animals [22].

Study design and treatment protocol

After recording the body weights, the rats were anesthetized with an intraperitoneal injection of ketamine hydrochloride (80 mg/kg, b.wt) and xylazine (20 mg/kg, b.wt). A midline incision was made in the neck and the trachea was exposed. A tracheal cannula was inserted under direct visualization, and a single intratracheal instillation of bleomycin BLM-A5 (5 mg/kg, b.wt) dissolved in sterile 0.9% NaCl was delivered on day 1 of the experiment for induction of pulmonary fibrosis as previously reported [23].

Rats were randomly allocated into six groups with fifteen animals in each group. Group I animals received intratracheal injection of physiological saline alone (0.2–0.3 mL) and served as control group; Group II animals were subjected to a single intratracheal instillation of BLM (5 mg/kg b.wt in sterile 0.9% NaCl); Group III animals received BLM in the same as group II and treated with DEX (1.4 mg/kg, i.v. injection via tail vein); Group IV animals received BLM in the same as group II along with low-dose SML (SM + L: 125 + 43.75 mg/kg, i.v. injection via tail vein); Group V animals received BLM as group II and supplemented with medium-dose SML (SM + L: 250 + 87.5 mg/kg, i.v. injection via tail vein); Group VI received BLM as group II and supplemented with high-dose SML (SM + L: 500 + 175 mg/kg, i.v. injection via tail vein). Rats in each group was further divided into three subgroups and were sacrificed on day 7, 14, and 28 after BLM instillation, respectively.

H&E and Masson's trichrome staining
The left lungs of rats were excised, fixed in 10% neutral buffered formalin and embedded in paraffin. The paraffin-embedded tissue samples were sectioned into 5-μm slices, then deparaffinized, and stained with H&E as well as Masson's trichrome to investigate the degree of lung tissue inflammation and fibrosis, respectively. The sections were examined and evaluated randomly using standard light microscopy (DP73, Olympus) by an experienced histologist, unaware of the treatment groups. The pulmonary fibrosis grade was scored by examining 10 randomly selected regions per sample at 200× magnification for fibrotic tissue and collagen and the scores were averaged per group. The criteria used for grading lung fibrosis were as follows: Grade 0, normal; Grade 1, minimal fibrous thickening of alveolar or bronchial walls; Grades 2–3, moderate thickening of walls without obvious lung damage; Grades 4–5, increased fibrosis with definite lung damage and formation of fibrous bands or small fibrous mass; Grades 6–7, severe distortion of structure and large fibrous areas or "honeycomb lung"; and Grade 8, total fibrous obliteration of the field [9, 23].

Immunohistochemical analysis
The lung tissue sections were deparaffinized in xylene and rehydrated using graded ethanol solutions. The endogenous peroxidase activity was quenched using 0.3% hydrogen peroxide in methanol for 15 min. To eliminate non-specific binding, the sections were blocked with 5% BSA, 0.1% Tween-20 in TBS and incubated for

1 h. Following blocking, the sections were rinsed with TBST buffer containing 0.1% Tween-20. The tissue sections were incubated with TNF-α, TGF-β1 and SMAD4 polyclonal antibodies (1:100 for both) overnight at 4 °C. The sections were re-equilibrated to room temperature and washed with TBS, followed by the incubation with streptavidin–biotin–peroxidase conjugated secondary antibody for 1 h at room temperature (Dako LSAB). Finally, reaction products were visualized with 3,3′-diaminobenzidine (DAB) and then counterstained with haematoxylin. Images were collected using the inversion fluorescence microscope (Leica DMIRB) and computer image acquisition software (Leica). The Graphic context analysis software (ImagePro plus 6.0) was used to analyze the pictures of immunohistochemistry. Five fields were chosen under the 200× microscope for each slice to record the positive staining for average integral optical density.

Quantification of serum TNF-α and TGF-β1 levels
The serum levels of TNF-α and TGF-β1 were determined using ELISA kits following the manufacturer's instruction.

Biochemical analysis of rat serum
On day 28th, rats were anaesthetized and blood were collected through cardiac punctuation. Serum were obtained for determination of alanine aminotransferase (ALT), aspartate aminotransferase (AST) and creatinine (Cre) on an Advia 2400 Clinical Chemistry System (Siemens Healthcare).

Statistical analysis
All the results were expressed as mean ± SD. Statistical analysis was performed with Graphpad Prism 7.0 using one-way or two-way ANOVA followed by Tukey's multiple comparisons test. The p value < 0.05 was considered as statistically significant.

Results
SML attenuated BLM-induced lung injury and inflammation
The histopathological alterations using H&E staining in different groups are depicted in Fig. 1a. The lung tissue sections of control rats showed normal architecture with intact alveolar epithelium, normal thickening of alveolar septa and no pathological changes such as alveolitis or interstitial pulmonary fibrosis (Fig. 1a, upper panel). Intratracheal administration of BLM led to abnormal lung morphologies, including significant interstitial infiltration of inflammatory cells, alveolar septal thickening and collapsed alveolar spaces (Fig. 1b, upper panel). Notably, treatment with dexamethasone or SML

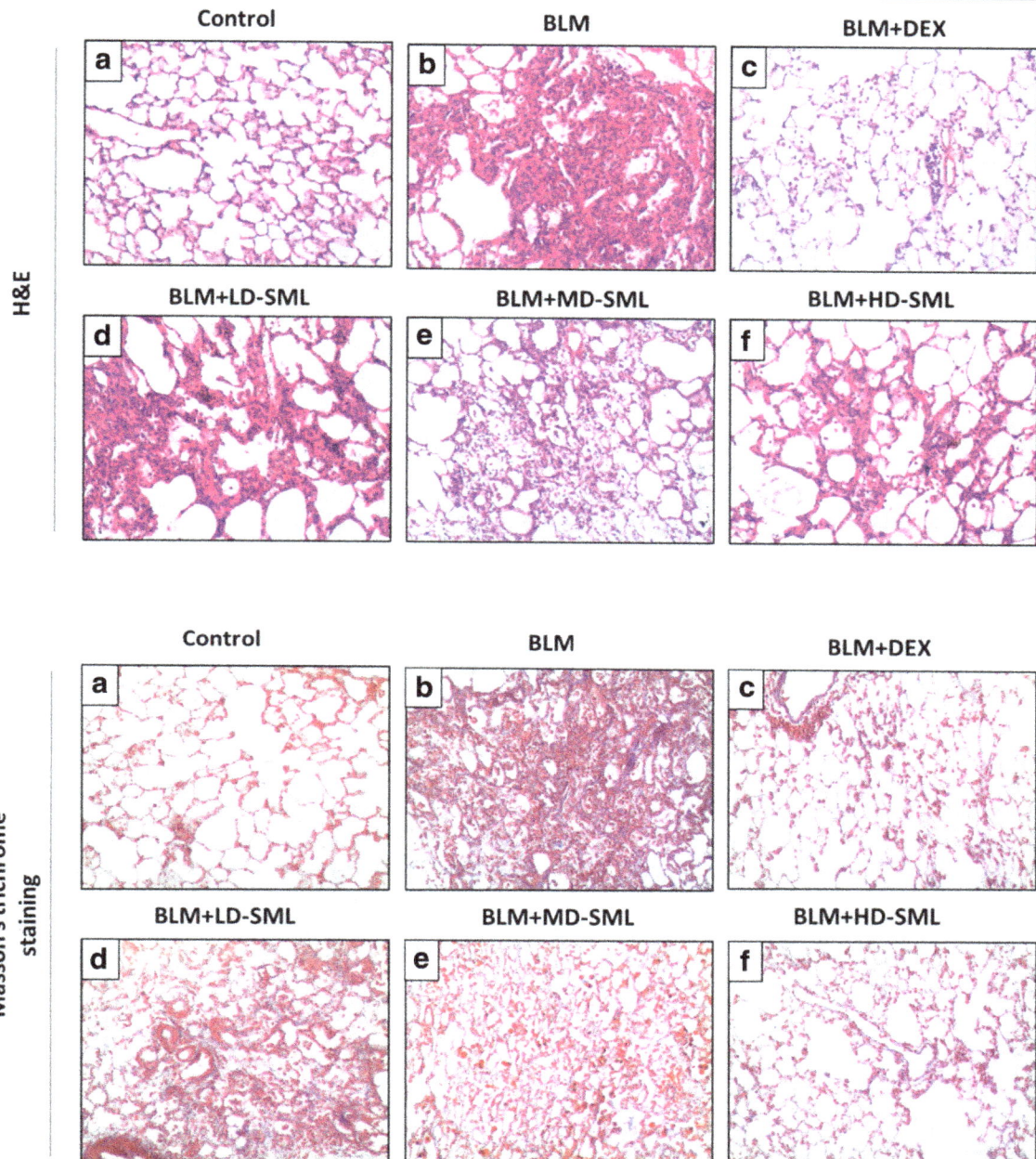

Fig. 1 Representative photographs for H&E (upper panel) and Masson's trichrome (lower panel) staining of rat lung tissues on the 28th day. H&E staining of lung tissue sections are shown in the upper panel: **a** control animals showing normal lung tissue morphology; **b** bleomycin treated animals showing distorted lung morphologies with inflammatory cell infiltration, thickened interalveolar septa, alveolar edema, alveolar exudate, collapsed alveolar spaces with inflammatory exudates; **c** dexamethasone treated rats with significant less inflammatory cell infiltration; **d–f** animals treated with low-dose (LD), medium-dose (MD) and high-dose (HD) SML showing less inflammation compared to bleomycin alone treated animals. Masson's trichrome staining for collagen assessment in lung tissues are shown in the lower panel: **a** lung tissue sections of control animals showing scarcely deposited collagen in the lung parenchyma; **b** BLM-induced animals showing dense collagen accumulations; **c** DEX-treated animals showing less collagen deposition as compared to BLM-induced group; **d–f** low-dose (LD), medium-dose (MD) and high-dose (HD) SML-treated animals showing improved collagen deposition compared to BLM-induced group

prominently reduced the lung damage induced by BLM, and the effect of SML was in a dose-dependent manner (Fig. 1c–f, upper panel). The low-dose SML treatment slightly ameliorated the BLM-induced pathological changes, while the medium- and high-dose SML significantly alleviated the lung damage as shown by decrease in infiltration of inflammatory cells and thin lined alveolar septa compared with BLM-induced animals (Fig. 1f, upper panel).

Alveolitis scoring was performed depending on the severity of inflammation. In BLM group, significant infiltration ($p < 0.05$) of inflammatory cells was observed on day 7 compared to control group, which gradually subsided on day 14 and 28. Whereas, in groups supplemented with medium- and high-dose SML, significant decrease ($p < 0.05$) in the infiltration of inflammatory cells were observed in the lung tissue on day 14 and 28 as demonstrated by lower alveolitis score compared to BLM-treated rats (Fig. 2). The low-dose SML slightly ameliorated the infiltration, but the value was not significant compared to that of BLM-group at day 14 and 28. It should be noted that the medium- and high-dose SML intervention showed comparable anti-fibrotic effect compared with the DEX treatment on day 14 and 28 according to the histological examination and alveolitis scores (Fig. 1, upper panel and Fig. 2).

SML reduced pathological collagen deposition in BLM-induced lung fibrosis

Fibrillar collagen deposition, an indicator of lung fibrosis, was determined by Masson's trichome staining (Fig. 1, lower panel). Injection of BLM increased collagen accumulation in the interstitial lung spaces with almost complete destruction of the alveolar architecture (Fig. 1b, lower panel). The collagen deposition was attenuated by administration of DEX or SML (Fig. 1c–f, lower panel),

which showed fewer and smaller fibrotic foci. The Ashcroft quantitative pathological scoring of Masson's trichrome staining is presented in Fig. 3. The fibrosis score was significantly higher ($p < 0.05$) in BLM-induced fibrotic rats compared with the negative control group at day 7, 14 and 28, while treatment of DEX or SML (medium and high-dose) significantly reduced the fibrosis score ($p < 0.05$). The low-dose SML showed no obvious anti-fibrotic effect. Of particular note, DEX and medium- or high-dose SML showed comparable extent of anti-fibrotic effect on day 14 and 28. These data supported the view that SML played an important role in reducing pathological collagen deposition and structural damage in the BLM-induced rat lung fibrosis model.

SML represses the expression of TNF-α, TGF-β1 and SMAD4 proteins in BLM-induced lung fibrosis

To demonstrate the anti-inflammatory and anti-fibrotic activity of SML, the levels of TNF-α, TGF-β1 and SMAD-4 were studied in different groups by immunohistochemical analysis. SMAD-4 plays an important role in the modulation of the TGF-β pathway. The results are displayed in Figs. 4 and 5. The lung tissue from the control rats showed less expression of TNF-α, TGF-β1 and SMAD4 compared with other groups. The expression of TNF-α, TGF-β1 and SMAD4 in the DEX group and low-, medium-, high-dose SML groups were significantly reduced compared with that in BLM-group (Fig. 4). Importantly, compared with DEX group, medium and high-dose SML showed more significantly reduced expression of TNF-α, TGF-β1and SMAD4 on day 7, 14 and 28 (Fig. 5; $p < 0.05$). In particular, on day 28, the relative expression of TNF-α was significantly reduced to 1.92 ± 0.17, and 1.83 ± 0.13 in medium-, and

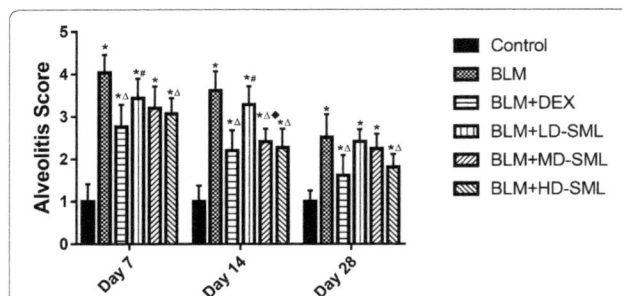

Fig. 2 Inflammatory (alveolitis) score in the control and experimental animals at 7, 14 and 28 days of treatment. Each value is expressed as mean ± S.D. (n = 5). Results are statistically significance at $p < 0.05$. *$p < 0.05$ vs control; $^\Delta p < 0.05$ vs BLM; $^\# p < 0.05$ vs BLM + DEX; ■$p < 0.05$ vs BLM + LD-SML, by two-way ANOVA followed by Tukey's multiple comparisons test. *LD* low-dose, *MD* medium-dose, *HD* high-dose

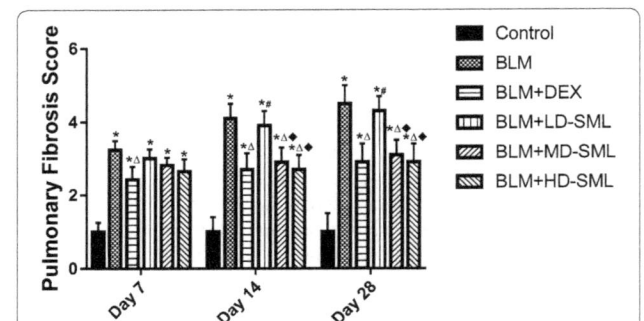

Fig. 3 Quantitative evaluation of fibrotic changes (fibrotic tissue and collagen) in the lung sections by Ashcroft scoring at 7, 14 and 28 days of treatment. Each value is expressed as mean ± S.D. (n = 5). Results are statistically significance at $p < 0.05$. *$p < 0.05$ vs control; $^\Delta p < 0.05$ vs BLM; $^\# p < 0.05$ vs BLM + DEX; ■$p < 0.05$ vs BLM + LD-SML, by two-way ANOVA followed by Tukey's multiple comparisons test. *LD* low-dose, *MD* medium-dose, *HD* high-dose

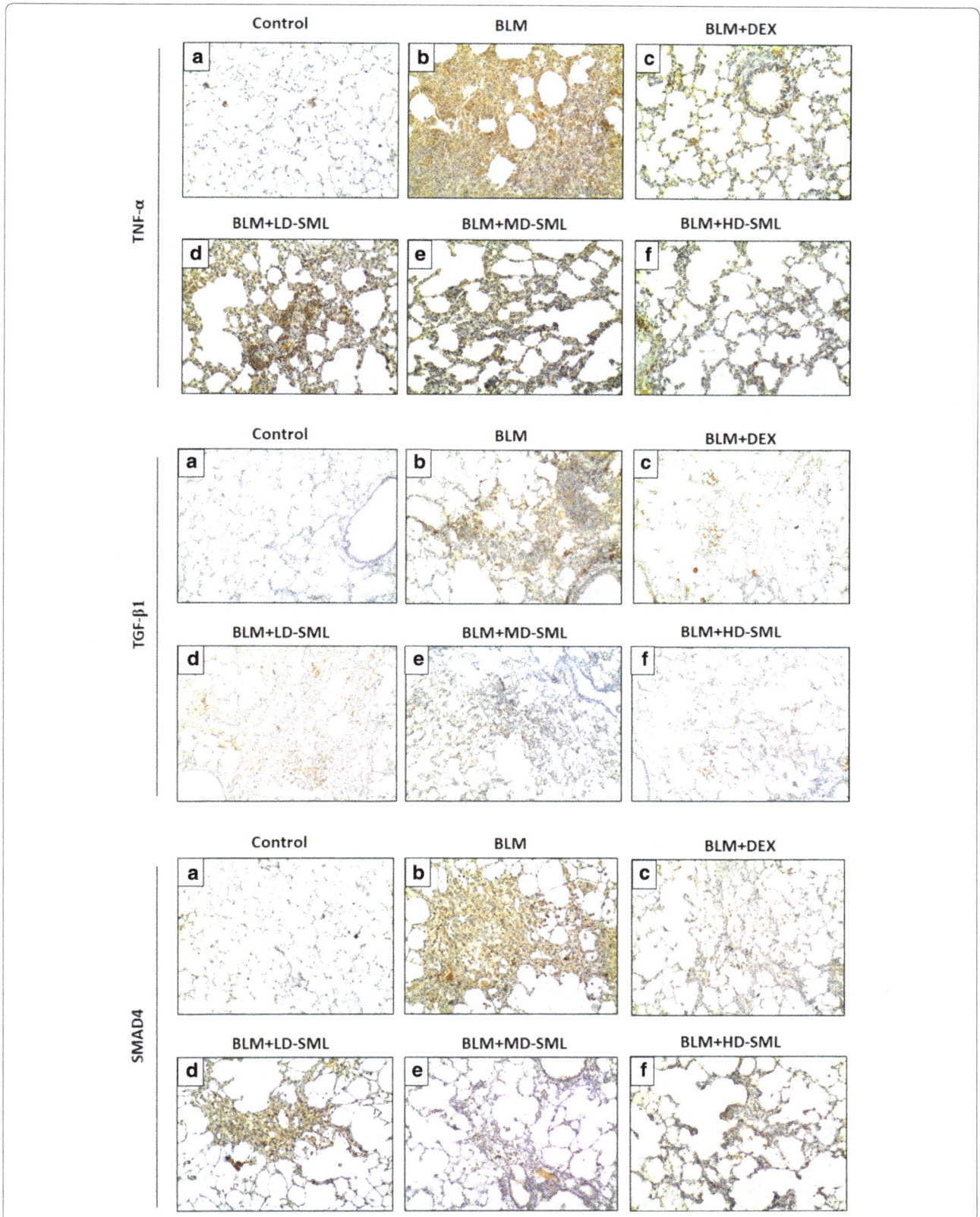

high-dose SML groups, respectively, while that in DEX group was 2.58 ± 0.14. Similarly, the relative expression of TGF-β1 protein in medium- and high-dose SML groups on day 28 was significantly reduced to 2.59 ± 0.33, and 2.46 ± 0.20, respectively, while that in DEX group was 3.07 ± 0.35. Moreover, compared to low-dose SML, treatment with medium- and high-dose of SML showed significant decrease in the expression of TNF-α, TGF-β1 and SMAD4 ($p < 0.05$). There is no significant difference between medium- and high-dose SML in the level of TNF-α, TGF-β1 and SMAD4 protein (Fig. 5).

The above results were further confirmed by quantitatively analysis of serum levels of TNF-α and TGF-β1 using ELISA kit. The data shown in Fig. 6 indicated that DEX and medium- and high-dose SML significantly decreased the serum concentrations of TNF-α and TGF-β1 at day 28 ($p < 0.05$). The medium- and/or high-dose SML showed a better effect than DEX to repress TNF-α and TGF-β1. Moreover, compared to the serum levels of TNF-α and TGF-β1 in medium- and high-dose of SML groups were lower than that in low-dose SML group ($p < 0.05$). These results indicated that SML treatment attenuated BLM-induced fibrosis via significantly reducing the expression of TNF-α and TGF-β1 in fibrotic lung tissues.

SML did not induce toxicity in rats

The serum levels of ALT, AST and Cre in rats on day 28th were determined to assess the safety of applying SML and DEX. ALT and AST are important indices commonly used for evaluating liver function, while Cre is one of the most critical indices to monitor kidney function. The results (Fig. 7) indicated that the serum levels of ALT, AST and Cre in all rats were within the normal physiological range, and no differences were found among different groups. This suggested that SML and DEX at the designed dosage did not induce significant toxicity in rats.

Discussion

IPF is a progressive fatal lung disease characterized by epithelial/fibroblastic disarray with excessive ECM deposition, which is due to injury to the alveolar epithelial cell, re-modelling of the ECM matrix, proliferation and accumulation of fibroblast, resulting in impaired lung

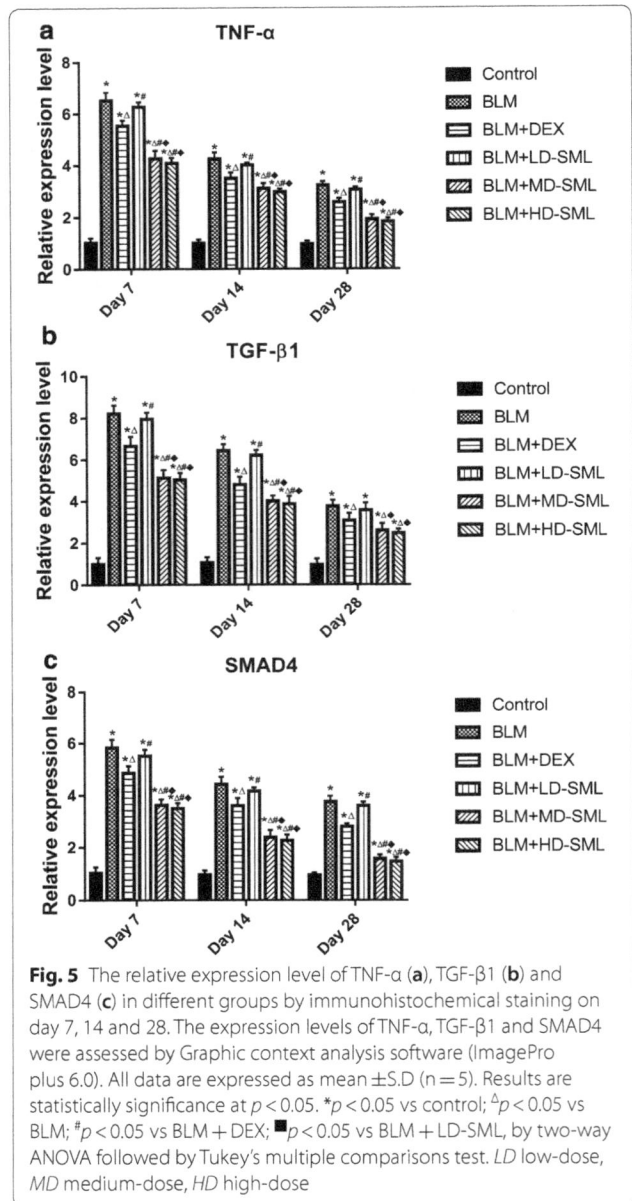

Fig. 5 The relative expression level of TNF-α (**a**), TGF-β1 (**b**) and SMAD4 (**c**) in different groups by immunohistochemical staining on day 7, 14 and 28. The expression levels of TNF-α, TGF-β1 and SMAD4 were assessed by Graphic context analysis software (ImagePro plus 6.0). All data are expressed as mean ±S.D (n = 5). Results are statistically significance at $p < 0.05$. *$p < 0.05$ vs control; $^\Delta p < 0.05$ vs BLM; $^\# p < 0.05$ vs BLM + DEX; $\blacksquare p < 0.05$ vs BLM + LD-SML, by two-way ANOVA followed by Tukey's multiple comparisons test. *LD* low-dose, *MD* medium-dose, *HD* high-dose

function and death. Currently, there is no complete cure for IPF, and the treatment options available are limited. This necessitates the need for developing new modalities for treating this devastating disorder. In this study,

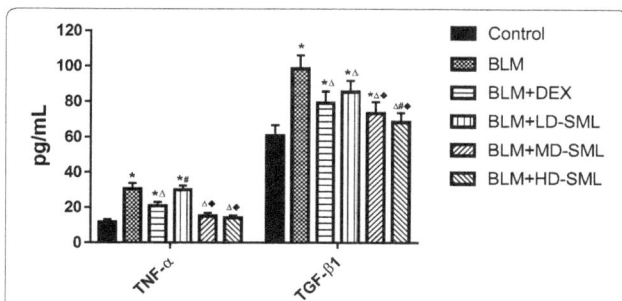

Fig. 6 The serum levels (pg/mL) of TNF-α and TGF-β1 in different groups by ELISA on day 28. All data are expressed as mean ± S.D. (n = 5). Results are statistically significance at $p < 0.05$. *$p < 0.05$ vs control; $^{\Delta}p < 0.05$ vs BLM; $^{\#}p < 0.05$ vs BLM + DEX; $^{\blacksquare}p < 0.05$ vs BLM + LD-SML, by one-way ANOVA followed by Tukey's multiple comparisons test. *LD* low-dose, *MD* medium-dose, *HD* high-dose

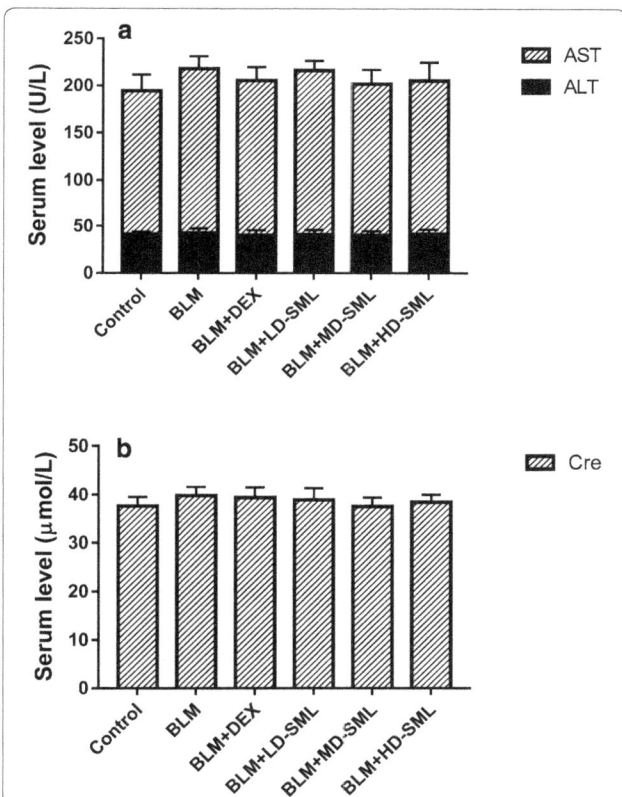

Fig. 7 The serum levels of ALT, AST and Cre in rats on day 28th. All data are expressed as mean ± S.D. (n = 5). Statistical analysis was performed by one-way ANOVA followed by Tukey's multiple comparisons test

the anti-fibrotic role of SML against BLM-induced pulmonary fibrosis was evaluated. We showed evidence that SML prevented BLM-induced fibrosis by attenuating inflammation and collagen deposition and modulating the expression of TNF-α and SMAD4.

BLM is a chemotherapeutic agent used in the management of various neoplastic diseases such as lymphomas, head and neck squamous cell carcinomas, testicular carcinomas, ovarian cancer and malignant pleural effusions [24]. The development of pulmonary fibrosis is the major dose-limiting side effect of this anticancer agent. Various methods to induce lung damage similar to human IPF are available by using chemicals (BLM, peplomycin, fluorescein isothiocyanate, vanadium pentoxide, trinitrobenzene sulfonic acid), growth factor gene over-expression (TGF-β, IL-1β, IL-13, etc.) and inorganic particles (silica, asbestos). Amongst all, BLM-induced pulmonary fibrosis is ideal, reproducible, consistent. The established animal model, as intratracheal instillation, mimics all the clinico-pathological features of human IPF [25]. BLM-induced pulmonary fibrosis consists of two phases. The first phase is characterized by predominant inflammatory component where activated inflammatory cells release increased amounts of ROS and RNS resulting in parenchymal injury, and this occurs in 2-weeks after BLM administration. The inflammatory phase is followed by late fibrotic phase between the 3rd and 4th week, and is characterized by intense deposition of ECM, resulting in fibrosis [24, 26]. In the present study, BLM caused distortion of lung morphology with interstitial infiltration of inflammatory cells, peribronchial and perialveolar septal thickening and collapsed alveolar spaces (Fig. 1, upper panel). Moreover, BLM administration increased collagen accumulation in the interstitial lung spaces. Treatment with DEX and SML significantly reduced the damage and attenuated the collagen deposition induced by BLM demonstrating the protective effect in BLM-induced fibrosis. This is also evident from the decreased alveolitis and fibrosis scores in SML-treated animals compared to BLM-group.

Cytokines play an important role in pathogenesis of pulmonary fibrosis [27]. Different cytokines interact with each other and forms a complicated network which play the key role in the pathogenesis of IPF. Many researchers investigated the effect of TNF-α in IPF, and found that TNF-α plays an important role in the development of interstitial inflammation and pulmonary fibrosis. TNF-α regulates the apoptosis of respiratory epithelial cells, induces the expression of other cytokines and inflammatory mediators [28]. Also, TNF-α up-regulates the expression of TGF-β1, activates NF-κB, and promotes the proliferation, differentiation of fibroblasts finally induces pulmonary fibrosis [8, 24]. Previous studies have demonstrated that infliximab, a TNF-α antagonist, improved the degree of pulmonary fibrosis induced by BLM in rats [12]. Moreover, a randomized, placebo-controlled, multicentred trial demonstrated that etanercept, another TNF-α antagonist, decreased the rate of disease progression in IPF patients [10]. In the present study, increased expression of TNF-α was observed in the lung tissues of BLM-treated rats. Treatment of SML attenuated the expression of TNF-α. Importantly, the medium- and high-dose SML showed much better activity than DEX on days 7, 14 and 28.

TGF-β, the pro-fibrotic cytokine, plays a key role in pulmonary fibrosis by inducing fibroblast activation, myofibroblast differentiation with increased αSMA expression and ECM accumulation. TGF-β1 signalling from the cell membrane to the nucleus occurs mainly via SMAD proteins. SMAD4 combines with the activated SMAD2/3 to form a tripolymer, which activates the promoter of ECM, like collagen, in the cell nucleus. This might be the process which explains the involvement of SMAD4 in the occurrence and progression of pulmonary fibrosis. Recent study has shown that pirfenidone, the anti-fibrotic agent, significantly repressed the TGF-β1 induced expression of SMAD2/4 proteins and prevented the nuclear accumulation and translocation of SMAD2 protein, thereby inhibiting proliferation, migration and differentiation of TGF-β1-stimulated murine mesenchymal stem cells [29]. In the present study, SML reduced the expression of both TGF-β1 and SMAD4. Similar to SML, many natural compounds including berberine [13], daidzein [30], and ginsenoside Rg1 [31] exerted protective effect by intervening the TGF-β/SMAD signalling pathway. The advantage of using natural products, including SML, is that they usually do not induce significant side effects in body even with a long-term application. In our study, it is found that both SML did not induce toxicity in rats, as evidenced by no significant changes in ALT, AST and Cre levels in serum. However, DEX, the typical immunosuppressive therapy, always leads to unwanted adverse effects on cardiac, digestive and skin systems. Taken together, in the present study, SML decreased the tissue expression of TNF-α and TGF-β1, and improved pulmonary fibrosis in rats, which was much effective at medium and high doses compared with DEX. Hence, the current study confirms that SML exhibits anti-fibrotic activity by repressing the expression of TNF-α and TGF-β1 proteins.

Conclusions

The present study demonstrated the anti-fibrotic effect of SML in BLM-induced pulmonary fibrosis as evidenced from the H&E and Masson's trichome staining, showing improved alveolitis and fibrosis scores. Furthermore, SML alleviates BLM-induced fibrosis by decreasing the expression of TNF-α, TGF-β1 and SMAD4 in the lung tissues. We also compared the anti-fibrotic effect of SML with DEX, a drug commonly used for IPF. SML at

the medium or high dose showed comparable or even higher extent of anti-fibrotic effect with that of DEX. These findings reveal the beneficial effect of SML against BLM mediated fibrotic challenge through suppressing TNF-α and TGF-β mediated fibrotic events. However, further research is warranted to elucidate the mechanisms regarding SML regulation on the profound cellular events of BLM-induced pulmonary fibrosis.

Abbreviations
ALT: alanine aminotransferase; AST: aspartate aminotransferase; BLM: bleomycin; Cre: creatinine; DEX: dexamethasone; ECM: excessive extracellular matrix; IPF: idiopathic pulmonary fibrosis; SML: combination of *Salvia miltiorrhiza* and ligustrazine.

Authors' contributions
CH and XF designed the study. XW, WW and FG conducted the literature search. XW, CH and SW drafted the manuscript and prepared tables and figures. XW, YC, BP and MZ contributed to revisions of the manuscript. All authors read and approved the final manuscript.

Author details
[1] Department of Respiratory Medicine II, The Affiliated Hospital of Southwest Medical University, Luzhou, Sichuan, China. [2] Laboratory of Molecular Pharmacology, Department of Pharmacology, School of Pharmacy, Southwest Medical University, Luzhou, Sichuan, China. [3] State Key Laboratory of Quality Research in Chinese Medicine, Institute of Chinese Medical Sciences, University of Macau, Macao, China.

Acknowledgements
The authors would thank Professor Xiaoqin Zhan for discussion and helpful suggestions. The authors acknowledge Dr. Lakshmi Narendra B for providing linguistic assistance in the preparation of the manuscript.

Competing interests
The authors declare that they have no competing interests.

Consent for publication
The manuscript is approved by all authors for publication.

Funding
The project was supported by grant received by Prof. Xianming Fan from Youth Science and Technology Fund of Sichuan Province (Grant No: 2009-04-395).

References
1. Ahluwalia N, Shea BS, Tager AM. New therapeutic targets in idiopathic pulmonary fibrosis. Aiming to rein in runaway wound-healing responses. Am J Respir Crit Care. 2014;190:867–78.
2. Sgalla G, Biffi A, Richeldi L. Idiopathic pulmonary fibrosis: diagnosis, epidemiology and natural history. Respirology. 2016;21:427–37.
3. Huang H, Peng X, Zhong C. Idiopathic pulmonary fibrosis: the current status of its epidemiology, diagnosis, and treatment in China. Intractable Rare Dis Res. 2013;2:88–93.
4. King TE, Pardo A, Selman M. Idiopathic pulmonary fibrosis. Lancet. 2011;378:1949–61.
5. Wuyts WA, Agostini C, Antoniou KM, Bouros D, Chambers RC, Cottin V, Egan JJ, Lambrecht BN, Lories R, Parfrey H. The pathogenesis of pulmonary fibrosis: a moving target. Eur Respir J. 2013;41:1207–18.

6. Coward WR, Saini G, Jenkins G. The pathogenesis of idiopathic pulmonary fibrosis. Ther Adv Respir Dis. 2010;4:367.
7. Song X, Liu W, Xie S, Wang M, Cao G, Mao C, Lv C. All-transretinoic acid ameliorates bleomycin-induced lung fibrosis by downregulating the TGF-β1/Smad3 signaling pathway in rats. J Wuhan Univ Sci Technol. 2013;93:1219–31.
8. Zhao Y, Tian B, Sadygov RG, Zhang Y, Brasier AR. Integrative proteomic analysis reveals reprograming tumor necrosis factor signaling in epithelial mesenchymal transition. J Proteomics. 2016;148:126–38.
9. Kabel AM, Omar MS, Elmaaboud MAA. Amelioration of bleomycin-induced lung fibrosis in rats by valproic acid and butyrate: role of nuclear factor kappa-B, proinflammatory cytokines and oxidative stress. Int Immunopharmacol. 2016;39:335–42.
10. Raghu G, Brown KK, Costabel U, Cottin V, Du BR, Lasky JA, Thomeer M, Utz JP, Khandker RK, Mcdermott L. Treatment of idiopathic pulmonary fibrosis with etanercept: an exploratory, placebo-controlled trial. Expert Opin Emerg Drugs. 2008;178:948.
11. Turgut NH, Haki K, Sahende E, Koksal D, Huseyin G, Emre A. The protective effect of naringin against bleomycin-induced pulmonary fibrosis in Wistar rats. Pulm Med. 2016;2016:1–12.
12. Altintas N, Erboga M, Aktas C, Bilir B, Aydin M, Sengul A, Ates Z, Topcu B, Gurel A. Protective effect of infliximab, a tumor necrosis factor-alfa inhibitor, on bleomycin-induced lung fibrosis in rats. Inflammation. 2016;39:65–78.
13. Chitra P, Saiprasad G, Manikandan R, Sudhandiran G. Berberine attenuates bleomycin induced pulmonary toxicity and fibrosis via suppressing NF-κB dependant TGF-β activation: a biphasic experimental study. Toxicol Lett. 2013;219:178–93.
14. Lei L, Wei L, Zhuang M, Zhenhua L. Oxymatrine attenuates bleomycin-induced pulmonary fibrosis in mice via the inhibition of inducible nitric oxide synthase expression and the TGF-β/Smad signaling pathway. Int J Mol Med. 2012;29:815.
15. Ti DY, Han YL, Yang GY, Yang XL. Clinical observation of efficacy of Danshen and ligustrazine on 86 patients with idiopathic pulmonary fibrosis. Heilongjiang Med J. 2010;23:102–3.
16. Guo F, Fan XM. Therapeutic effect of Danshen and ligustrazine for fibrosis. Med Recapitulate. 2010;16:2087–90.
17. Pan Y, Fu H, Kong Q, Xiao Y, Shou Q, Chen H, Ke Y, Chen M. Prevention of pulmonary fibrosis with salvianolic acid a by inducing fibroblast cell cycle arrest and promoting apoptosis. J Ethnopharmacol. 2014;155:1589–96.
18. Lu SJ, Liu YN. Study of *Salvia miltiorrhiza* on bleomycin-induced pulmonary fibrosis in mice. Chin J Clin Pharmacol Ther. 2005;10:514–7.
19. Liu M, Xu H, Zhang L, Zhang C, Yang L, Ma E, Liu L, Li Y. Salvianolic acid B inhibits myofibroblast transdifferentiation in experimental pulmonary fibrosis via the up-regulation of Nrf2. Biochem Biophys Res Commun. 2018;495:325–31.
20. Li YF, Yu Y. Effect of ligustrazine on pulmonary fibrosis caused by hyper-oxia in neonatal rats. J Appl Clin Pediatr. 2009;24:126–8.
21. Zhao J, Wang HM, Wang HZ. The protective effect of ligustrazine on bleomycin-induced pulmonary fibrosis. J Liaoning Med Univ. 2006;27:11–3.
22. Wu X, Zhang F, Xiong X, Lu C, Lian N, Lu Y, Zheng S. Tetramethylpyrazine reduces inflammation in liver fibrosis and inhibits inflammatory cytokine expression in hepatic stellate cells by modulating NLRP3 inflammasome pathway. IUBMB Life. 2015;67:312–21.
23. Mai AZ, Zaki HF, El-Brairy AI, Kenawy SA. Pyrrolidinedithiocarbamate attenuates bleomycin-induced pulmonary fibrosis in rats: modulation of oxidative stress, fibrosis, and inflammatory parameters. Exp Lung Res. 2016;42:408–16.
24. Della LV, Cecchettini A, Del RS, Morales MA. Bleomycin in the setting of lung fibrosis induction: From biological mechanisms to counteractions. Pharmacol Res. 2015;97:122–30.
25. Kandhare AD, Bodhankar SL, Mohan V, Thakurdesai PA. Effect of glyco-sides based standardized fenugreek seed extract in bleomycin-induced pulmonary fibrosis in rats: decisive role of Bax, Nrf2, NF-κB, Muc5ac, TNF-α and IL-1β. Chem Biol Interact. 2015;237:151–65.
26. Tian K, Lin L, Jia Z, Guo X, Zhang L. Preventive effect of chrysin on bleomycin-induced lung fibrosis in rats. Inflammation. 2014;37:2116–24.
27. Antoniou KM, Alexandrakis MG, Siafakas NM, Bouros D. Cytokine network in the pathogenesis of idiopathic pulmonary fibrosis. Sarcoidosis Vasc Diffuse Lung Dis. 2005;22:91–104.
28. Carré P, Léophonte P. Cytokines and pulmonary fibroses. Rev Mal Respir. 1993;10:193–207.
29. Jin SF, Ma HL, Liu ZL, Fu ST, Zhang CP, He Y. XL413, a cell division cycle 7 kinase inhibitor enhanced the anti-fibrotic effect of pirfenidone on TGF-β1-stimulated C3H10T1/2 cells via Smad2/4. Exp Cell Res. 2015;339:289–99.
30. Soumyakrishnan S, Divya T, Kalayarasan S, Sriram N, Sudhandiran G. Daidzein exhibits anti-fibrotic effect by reducing the expressions of proteinase activated receptor 2 and TGFβ1/smad mediated inflammation and apoptosis in bleomycin-induced experimental pulmonary fibrosis. Biochimie. 2014;103:23–36.
31. Zhan H, Huang F, Ma W, Zhao Z, Zhang H, Zhang C. Protective effect of ginsenoside rg1 on bleomycin-induced pulmonary fibrosis in rats: involvement of caveolin-1 and TGF-β1 signal pathway. Biol Pharm Bull. 2016;39:1284–92.

6

A research on syndrome element differentiation based on phenomenology and mathematical method

Enliang Yan[1], Jialin Song[1], Chaonan Liu[2] and Wenxue Hong[1,2]*

Abstract

Background: As an empirical medical system independent of conventional Western medicine (CWM), over thousands of years, traditional Chinese medicine (TCM) has established its own unique method of diagnosis and treatment. The perspective of holism and system in TCM is essentially different from the view of Reductionism in CWM. With the development of modern science and technology, the restriction of reductionism is more and more prominent, and researchers begin to pay more attention to holistic thinking in TCM. Confronted with the above situation, there is an urgent need to explore the diagnosis of TCM by the techniques of modern science.

Methods: To explore the feasibility of using modern science to describe and realize the diagnosis of TCM, in this paper, a method of syndrome element differentiation based on phenomenology is proposed. The proposed method is implemented by mathematical mapping, and then it is testified through analysis of 670 medical records: Based on the original mapping data between two data sets (set of syndrome elements and set of clinical manifestations), new mapping data is generated, and thus the corresponding quantitative diagnostic results are calculated and evaluated. Finally, knowledge discovery of the diagnosis results based on attribute partial-ordered structure diagram is conducted.

Results: The value order's matching results between original and new results show that the matched degree of each record is no less than 65%, while there are at least 87% records whose matched degree is more than 80%. In addition, the knowledge discoveries of new results are basically identical with the ones of original results as well.

Conclusion: Using phenomenology to describe syndrome differentiation should be feasible, and further research on mapping relations between various sets (symptoms, formulas, drugs) of TCM should be conducted and evaluated through clinical trials in future.

Keywords: Syndrome element, Syndrome differentiation, Traditional Chinese medicine, Mathematical mapping, Phenomenology, Attribute partial-ordered structure diagram

Background

With the development of science and the change of living environment, people's cognition of health has deepened, and the focus of medical science has gradually shifted from disease treatment to prevention and healthcare. Therefore, it has been an urgent issue to evaluate health state objectively and accurately. As an important and

irreplaceable constitution of modern medicine, over the past decades, traditional Chinese medicine (TCM) has gained wide attention in the medical field of both domestic and abroad. In terms of both theory and practice, TCM provides an essentially distinct medical approach compared to conventional Western medicine (CWM). Taking holism as core, TCM has unique advantages in the aspects of health maintenance and disease prevention. Meanwhile, with the dramatic increase in prevalence of chronic diseases, the treatment of CWM has begun to be stretched, while the natural medicine and

*Correspondence: 844353390@qq.com
[1] Institute of Electrical Engineering, Yanshan University, No. 438, Hebei Avenue, Qinhuangdao 066004, Hebei, People's Republic of China

therapy of TCM can contribute a lot to this condition. Therefore, TCM has attracted unprecedented expectations and attention [1]. However, despite the great advantages, the understanding, education and application of TCM is relatively insufficient, the main reason of which may be that the diagnosis of TCM is equivocal in the perspective of modern science. Therefore, using methods of modern science to describe and realize the diagnosis of TCM has been an urgent issue.

Over the past decades, with the goal of modernization, research on TCM diagnosis has attracted significant attention. Wang constructed a quantitative system for pulse diagnosis [2] and proposed a quantitative method for syndrome differentiation [3] based on Bayesian networks. Wang also proposed a method based on decision tree to explore the quantitative recognition of pulse strength [4]. To make both qualitative and quantitative analysis for analysis for facial complexion, Zhao [5] proposed a feature representation of facial complexion from whole face of patients. Using multi-class support vector machine, Li [6] designed a computer-assisted classification method for syndrome diagnosis based on lip images. Liu [7] explored a multi-label learning technique to do inquiry diagnosis for CHD in TCM. Su [8] reviewed the technologies and methods and their application in syndrome differentiation for TCM.

These studies provide valuable experience and guidance for the research of syndrome differentiation in TCM. However, even a large amount of TCM diagnosis system is developed by computational methods, and most of them claimed that their methods or systems could analyze TCM data from a quantitative perspective. Actually none of them could quantize their diagnostic data with meaningful implications corresponding to TCM theory, as the clinical indicators from the perspective of CWM. If this situation could not be improved, the establishment of quantitative diagnosis of TCM may be very difficult [9]. As was Prof. Qian said, the theory of TCM is not natural science, while it is natural philosophy which is based on phenomenological cognition [10], that's why the classical methods for CWM are not suitable for TCM. Therefore, it is still a challenging issue to develop an approach which can both realize the quantitative diagnosis of TCM in modern science and be consistent with the phenomenological cognition of TCM.

In view of the above situation, to explore the feasibility of using modern science to describe and realize the diagnosis of TCM, a method of syndrome differentiation, which is based on phenomenology TCM, is proposed in this article. The approach can realize the quantitative diagnosis of TCM, and it is implemented by mathematical mapping.

This paper is organized as follows: "Background" introduces the research background and the motivation of the study. "Theories" describes the theories adopted in this paper, including phenomenology, syndrome element differentiation and attribute partial-ordered structure diagram. "Methods" explains the methods of clinical data acquisition, mapping data reconstruction, matching, evaluation and knowledge discovery of results. "Results" shows the results of data processing and knowledge discovery. "Discussion" discusses the results of the research. "Conclusion" draws the conclusion of the study.

Theories
Theory of phenomenology
Phenomenology, proposed by philosopher Edmund Husserl, is a philosophical methodology [11]. Phenomenological researchers believe that people usually cognitive the world through direct experience and ideological processing, which is called 'phenomenological method' in the field of physics. In the perception of phenomenology, the microscopic cause of phenomenon is not so important, while associations between diverse phenomena are the key points, and these associations can be acquired by summing up experience and summarizing experimental facts.

To sum up, concentrating on the research of 'phenomena': appearances of things, or things as they appear in our experience, or the ways we experience things [12], phenomenology refers to the system theory which analyzes, induces and summarizes the essence of things by the phenomenon, which happens to be consistent with the thought of TCM. TCM is also a qualitative theory which uses a summarization of the associations between phenomena or functions, not detail description of concrete mechanism [13]. Therefore, using phenomenology to describe the diagnosis of TCM should be feasible in theory.

Figure 1 shows the mathematical description of phenomenology. As shown in the figure, the appearance of things can be regarded as a source domain set, while the essence of things can be seen as an image domain set, and the relations between appearance and essence can be described by generalized mapping. As philosophers say, our conception (phenomenon) of natural laws (mapping) depend on our approach to understanding reality (essence), there is no theory-independent concept of reality, and every law (mapping) we acquired is only an approximation of reality. In real life, the approximation of mapping between appearance and essence can be acquired by observation, induction, deduction and many other kinds of machine learning methods.

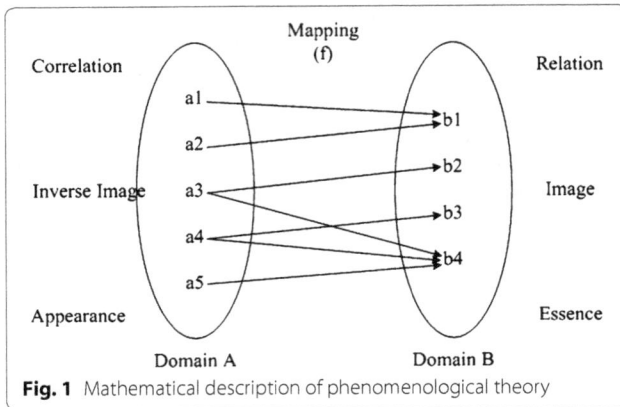

Fig. 1 Mathematical description of phenomenological theory

Theory of syndrome element differentiation

As a peculiar rational concept in TCM, syndrome is the combination of philosophy, epistemology, medical theory and clinical practice. It is a physiological or pathological generalization of the overall health state of a body at a given stage. Syndrome usually consists of two parts: location and essence. Syndrome differentiation is the process of obtaining the location and essence of syndrome through overall analysis of clinical manifestations acquired from patient by four examinations and achieving a syndrome name which can represents the health state of the patient. In TCM, for the diagnosis and treatment of disease, it is essential to identify the syndrome accurately and precisely [14].

Syndrome element differentiation is a method of syndrome differentiation proposed by Prof. Zhu [15], and in his theory, the process of syndrome differentiation is divided into two parts: quantification of syndrome elements according to clinical manifestations and syndrome

matching based on the quantification of syndrome elements [16].

Figure 2 shows the mathematical description of syndrome element differentiation. From the perspective of phenomenology, the process of syndrome element differentiation can be regarded as two mappings between three domain sets, and the key to syndrome differentiation is to discover these two mapping relations.

With years of research, extracting from classical literature and clinical records, Prof. Zhu has given out the original mapping data between clinical manifestations and syndrome elements [16].

Theory of attribute partial-ordered structure diagram (APOSD)

APOSD, which can extract knowledge from formal context and visualize the results in intelligible diagram, is a method of knowledge discovery proposed by Prof. Hong [17]. APOSD stems from formal concept analysis (FCA), partial order of mathematics is its basis of data analyzing and the generation of APOSD is identical with the philosophical principle of human cognition of things [18].

Formal context is the data basis of APOSD. A formal context $K = (U, M, I)$ consists of two sets $U = \{u1, u2, \ldots, un\}$ and $M = \{m1, m2, \ldots, mk\}$ and a relation I between U and M. The elements of U are called the objects and the elements of M are called the attributes of the context. The data shown in Table 1 is a classical example of formal context.

As shown in Table 1, the data in the first row is the set of attributes, while the data in the first column is the set of objects, and the number '1' in the intersection of object and attribute means the object has the attribute, or the attribute belongs to the object.

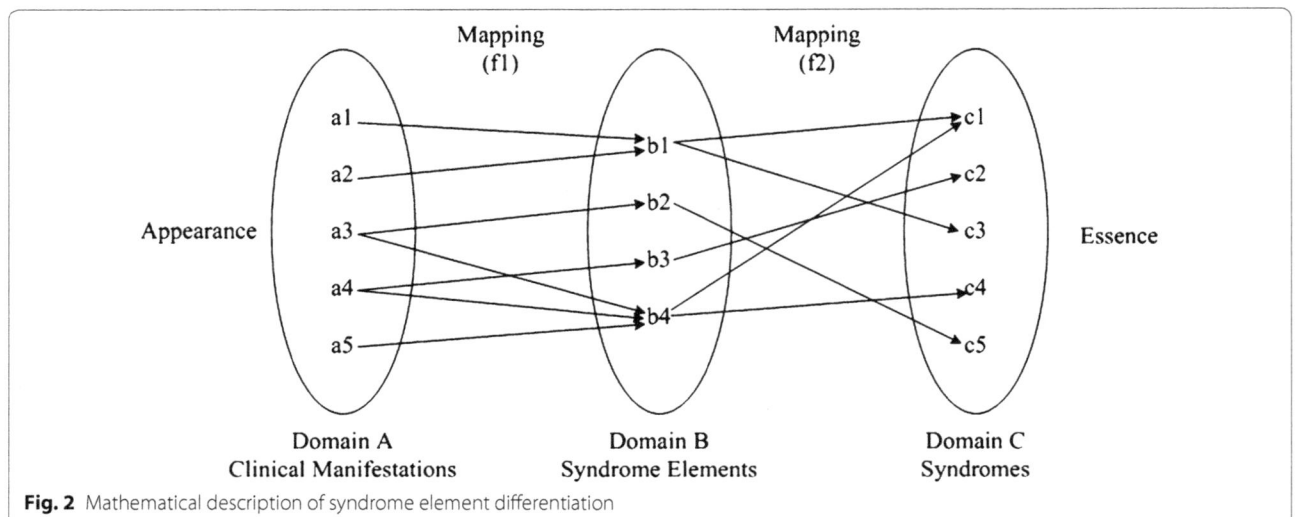

Fig. 2 Mathematical description of syndrome element differentiation

Table 1 Formal context of example

	a1	a2	a3	a4	a5	a6	a7	a8	a9
o1	1	1					1		
o2	1	1					1	1	
o3	1	1	1				1	1	
o4	1		1				1	1	1
o5	1	1		1		1			
o6	1	1	1	1		1			
o7	1		1	1	1				
o8	1		1	1		1			

Similar to formal concept analysis (FCA), APOSD emphasizes cognitive ability and concentrates on the relation between different data sets. The difference between FCA and APOSD is that FCA focuses on the generation and analysis of concept and concept lattice, while APOSD concentrates on the study of attributes' feature. Based on the formal context in Table 1, using the definition of attributes' feature [19] and the method of data processing [17], the APOSDs shown in Fig. 3 are generated.

As shown in Fig. 3, APOSD can be presented in three styles: star [20], annular and tree. In APOSD, sequential structure visualization model is adopted. From top to bottom (tree style), or from inner to outer (star and annular style), the nodes of attributes represent the constitution of the corresponding object and the layer each attribute node located in shows the universal degree of the attribute. The attribute located in the innermost (toppest) layer has the highest university (covering the most objects).

Over the past decade, APOSD has been widely employed in the knowledge discovery for TCM, and it proved effective in the field of TCM [21–24]. Therefore, APOSD is adopted to analyze the combination structure of syndrome elements based on the quantitative results of 670 medical records.

Methods

The minimum standards of reporting checklist contains details of the experimental design, and statistics, and resources used in this study (Additional file 1).

Acquisition of clinical records
System design of data acquisition
Based on the theory of syndrome element differentiation, with the support of National Science Foundation of China (NSFC, No. 61074130), a prototype system (Fig. 4) of syndrome element measurement was designed by the team of Prof. Hong [25].

In the system, for the clinical manifestations mapping to syndrome elements, 177 inquiry questions (related to symptoms or signs common in clinical diagnosis) are designed for male, while 194 inquiry questions are designed for female. According to the severity and frequency of each symptom or sign, the answer to the corresponding question can be divided into four levels (Fig. 4a; Table 2).

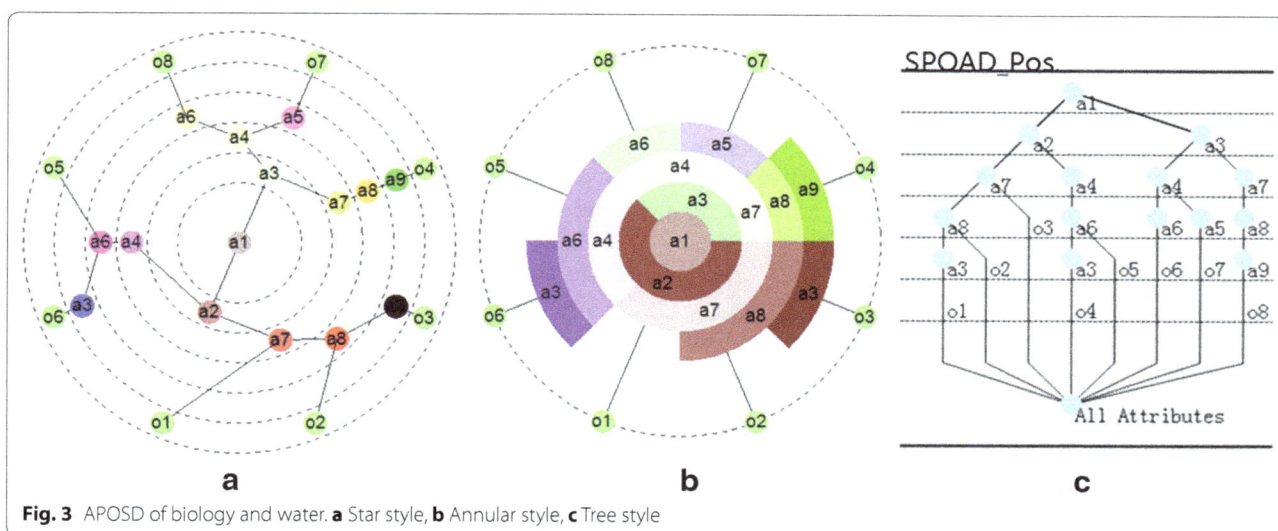

Fig. 3 APOSD of biology and water. a Star style, b Annular style, c Tree style

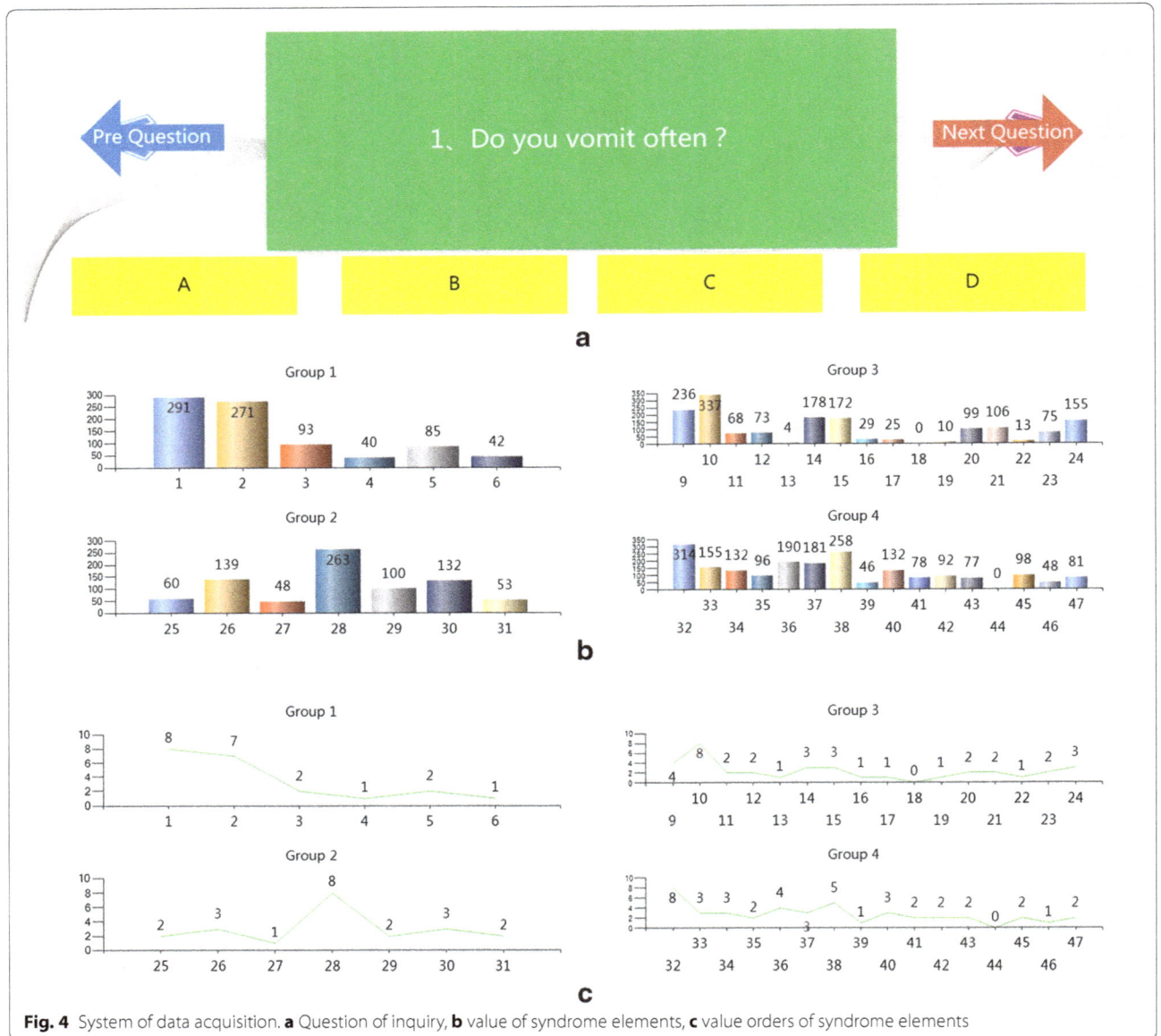

Fig. 4 System of data acquisition. **a** Question of inquiry, **b** value of syndrome elements, **c** value orders of syndrome elements

The output quantitative values (Fig. 4b) and value orders (Fig. 4c) of 47 syndrome elements (divided into four groups, Table 3) are acquired from clinical input data (answers to symptoms and signs) and the corresponding mapping data between syndrome elements and clinical manifestations.

Table 2 List of input answers

No	Label	Severity	Frequency	Weight
5	A	Severe	Always	1
4	B	A little severe	Sometimes	0.618
3	C	Not severe	Seldom	0.382
0	D	None	Never	0

Clinical evaluation of prototype system

The clinical evaluation of the prototype was conducted at the first affiliated hospital of Guangzhou University of Chinese Medicine in 2013. In May and November, the double blind comparative trial between diagnosis of prototype system and TCM expert was carried out twice. Through the clinical trial, 312 valid medical records were collected. Through comparative analysis of diagnosis of 312 records, the matching results are: there are 171 (54.81%) records whose matched

Table 3 List of syndrome elements

Group	No	Syndrome element	Group	No	Syndrome element
Eight principle syndrome differentiation (group 1)	1	Yang deficiency	Disease cause syndrome differentiation (group 2)	25	External wind
	2	Yin deficiency		26	Cold
	3	Yang hyperactivity		27	Summerheat
	4	Yang floating		28	Dampness
	5	Exterior		29	Dryness
	6	Half-exterior half-interior		30	Fire-heat
	7	Deficiency		31	Food accumulation
	8	Excess			
Qi–blood–fluid–humor syndrome differentiation (group 3)	9	Qi deficiency	Visceral syndrome differentiation (group 4)	32	Liver
	10	Qi stagnation		33	Gallbladder
	11	Qi sinking		34	Lung
	12	Insecurity of qi		35	Large intestine
	13	Qi counterflow		36	Spleen
	14	Blood deficiency		37	Stomach
	15	Blood stasis		38	Kidney
	16	Blood heat		39	Bladder
	17	Blood cold		40	Heart
	18	Stirring blood		41	Small intestine
	19	Stirring wind		42	Heart spirit
	20	Phlegm		43	Chest and diaphragm
	21	Retained fluid		44	Uterus
	22	Water retention		45	Sinew and bone
	23	Fluid depletion		46	Skin
	24	Essence deficiency		47	Meridian–collateral

degree is more than 80%, while there are only 6 (1.92%) records whose matched degree is less than 50% [25, 26].

In addition, through the analysis of combination structure of syndrome elements, the structures found from the 312 collected records, are basically identical with the discoveries of Prof. Wang (973 program No. 2003CB517100) [27].

Therefore, it can be concluded that the prototype system of syndrome element measurement is effective in clinical practice.

Collection and screening of clinical records

After the clinical evaluation, during the period of 2013–2017, according to the following criteria, the prototype system was used to collect data at school, exhibition, and hospital.

Inclusion criteria (a) People who are willing to detect the health state by the prototype system of syndrome elements measurement; (b) people who can express his feelings clearly; (c) people who can complete the inquiry finally.

Exclusion criteria (a) Records without any symptoms; (b) records whose inquiry time is too much shorter than the normal standard; (c) records whose answers to all inquiry questions are identical.

Finally, including the previous 312 records for clinical trials, 670 (301 males and 369 females) records have been collected for the following analysis.

Generation of mapping weights

According to the theory of syndrome element differentiation, the quantitative value of syndrome elements can be acquired based on the model shown in Fig. 5. Through the inquiry of system, clinical input data (matrix of answers to symptom-related questions) can be obtained, and then according to the obtained matrix of inquiry answers, the quantitative values of syndrome elements can be acquired based on the matrix of mapping weights.

Therefore, the key to the quantification of syndrome elements is the matrix of mapping weights between clinical input data and syndrome elements. The original matrix of mapping weights of this paper is mainly from Prof. Zhu [16]. Effective as the original mapping data is, there are still several issues unresolved:

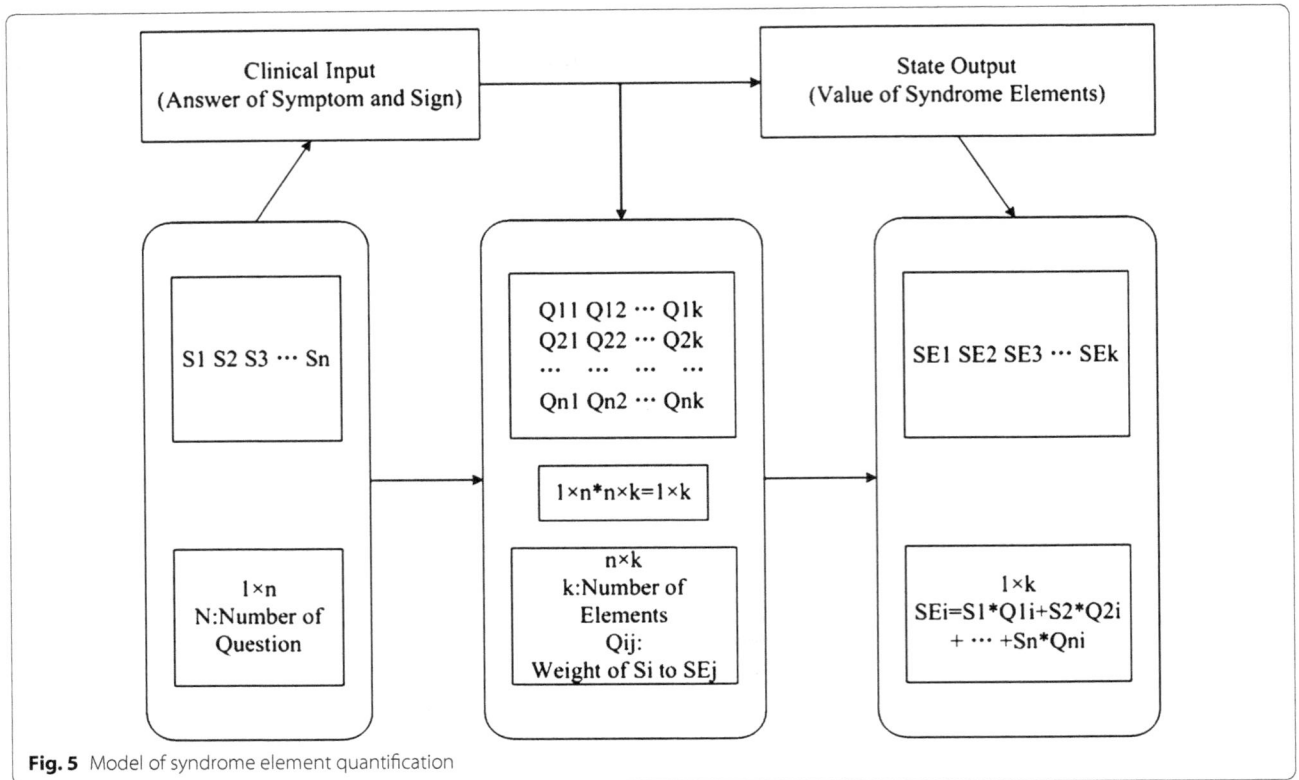

Fig. 5 Model of syndrome element quantification

a. The original mapping data is from statistical analysis of large amounts of clinical records, however it is difficult to explain the meaning of mapping data in the perspective of TCM;

b. The original mapping data only gives the mapping weights between set of clinical manifestations and set of syndrome elements, while the mapping relations between other sets of TCM (such as symptoms and formulas) are still uncertain.

In order to resolve these issues, this paper attempts to convert the original mapping weights into condensed ones, which have corresponding meanings in TCM.

Table 4 shows the generation rules of new condensed mapping weights.

In the generation of new weights, to explore whether or not the association between different symptoms should be considered, two different generation rules are proposed: *Symptom* and *Element*. Type of *Symptom* refers to the generation of new weights only considers the mapping data of one symptom, while type of *Element* means that the generation of new weights should consider all of the symptoms which are related with one specific syndrome element.

In addition, to explore which granularity level of new weights is more effective, two types of new weights are proposed: *Normal* and *Fuzzy*. *Normal* type means that, according to the mapping correlation compactness between symptom and syndrome element, the new weight data is divided into 4 levels, which are corresponding to the qualitative definition of correlation degree in TCM: 10 (maximum correlation), 2 (minimum correlation), 8 and 6 (medium correlation), while the new weights of *Fuzzy* type are more refined.

Therefore, combining two types of generation methods and two kinds of granularity level of new weights, there are four types of generation rules of new weight: Symptom_Normal, Symptom_Fuzzy, Element_Normal, and Element_Fuzzy.

The new weights generation of Symptom_Normal type is simple:

1. Listing all weight values of one symptom from matrix of original weights;
2. According to the value range of each original weight, generating a new weight value;
3. Integrating the new weight values of the symptom together;

Table 4 Generation of new weights

Type	Original range (value)	New weight	Type	Original range (ratio)	New weight
Symptom_Normal	[40, 100)	10	Element_Normal	[0.6, 1]	10
	[25, 40)	6		[0.4, 0.6)	6
	[10, 25)	4		[0.2, 0.4)	4
	(0, 10]	2		(0, 0.2)	2
Symptom_Fuzzy	[45, 100)	10	Element_Fuzzy	[0.65, 1]	10
	[40, 45)	8		[0.6, 0.65)	8
	[35, 40)	8		[0.55, 0.6)	8
	[30, 35)	6		[0.45, 0.55)	6
	[25, 30)	5		[0.4, 0.45)	5
	[20, 25)	5		[0.35, 0.4)	5
	[12, 20)	4		[0.25, 0.35)	4
	(10, 12)	3		(0.2, 0.25)	3
	(8, 10]	3		(0.15, 0.2]	3
	(0, 8]	2		(0, 0.15]	2

4. Repeating the first three steps, generating new weight values of all symptoms (177 for male and 194 for female);
5. Composing a matrix of new weight values.

Compared with Symptom_Normal type, the new weights generation of Symptom_Fuzzy type is a little complicated:

1. Listing all weight values of one symptom from matrix of original weights;
2. According to the value range of each original weight, generating a new weight value;
3. If the value of original weight is close to the boundary of range, a new secondary weight value (8, 5, and 3) will be generated according to the secondary range;
4. Integrating the new weight values of the symptom together;
5. Repeating the first four steps, generating new weight values of all symptoms (177 for male and 194 for female);
6. Composing a matrix of new weight values.

Compared with type of Symptom_Normal and Symptom_Fuzzy, the new weights generation of Element_Normal type is more complicated:

1. Listing all weight values of one syndrome element from matrix of original weights;
2. Finding the maximum weight value of the syndrome element, and calculating the ratio of each weight value to the maximum value;

3. According to the ratio range of each weight value, generating a new weight value;
4. Integrating the new weight values of the syndrome element together;
5. Repeating the first four steps, generating new weight values of all syndrome elements listed in Table 3;
6. Composing a matrix of new weight values.

Compared with type of Symptom_Normal, Symptom_Fuzzy, Element_Normal, the new weights generation of Element_Fuzzy type is the most complicated:

1. Listing all weight values of one syndrome element from matrix of original weights;
2. Finding the maximum weight value of the syndrome element, and calculating the ratio of each weight value to the maximum value;
3. According to the ratio range of each weight value, generating a new weight value;
4. If the ratio of original weight is close to the boundary of range, a new secondary weight value (8, 5, and 3) will be generated according to the secondary range;
5. Integrating the new weight values of the syndrome element together;
6. Repeating the first five steps, generating new weight values of all syndrome elements listed in Table 3;
7. Composing a matrix of new weight values.

Evaluation of mapping weights

To evaluate the effectiveness of new weights, the four kinds of new weights will be used to approximate the results of the original mapping data. Figure 6 shows the evaluation model of mapping weights.

The process of evaluation can be divided into several steps:

1. Based on the clinical input data, calculating the quantitative values of syndrome elements according to the corresponding matrix of mapping weights;
2. According to the quantitative values of syndrome element and the group it belongs to, based on specified rules (Table 5), calculating the value order of each syndrome element.
3. Taking the value orders of original weights as standard, calculating the matched degree of each syndrome differentiation group based on the value order of each syndrome element.

$$MDG = (CG - \sum SE\_N*SE\_W)/CG \qquad (1)$$

Table 5 Rules of value order

Value order	Ratio (value/maxvalue of group)	Weight
8	[0.95, 1]	1
7	[0.9, 0.95)	0.95
6	[0.85, 0.9)	0.9
5	[0.8, 0.85)	0.8
4	[0.6, 0.8)	0.7
3	[0.4, 0.6)	0.6
2	[0.2, 0.4)	0.4
1	(0, 0.2)	0.2

MDG: matched degree of the syndrome differentiation group; CG: count of syndrome element in the syndrome differentiation group; SE_N: the syndrome

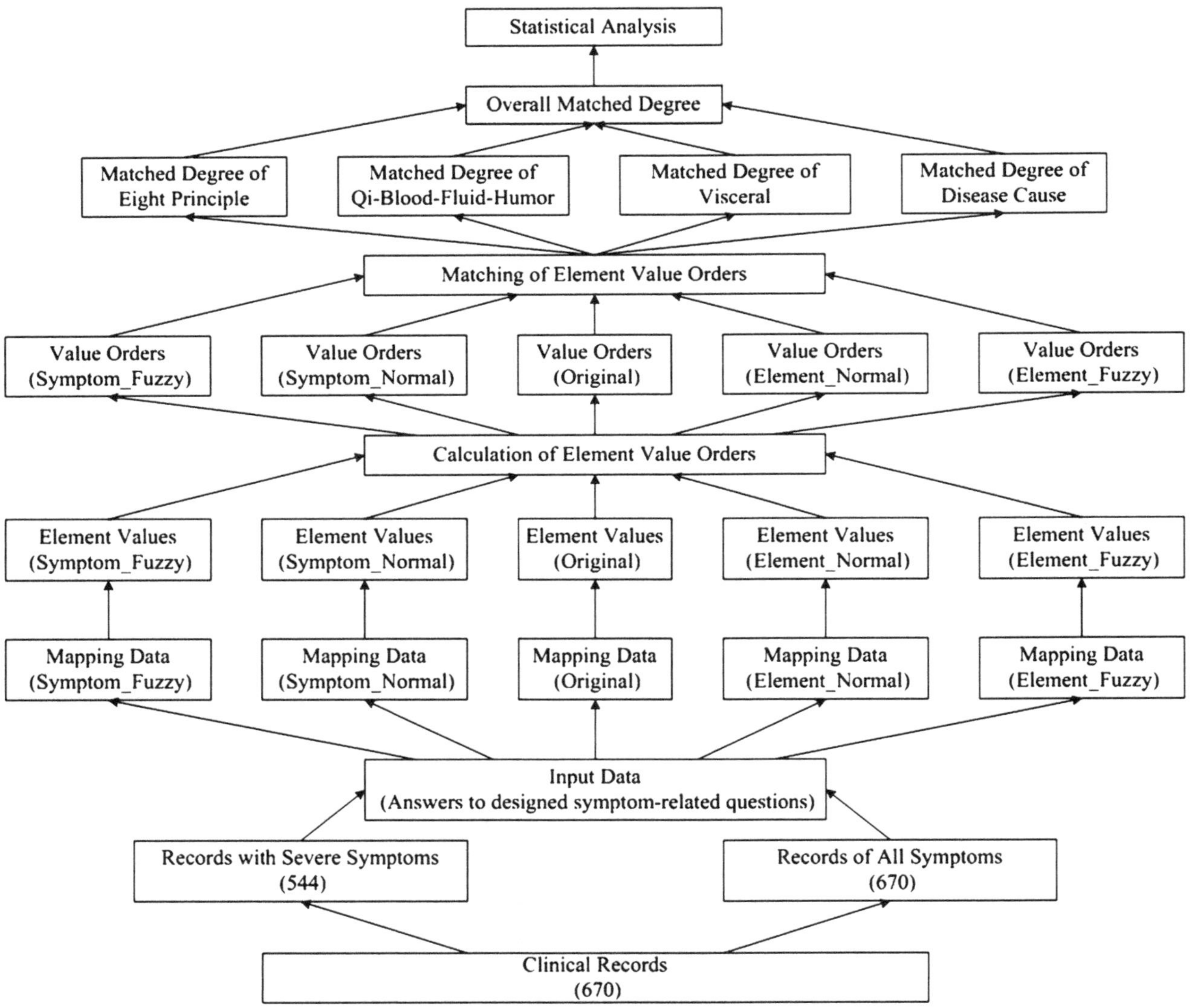

Fig. 6 Evaluation model of mapping weights

element whose value order is not consistent with real value order; SE_W: the weight of syndrome element.

4. Calculating the integrated matched degree according to the matched degree of each syndrome differentiation group.

$$MD = \sum (MDG * CG/CT) \qquad (2)$$

MD: matched degree of the integrated syndrome differentiation; MDG: matched degree of specific syndrome differentiation group; CG: count of syndrome element in specific syndrome differentiation group; CT: count of syndrome element in all groups.

5. Statistical analysis of all records according to the matched degree of each record.
6. Evaluation of four kinds of new mapping weights based on the statistical distribution of matched degree.

In addition, for a more obvious contrast, results calculated from all symptoms (*overall health state*) and results acquired from severe symptoms (*major health state*) are evaluated together. As excess (No. 8 element) and deficiency (No. 7 element) are not calculated directly from input answers, so they are excluded during evaluation.

Knowledge discovery

In this part, APOSD will be adopted to analyze and visualize the combination structure of syndrome elements based on 670 medical records. The process can be divided into several steps:

1. Extracting the syndrome elements whose value order is at the highest level from the 670 collected medical records;
2. Taking syndrome elements extracted from the first step as attributes, and using the medical records as objects, establishing formal context of the 670 medical records;
3. Based on the formal context, generating the corresponding APOSD;
4. Discovering combination structure of syndrome elements from the APOSD.

The knowledge discovered from different types of results will be compared to verify whether they are consistent.

Results

Results of weights generation

Figure 7 shows the contrast examples of mapping weights of different types.

In the mapping figure of asthma (Fig. 7a), the labels of X axis represent the numbers of syndrome elements this symptom is mapping to, while the values of Y axis express the correlation degree of the mapping. In the mapping figure of yang hyperactivity (Fig. 7b), the labels of X axis represent the numbers of symptoms this element is related to, while the values of Y axis express the correlation degree of the relation.

As shown in the figure, despite the weight deviations between different types, the changing trend of the values is consistent, which means that the qualitative mapping relations between medical manifestations and syndrome elements have not changed.

Results of weights evaluation

Figure 8 shows the values and value orders contrast of syndrome elements calculated from the input answers of one example record. As shown in the figure, the value orders of the five types are basically consistent, which means that the corresponding qualitative diagnosis results are consistent as well.

Table 6 shows the statistical distribution of matched degree (eight principle, disease cause, qi–blood–fluid–humor, visceral and integrated differentiation) calculated from the 670 records.

As shown in the Table 6, for the Symptom_Normal type results of 670 all records, the numbers of records whose matched degree is no less than 80% are 615 (91.8% for eight principle group), 647 (96.5% for qi–blood–fluid–humor group), 620 (92.5% for disease cause group), 658 (98.2% for visceral) and 670 (100% for integrated group).

For the Symptom_Normal type results of 544 records with severe symptoms, the numbers of records whose matched degree is no less than 80% are 473 (86.9% for eight principle group), 522 (95.9% for qi–blood–fluid–humor group), 472 (86.7% for disease cause group), 529 (97.2% for visceral) and 538 (98.9% for integrated group).

To sum up, for the integrated syndrome differentiation of 670 records, the matched degree of each record is no less than 65%, while there are at least 87% records whose matched degree is more than 80%.

Results of knowledge discovery

Among the four new types of mapping weights, the matching result of Symptom_Normal type is the best. Therefore, in this part, the APOSD of Symptom_Normal type is used to compare with the APOSD of original results. In this part, only the annular style of APOSD is adopted. In addition, the outermost circle of objects is removed because of the excessive objects. In the

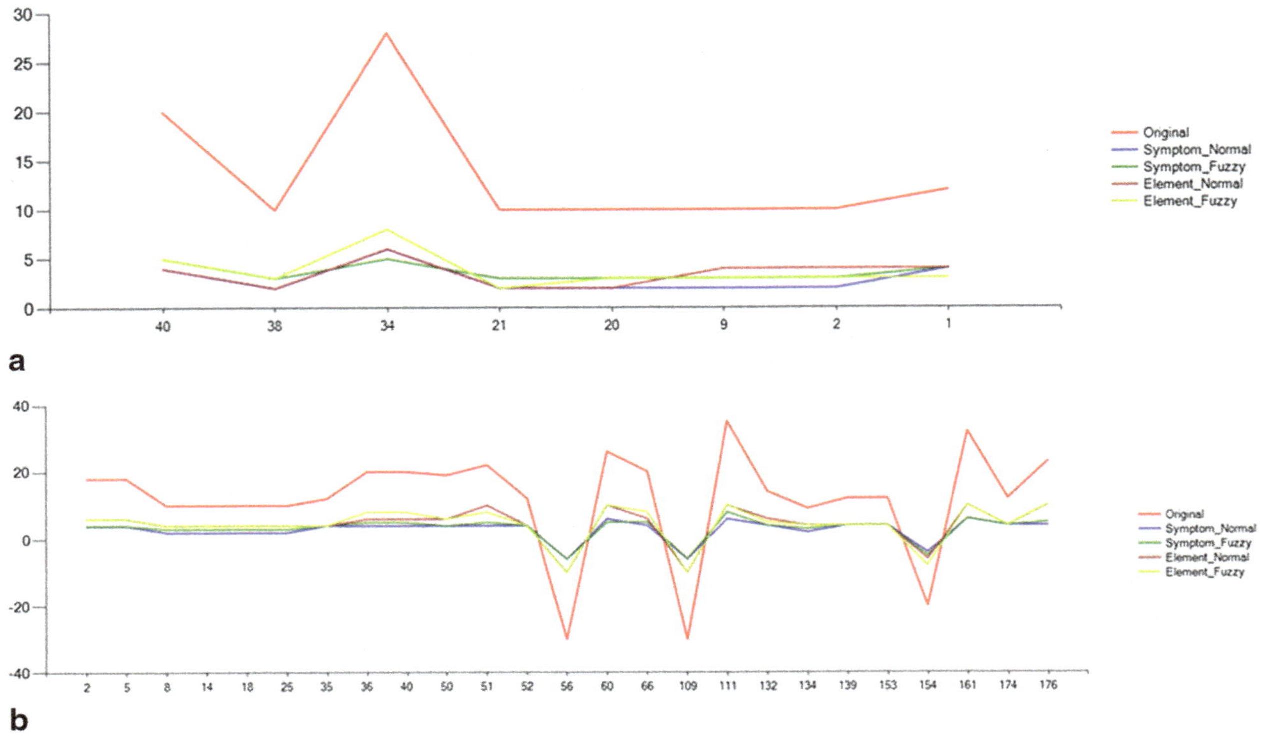

Fig. 7 Contrast of mapping weights. **a** Mapping weights of asthma (symptom), **b** mapping weights of yang hyperactivity (element)

diagrams, the labels are used to represent the syndrome elements (e.g.: '*e1*' represents the syndrome elements whose No. listed in Table 3 is 1).

Figure 9 shows the hierarchical structure of APOSD generated from the original results of 670 medical records. As shown in the figure, in the innermost layer, {e28 = dampness} is the biggest arc, which means that dampness is the most common syndrome element among the 670 records. Under the arc of {e28 = dampness}, in the second layer, the diagram is divided into two big arcs: {e1 = yang deficiency} and {e2 = yin deficiency}. In the third layer, there are some big arcs for three syndrome elements: {e9 = qi deficiency}, {e10 = qi stagnation} and {e14 = blood deficiency}. In the fourth layer, there are several big arcs for syndrome elements of location: {e36 = spleen}, {e32 = liver} and {e38 = kidney}.

It can be concluded from the APOSD (Fig. 9) that, among the 670 medical records, the most common syndrome elements of location are: spleen, liver and kidney, while the most frequent syndrome elements of nature are: dampness, yang deficiency, yin deficiency, qi deficiency, qi stagnation and blood deficiency.

Figure 10 shows the hierarchical structure of APOSD generated from the Symptom_Normal type results of 670

medical records. As shown in the figure, in the innermost layer, {e28 = dampness} is also the biggest arc. Under the arc of {e28 = dampness}, in the second layer, the diagram is also divided into two big arcs: {e1 = yang deficiency} and {e2 = yin deficiency}. In the third layer, there are also some big arcs for three syndrome elements: {e9 = qi deficiency}, {e10 = qi stagnation} and {e14 = blood deficiency}. In the fourth layer, there are also several big arcs for syndrome elements of location: {e36 = spleen}, {e32 = liver} and {e38 = kidney}.

It can be concluded from the APOSD (Fig. 10) that, among the 670 medical records, the most common syndrome elements of location are: spleen, liver and kidney, while the most frequent syndrome elements of nature are: dampness, yang deficiency, yin deficiency, qi deficiency, qi stagnation and blood deficiency.

From the APOSD, the common combinations of syndrome elements can also be discovered. Table 7 shows the knowledge discovered from the APOSDs of original results (Fig. 9) and Symptom_Normal type results (Fig. 10).

Through the knowledge discovery, it can be concluded that, despite the differences of details between the APOSDs of original and Symptom_Normal type

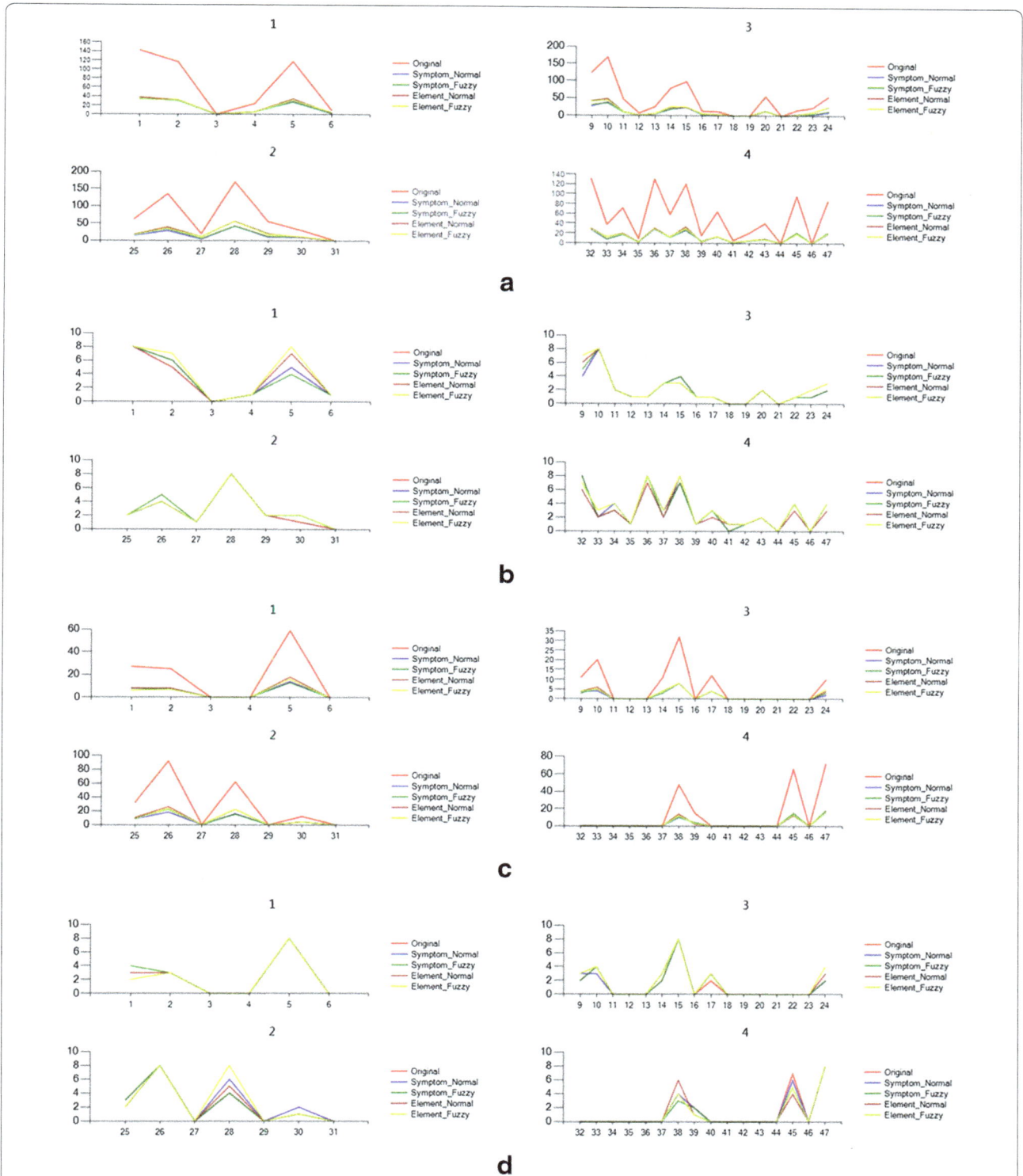

Fig. 8 Contrast of values and value orders of syndrome elements. **a** Values of elements calculated from all symptoms, **b** value orders of elements calculated from all symptoms, **c** values of elements calculated from severe symptoms, **d** value orders of elements calculated from severe symptoms

Table 6 Statistical analysis of matched degree

Group	Matched degree (%)	All samples (670)				Samples with severe symptoms (544)			
		Symptom_ Normal	Symptom_ Fuzzy	Element_ Normal	Element_ Fuzzy	Symptom_ Normal	Symptom_ Fuzzy	Element_ Normal	Element_ Fuzzy
Eight principle syndrome differentiation	[95, 100]	322	258	167	84	264	265	229	203
	[90, 95)	110	103	112	116	80	84	98	100
	[85, 90)	116	142	83	77	93	94	66	65
	[80, 85)	67	93	114	139	36	38	51	52
	[75, 80)	29	42	98	122	27	29	35	41
	[70, 75)	16	19	58	60	18	16	24	32
	[65, 70)	8	8	20	32	14	9	16	20
	[60, 65)	0	4	12	18	4	1	12	12
	[0, 60)	2	1	6	22	8	8	13	19
Qi–blood–fluid–humour syndrome differentiation	[95, 100]	227	238	24	29	247	248	142	152
	[90, 95)	208	212	86	97	139	156	125	132
	[85, 90)	155	140	144	189	97	85	119	121
	[80, 85)	57	61	172	173	39	35	80	79
	[75, 80)	18	13	124	109	16	14	49	38
	[70, 75)	3	6	86	50	4	5	21	11
	[65, 70)	2	0	25	15	2	1	5	7
	[60, 65)	0	0	6	7	0	0	3	4
	[0, 60)	0	0	3	1	0	0	0	0
Disease cause syndrome differentiation	[95, 100]	318	296	130	92	265	268	195	190
	[90, 95)	173	190	165	139	93	100	121	101
	[85,90)	81	88	159	130	76	62	66	76
	[80, 85)	48	47	94	125	38	46	45	53
	[75, 80)	19	18	48	83	24	35	44	39
	[70, 75)	11	15	39	46	28	18	29	35
	[65, 70)	11	8	15	24	12	5	13	19
	[60, 65)	8	5	11	13	4	4	17	12
	[0, 60)	1	3	9	18	4	6	14	19
Visceral syndrome differentiation	[95, 100]	245	173	118	127	253	240	224	261
	[90, 95)	209	199	163	173	153	146	146	139
	[85, 90)	142	177	172	192	70	90	92	83
	[80, 85)	62	80	109	113	53	52	46	36
	[75, 80)	9	37	70	45	13	13	25	15
	[70, 75)	3	4	30	19	2	3	11	9
	[65, 70)	0	0	5	1	0	0	0	1
	[60, 65)	0	0	2	0	0	0	0	0
	[0, 60)	0	0	1	0	0	0	0	0
Integrated syndrome differentiation	[95, 100]	153	98	4	2	163	169	108	125
	[90, 95)	333	333	102	91	224	233	170	167
	[85, 90)	156	201	258	293	130	117	154	147
	[80, 85)	28	35	224	204	21	22	92	88
	[75, 80)	0	3	70o	70	5	3	17	15
	[70, 75)	0	0	12	10	1	0	3	1
	[65, 70)	0	0	0	0	0	0	0	1
	[0, 65)	0	0	0	0	0	0	0	0

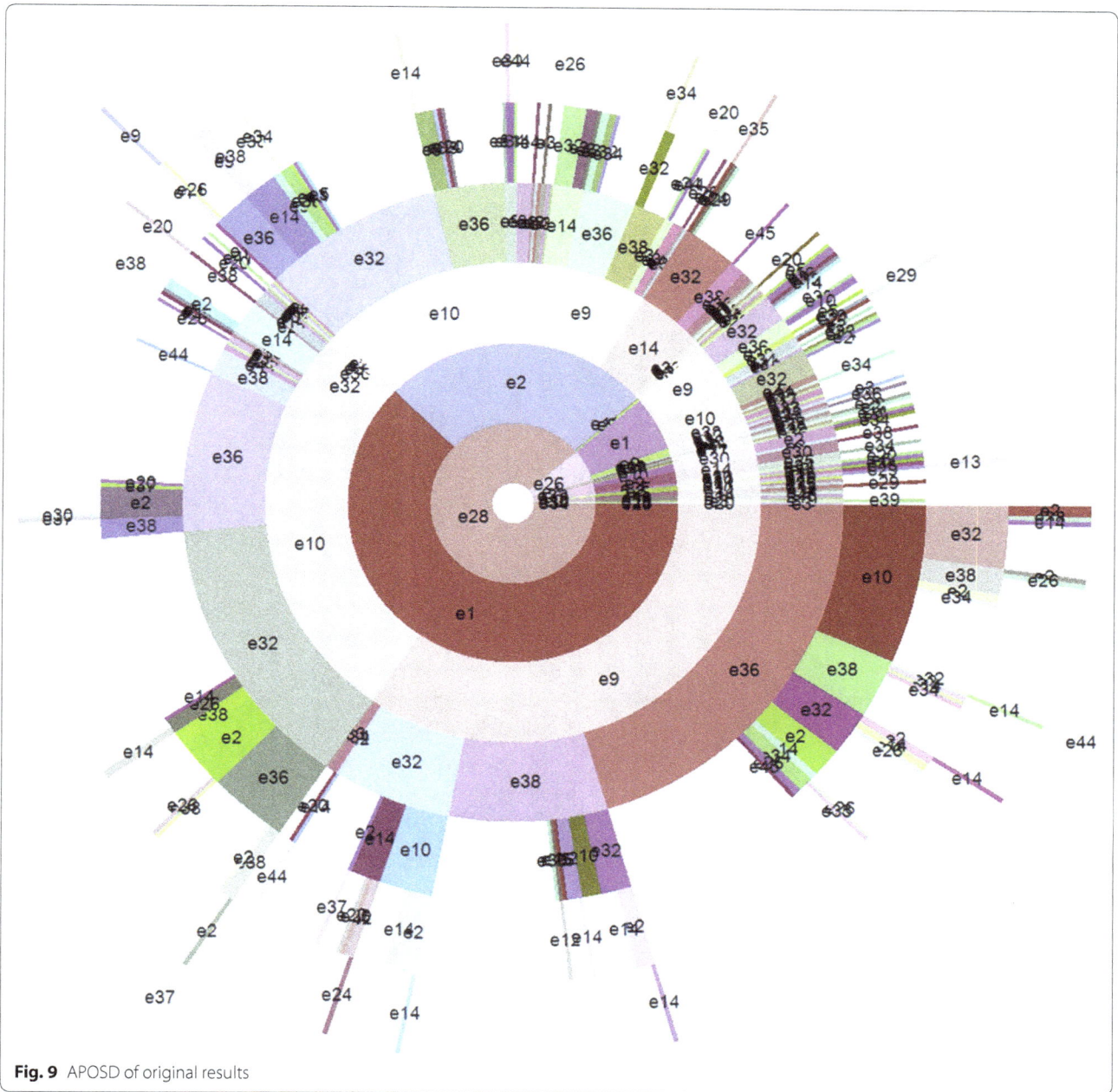

Fig. 9 APOSD of original results

results, the knowledge discovered from them is basically identical.

Discussion

In the history of TCM, methods of syndrome differentiation are diverse: eight principle, disease cause, visceral, qi–blood–fluid–humor, six-meridian, triple energizer, and defense-qi-nutrient-blood. These methods provide various cognitions of syndrome from different perspectives. Each of these methods has its own characteristics and scope of application, while all of them are incomplete and need complement of each other. In clinical practice of TCM, the combination of several methods of syndrome differentiation is frequently needed. The coexistence of multiple methods of syndrome differentiation has brought great difficulties to clinical application, teaching and research of TCM.

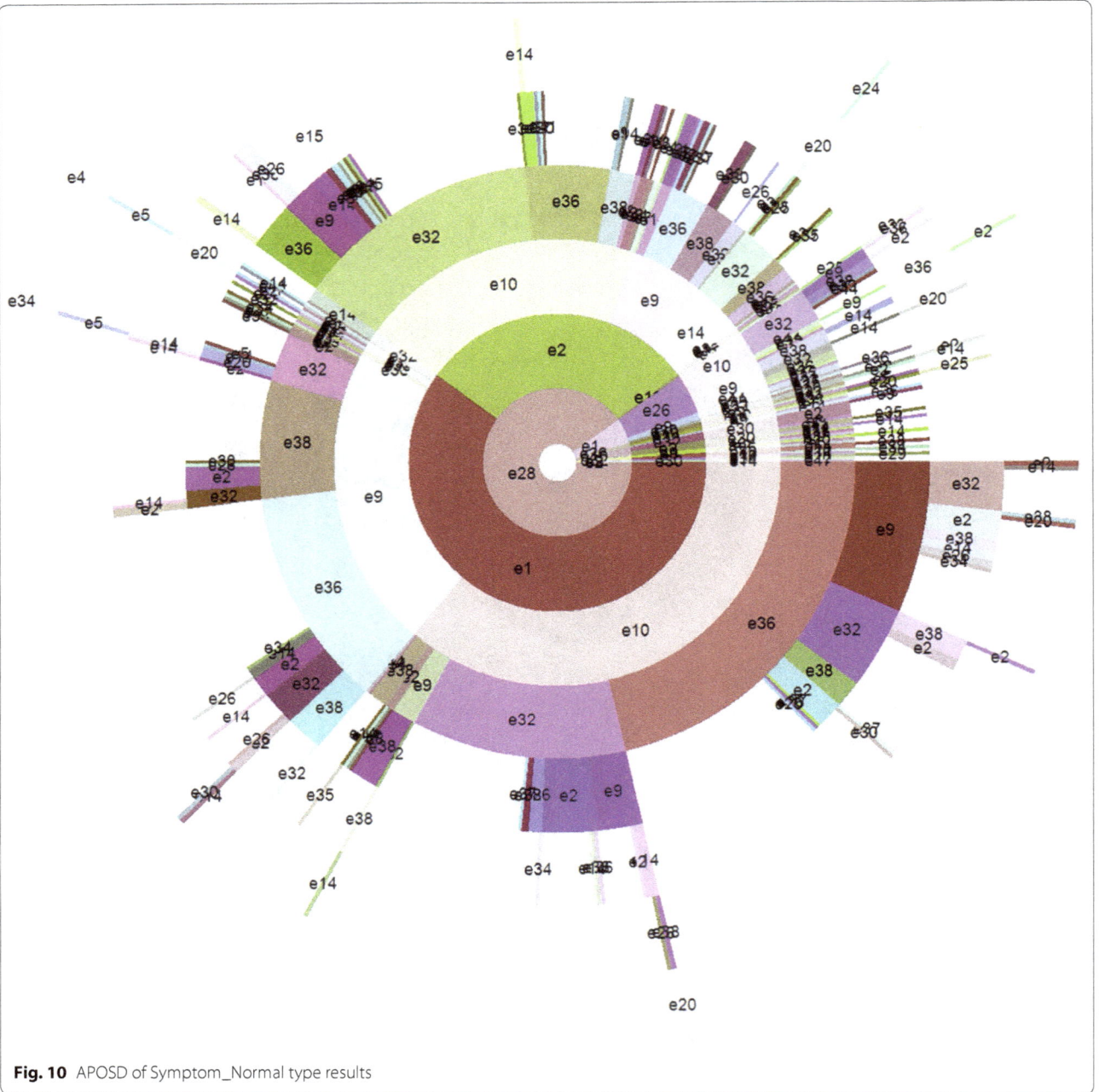

Fig. 10 APOSD of Symptom_Normal type results

In view of the above situation, based on the integration of these ancient methods, theory of syndrome element differentiation has been established by Prof. Zhu. Subsequently, in the light of Prof. Zhu's theory of syndrome element differentiation, based on phenomenology and mathematical mapping, a prototype system of syndrome element measurement has been designed by the team of Prof. Hong. Through clinical evaluation of the prototype system, the mapping data given by Prof. Zhu proved effective. However, the meaning of mapping data is hard to explain in the perspective of TCM and it is difficult to be used for the other sets of TCM.

Therefore, combining phenomenology, mathematical mapping and theory of TCM, four kinds of new mapping

Table 7 Results of knowledge discovery

	Original	Symptom_Normal		Original	Symptom_Normal
Common combinations of syndrome elements	e28-e1-e9-e36	e28-e1-e9-e36	Common syndrome elements	Essence	
	e28-e1-e9-e38	e28-e1-e9-e38		Dampness (e28)	Dampness (e28)
	e28-e1-e9-e32	e28-e1-e9-e32		Yang deficiency (e1)	Yang deficiency (e1)
	e28-e1-e10-e32	e28-e1-e10-e32		Yin deficiency (e2)	Yin deficiency (e2)
	e28-e1-e10-e36	e28-e1-e10-e36		Qi deficiency (e9)	Qi deficiency (e9)
	e28-e2-e10-e32	e28-e2-e10-e32		Qi stagnation (e10)	Qi stagnation (e10)
	e28-e2-e10-e36	e28-e2-e10-e36		Blood deficiency (e14)	Blood deficiency (e14)
	e28-e2-e9-e14			Location	
		e28-e2-e9-e38		Spleen (e36)	Spleen (e36)
	e28-e2-e9-e36	e28-e2-e9-e36		Liver (e32)	Liver (e32)
	e28-e2-e14-e32	e28-e2-e14-e32		Kidney (e38)	Kidney (e38)

weights have been constructed to approximate the results calculated from original mapping data.

"Results" shows the approximation results of all syndrome differentiation groups, and Fig. 11 shows the statistical pie charts of matched degree under the group of integrated syndrome differentiation.

As shown in the figure, for the Symptom_Normal type results of overall health state (calculated from all symptoms), the matched degrees of all of the 670 records are higher than 80%. For the Symptom_Normal type results of major health state (acquired only from severe symptoms), among the 544 records with severe symptoms, there are 99% records whose matched degree is no less than 80%.

For the results of the other three types (Symptom_Fuzzy, Element_Normal and Element_Fuzzy), the approximation effects are worse than that of Symptom_Normal type.

Therefore, for both overall health state (calculated from all symptoms) and major health state (acquired only from severe symptoms), compared with the approximation results of other three types, the approximation results of Symptom_Normal type are the best. In addition, the matched results of fuzzy types are not higher than that of normal types. Therefore, four levels of mapping weights are already enough, and there is no need to consider smaller granularity.

Conclusion

In this paper, a new approach to describe and realize the quantitative diagnosis of TCM based on phenomenology is proposed and it is testified through the syndrome element differentiation and knowledge discovery of 670 clinical records. The analyses show that new results of new mapping weights can approximate the results calculated from original mapping data. Therefore, using phenomenology and mathematical mapping to realize the quantitative diagnosis of TCM should be feasible, and mapping data between other sets of TCM can also be determined by the method proposed in this paper.

However, there are still several issues or limitations to be resolved:

1. The evaluation of the new mapping data is mainly based on the research of Prof. Zhu, which is insufficient to some extent. Consequently, further evaluation by clinical experts of TCM should be conducted in future.

2. The original mapping data between clinical manifestations and syndrome elements are static. To achieve self-renewal of the mapping data with the accumulation of medical records, research that using machine learning methods to approximate the mapping relations of TCM should be conducted in future.

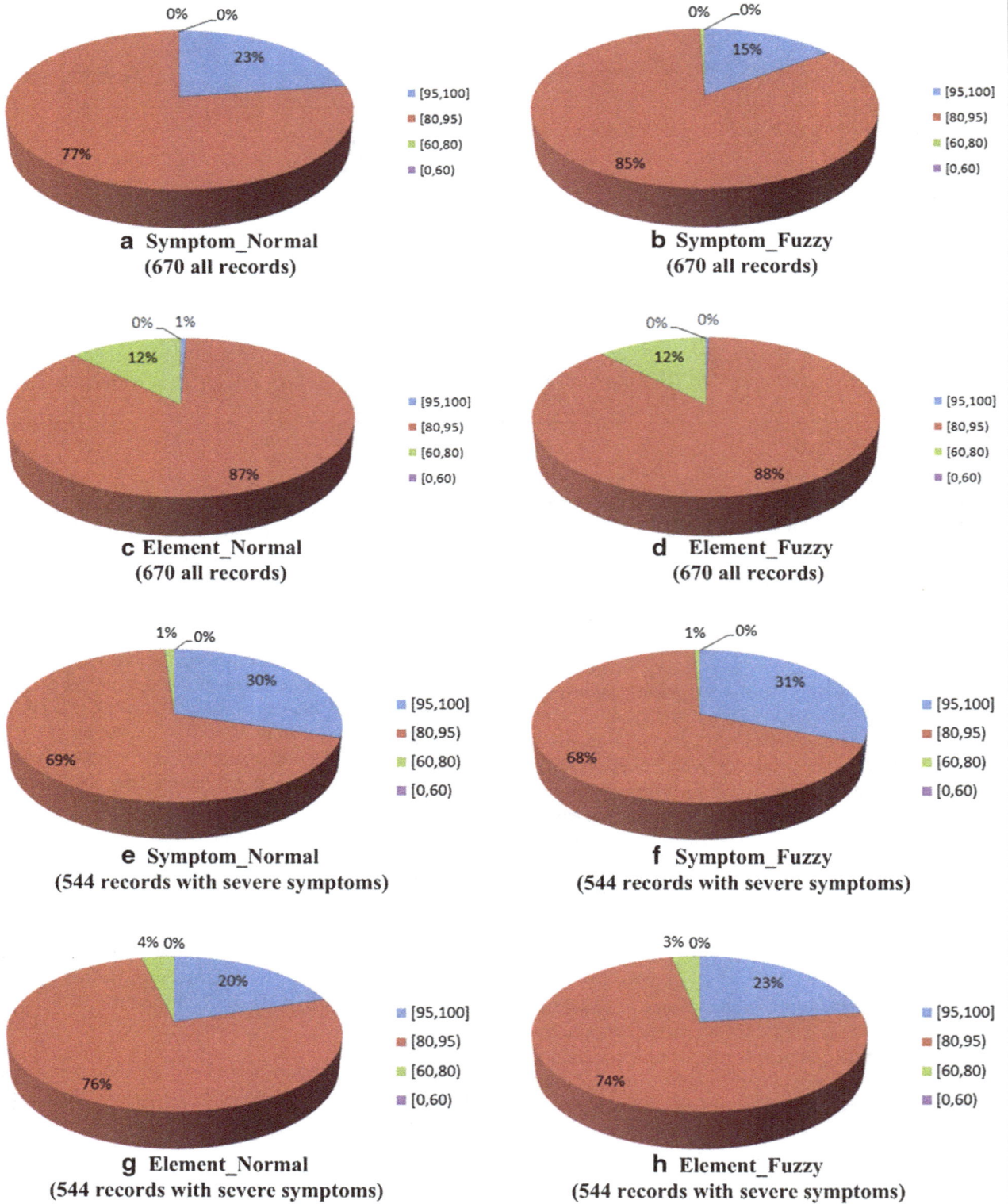

Fig. 11 Statistical pies of integrated matched degree

Abbreviations
TCM: traditional Chinese medicine; CWM: conventional Western medicine; APOSD: attribute partial-ordered structure diagram; FCA: formal concept analysis.

Authors' contributions
WH proposed the thought and framework of this paper. EY implemented the thought with software, analyzed the data and wrote this paper. JS and CL provided medical guidance of this paper. All authors read and approved the final manuscript.

Author details
[1] Institute of Electrical Engineering, Yanshan University, No. 438, Hebei Avenue, Qinhuangdao 066004, Hebei, People's Republic of China. [2] Guangzhou University of Chinese Medicine, Guangzhou, Guangdong 510405, People's Republic of China.

Acknowledgements
This work is supported by National Science Foundation of China (NSFC) under Grant Nos. 61273019, 31273740, 81373767, 61201111 and 61501397. It is also supported by Science Foundation of Hebei Province under Grant No. F2016203443. The authors gratefully acknowledge the supports. The authors are grateful to the reviewers of the paper for their helpful comments and suggestions.

Competing interests
The authors declare that they have no competing interests.

Funding
National Science Foundation of China (NSFC) under Grant Nos. 61273019, 31273740, 81373767, 61201111 and 61501397. Science Foundation of Hebei Province under Grant No. F2016203443.

References
1. Feng Y, Wu Z, Zhou X, et al. Knowledge discovery in traditional Chinese medicine: state of the art and perspectives. Artif Intell Med. 2006;38(3):219–36.
2. Wang H, Cheng Y. A quantitative system for pulse diagnosis in traditional Chinese Medicine. International Conference of the IEEE engineering in medicine and biology society; 2005. p. 5676.
3. Wang H, Wang J. A quantitative diagnostic method based on Bayesian networks in traditional Chinese Medicine. International Conference neural information processing, ICONIP, DBLP, Hong Kong, China, October 3–6, 2006; 2006. p. 176–83.
4. Wang H. A quantitative method for pulse strength classification based on decision tree. International Symposium on information science and engineering. IEEE; 2008. p. 111–15.
5. Zhao C, Li G, Li F, et al. Qualitative and quantitative analysis for facial complexion in traditional Chinese Medicine. Biomed Res Int. 2014;2014(3):207589.
6. Li F, Zhao C, Xia Z, et al. Computer-assisted lip diagnosis on Traditional Chinese Medicine using multi-class support vector machines. BMC Complement Altern Med. 2012;12(1):127.
7. Liu G, Li G, Wang Y, et al. Modelling of inquiry diagnosis for coronary heart disease in traditional Chinese medicine by using multi-label learning. BMC Complement Altern Med. 2010;10(1):37.
8. Su S. Recent advances in ZHENG differentiation research in traditional Chinese Medicine. Int J Integr Med. 2013:1.
9. Zhao C, Li G, Wang C, et al. Advances in patient classification for traditional Chinese Medicine: a machine learning perspective. Evid-based Complement Altern Med. 2015;2015(5):376716.
10. Yang X. Chinese traditional medicine: the nature and the roadmap to modernization. Smart Healthc. 2015;1(1):60–4.
11. Corby D, Taggart L, Cousins W. People with intellectual disability and human science research: a systematic review of phenomenological studies using interviews for data collection. Res Dev Disabil. 2015;47:451–65.
12. Kaivo-Oja J. Towards better participatory processes in technology foresight: how to link participatory foresight research to the methodological machinery of qualitative research and phenomenology. Futures. 2017;86:94–106.
13. Xutian S, Cao D, Wozniak J, et al. Comprehension of the unique characteristics of traditional Chinese medicine. Am J Chin Med. 2012;40(2):231–44.
14. Wang Y, Xu A. Zheng: a systems biology approach to diagnosis and treatments. Science. 2014;346(6216):S13–5.
15. Zhu W. Establishing a new system of syndrome differentiation with syndrome element as core. J Hunan Univ Chin Med. 2004;24(6):38–9.
16. Zhu W. Study of syndrome elements differentiation. Beijing: People's Medical Publishing House; 2008.
17. Hong W, Li S, Yu J, et al. A new approach of generation of structural partial-ordered attribute diagram. ICIC Express Lett Part B: Appl. 2012;3(4A):823–30.
18. Yu J, Hong W, Qiu C, et al. A new approach of attribute partial order structure diagram for word sense disambiguation of english prepositions. Knowl-Based Syst. 2016;95(C):142–52.
19. Luan J, Hong W, Liu J, et al. The complete definitions of object and abstract description of object features of the formal context. ICIC Express Lett. 2013;4(3):1065–72.
20. Hong W, Sun F, Li S, et al. Partial ordered structure radial tree: a new method for big data visualization. ICIC Express Lett. 2016;10(5):1181–6.
21. Fan F, Hong W, Song J, et al. Visualization method and knowledge discovery of prescription composition. Chin J Biomed Eng. 2016;35(6):764–8.
22. Fan F, Hong W, Song J, et al. A method of attribute partial-ordered structure diagram for the composition structures of prescription and knowledge discovery. ICIC Express Lett. 2016;10(3):593–600.
23. Song J, Yu J, Yan E, et al. Syndrome differentiation of six meridians for warm disease based on structural partial-ordered attributes diagram. ICIC Express Lett. 2013;7(3B):947–52.
24. Liu C, Xu S, Li S, et al. Knowledge discovery of formula classification according to therapies in Shanghanlun based on representation method of multi-layer complex concept network. J Beijing Univ Tradit Chin Med. 2014;37(7):452–7.
25. Luan J. A research about syndrome differentiation assistant system of traditional Chinese medicine based on structural partial-ordered attribute theory. Yanshan University; 2014 (Ph.D. Thesis).
26. Hong W, Zhang Z, Luan J, et al. A research about value order measurement system of traditional Chinese Medicine syndrome elements. International Conference on medical biometrics. IEEE; 2014. p. 74–9.
27. Hong W, Song J, Zheng C, Luan J, et al. Comparative study on pattern discovery of traditional Chinese medicine common syndrome elements. International Conference on medical biometrics. IEEE; 2014. p. 68–73.

7

Effects of different principles of Traditional Chinese Medicine treatment on TLR7/NF-κB signaling pathway in influenza virus infected mice

Ying-Jie Fu[1][†] , Yu-Qi Yan[1][†], Hong-Qiong Qin[1], Sha Wu[1], Shan-Shan Shi[1], Xiao Zheng[1], Peng-Cheng Wang[1], Xiao-Yin Chen[2]*, Xiao-Long Tang[3]* and Zhen-You Jiang[1]*

Abstract

Background: Influenza virus is a single-stranded RNA virus that causes influenza in humans and animals. About 600 million people around the world suffer from influenza every year. Upon recognizing viral RNA molecules, TLR7 (Toll-like receptor) initiates corresponding immune responses. Traditional Chinese Medicines (TCMs), including Yinqiao powder, Xinjiaxiangruyin and Guizhi-and-Mahuang decoction, have been extensively applied in clinical treatment of influenza. Although the therapeutic efficacy of TCMs against influenza virus in vivo was reported previously, its underlying mechanisms are not clearly understood. This study aimed to investigate the immunological mechanisms in the treatment of influenza virus infected mice with three Chinese herbal compounds as well as the effect on TLR7/NF-κB signaling pathway during recovery.

Methods: Wild type and TLR7 KO C57BL/6 mice were infected with influenza virus FM1 and then treated with three TCMs. The physical parameters of mice (body weight and lung index) and the expression levels of components in TLR7/NF-κB signaling pathway were evaluated.

Results: After viral infection, Guizhi-and-Mahuang decoction and Yinqiao powder showed better anti-viral effect under normal condition. Compared to the viral control group, expression levels of TLR7, MyD88, IRAK4 and NF-κB were significantly reduced in all treatment groups. Furthermore, the three TCM treatment groups showed poor therapeutic efficacy and no difference in viral load compared to the viral control group in TLR7 KO mice.

Conclusion: Our study indicated that Guizhi-and-Mahuang decoction and Yinqiao powder might play a crucial role of anti-influenza virus by regulating TLR7/NF-κB signal pathway.

Keywords: Influenza virus, Traditional Chinese Medicine, TLR7/NF-κB signaling pathway, TLR7 gene knockout, Guizhi-and-Mahuang decoction, Yinqiao powder, Xinjiaxiangruyin

*Correspondence: tchenxiaoyin@jnu.edu.cn; xltang@aust.edu.cn; tjzhy@jnu.edu.cn
[†]Ying-Jie Fu and Yu-Qi Yan are co-first authors
[1] Department of Microbiology and Immunology, School of Basic Medical Sciences, Jinan University, Guangzhou 510632, Guangdong, China
[2] College of Traditional Chinese Medicine, Jinan University, Guangzhou 510632, Guangdong, China
[3] Medical College, Anhui University of Science & Technology, Huainan 232001, Anhui, China

Background

Influenza virus causes seasonal epidemics and occasional pandemics in human beings and presents serious public health and economic problems [1]. Influenza viruses belong to the *Orthomyxoviridae* family, and are classified into three types, A, B, and C, in which type A virus (influenza A virus) is a major zoonotic pathogen [2]. Influenza A (H1N1) causes an acute respiratory infectious disease with symptoms including fever, cough, diarrhea or vomiting, muscle pain or fatigue, redness of eyes and even death [3]. The most effective means of protection against influenza is vaccination, but its effectiveness has been limited because etiological influenza A and B viruses constantly undergo antigenetic changes [4]. Several anti-influenza drugs have been developed, including M2 protein inhibitors and neuraminidase inhibitors (NAIs). However, nearly all influenza A (H3N2) viruses and part of influenza A (H1N1) viruses are adamantane resistant nowadays, which leaves NAIs the only option for the infection with these viruses [5]. Two NAIs, oseltamivir and zanamivir, are FDA approved for use against type A and type B influenza infections [6]. However, during the 2007–08 influenza season, emergence and transmission of oseltamivir-resistant type A (H1N1) viruses, with an H274Y mutation in the neuraminidase, were observed in several countries in the Northern Hemisphere and then spread globally [7]. In recent years, researchers have also identified oseltamivir resistant influenza type A (H5N1) and type B viruses [5], which makes it urgent for the research and development of new and effective anti-influenza drugs.

Traditional Chinese Medicine (TCM) is an important means to prevent and control influenza in China. Yinqiao powder is a classic prescription from "Wen Bing Tiao Bian", a TCM compound created by Jutong Wu in Qin Dynasty. As a representative of cool acrid exterior-resolving method of TCM, Yinqiao powder is effective in preventing and treating viral infection diseases, which belong to the category of TCM warm diseases, for its antipyretic and anti-inflammatory effect. Yinqiao powder is commonly used for the prevention of influenza in clinic, and has been widely used in the treatment of influenza A [8]. As a recommended drug against wind-heat offender, heat-infected lung influenza, it was included in the latest Influenza Diagnosis and Treatment Program (2018 edition) by the Chinese National Health and Family Planning Commission. Researches have confirmed that Yinqiao powder contains chlorogenic acid [9], phillyrin [10, 11] and arctiin [12, 13], which showed pharmacological effects of anti-influenza virus.

Xinjiaxiangruyin is also a TCM compound from "Wen Bing Tiao Bian" to prevent dampness and heat, and is mainly used for the treatment of summer fever and heat stroke etc. Some scholars used Xinjiaxiangruyin to treat influenza virus infected mice in hot and humid environment, and found that it had remarkable anti-viral effect [14]. Although it consists of five herbs, Xinjiaxiangruyin has a precise combination, in which elsholtzia mainly contains flavonoids and coumarin compounds, which show heat-clearing dampness, anti-bacterial, anti-inflammatory and other pharmacological effects [15]. In addition, magnolol, the main component of Cortex Magnoliae Officinalis, has antioxidative [16, 17], inflammation regulation [18], cancer cell inhibition [19] and other effects. At the same time, honokiol also has an anti-viral activity [20, 21].

Guizhi-and-Mahuang decoction is from classic Chinese medicine works "typhoid fever" written by Mr. Zhang Zhongjing and has acrid-warm herbs for relieving superficies and sweating slightly. Modern pharmacological studies suggest that Guizhi-and-Mahuang decoction has the functions of anti-influenza virus [22], antipyretic analgesia [23], and anti-inflammatory and asthma [24]. Ephedrine has been used in clinic in the past hundreds of years since its discovery. The studies show that ephedrine plays a role in many organs and tissues, and its mechanism is complex, which involves various types of adrenergic receptors [25]. Cinnamon aldehyde contained in Ramulus Cinnamomi can inhibit the infection of influenza A/PR/8 virus [26] and viral myocarditis [27]. However, although these three Chinese herbal compounds can be used for anti-influenza therapy, the molecular signaling pathway involved remains to be clarified.

It is well established that Toll-like receptors (TLRs) are a major family of pattern recognition receptors [28] and play a crucial role in the recognition of microbial pathogens, thereby inducing innate immune responses in mammalian hosts [29]. Toll-like receptor 7 (TLR7) is expressed within intracellular vesicles [30] and recognizes the single-stranded RNA viruses, like vesicular stomatitis virus and influenza virus [31, 32]. It's highly expressed by plasmacytoid dendritic cells (DCs) and B cells [32], and involves in the pathways used by the innate immune cells in the recognition of viral pathogens [31]. The TLRs signaling can be divided into two signal transduction pathways [33]. First, myeloid differentiation primary response 88 (MyD88) associates with TLRs through TIR (Toll/IL1-receptor homologous region) to form a complex that recruits the downstream signal molecule interleukin-1 receptor-associated kinase 4 (IRAK4). Phosphorylation of IRAK4 activates interleukin-1 receptor-associated kinase 1 (IRAK1), which subsequently promotes the activation of TNF receptor associated factor 6 (TRAF6). Activated TRAF6 binds to ubiquitin conjugating enzyme (E2) to degrade IKK-gamma and activate TGF-beta activated kinase 1 (TAK1). Activated TAK1 catalyzes the phosphorylation of IKK- beta protein and forms a complex. The phosphorylation results in translocation of nuclear factor kappa-light-chain-enhancer of activated B cells (NF-κB) related gene from cytoplasm into nucleus and activates the downstream mitogen-activated protein kinases (MAPK) pathway, thereby inducing the formation of activator protein-1 (AP-1), and production of inflammatory cytokines such as interleukin-6 (IL-6), interleukin-12 (IL-12) and Tumor Necrosis Factor-α (TNF-α) [34]. Since NF-κB is activated by a large number of stimuli, tight molecular feedback loops normally prevent sustained cellular responses and excessive inflammation. During infection, some influenza viral particles are degraded by endosomal proteases, releasing the viral genome RNA and initiating TLR7 signaling [35, 36].

In this study, we first confirmed that influenza virus infection indeed activated the TLR7/NF-κB signaling pathway. We then infected the wild type and TLR7 KO mice with influenza virus, and applied three TCMs to evaluate their effects on lung injury recovery. Furthermore, expression levels of components in TLR7/NF-κB pathway were detected and the possible immunological mechanisms were explored.

Methods
Information of experimental design and resources
The information regarding the experimental design, statistics, and resources used in this study are attached in the minimum standards of reporting checklist (Additional file 1).

Drug preparation and HPLC establishment
Yinqiao powder (15 g Fructus Forsythiae, 15 g Flos Lonicerae, 9 g Radix Platycodonis, 9 g Herba Menthae, 6 g Herba Lophatheri, 5 g Radix Glycyrrhizae, 6 g Herba Schizonepetae, 6 g Fermented soybean, 6 g Fructus arctii, 10 g Rhizoma Phragmitis); Xinjiaxiangruyin (6 g Herba Moslae, 9 g Flos Lonicerae, 9 g Dolichos, 6 g Cortex Magnoliae Officinalis, 6 g Fructus Forsythiae). Guizhi-and-Mahuang decoction contained equal part of Mahuang Tang (9 g Herba Ephedrae, 6 g Ramulus Cinnamomi, 9 g Semen Armeniacae Amarum, 6 g Radix glycyrrhizae preparata) and Guizhi Tang (9 g Ramulus Cinnamomi, 9 g Radix Paeoniae Alba, 6 g Radix Glycyrrhizae, 9 g Rhizoma Zingiberis Recens, 3 g Jujube), which were dissolved in water and combined; These three drugs were all Chinese patented granules, which were purchased from China Resources Sanjiu Medical & Pharmaceutical Co., Ltd. (Table 1). Oseltamivir Phosphate Capsules was obtained from Yichang Yangtze River East Sunshine pharmaceutical Ltd (Lot H20065415). 3,4-dihydroxybenzoic acid (Lot 170707); chlorogenic acid (Lot 171110); liquiritin (Lot 171222); forsythin (Lot 171103); arctiin (Lot 180207); thymol (Lot 171210); magnolol (Lot 171126);

amygdalin (Lot 170902); paeoniflorin (Lot 180124) were purchased from Beijing Shengshi Kangpu Chemical Engineering Technology Institute, Ephedrine Hydrochloride (Lot: 171241–201508) was purchased from China Research Institute of Food and Drug Verification. 500 mg of fine particles of each TCM was dissolved in 25 mL of 50% methanol solution, ultrasonic cleaning for 30 min, and filtered with 0.45 μm microporous filters. High performance liquid chromatography (HPLC) was performed to identify the main chemical constituents in the TCMs. Fingerprints of TCMs were read, and some chemical constituents of TCMs were identified according to the spectrograms and retention times of their standards (Fig. 1).

Animals
C57BL/6 wild type (WT) mice of SPF grade were purchased from Medical Animal Experiment Center of Guangdong Province (animal license #: SCXK 2013-0002). TLR7 knockout (TLR7 KO) mice were provided by the Jackson Laboratory (USA) and all the knockout mice were returned to C57BL/6 mice over ten generations. The breeding and feeding of TLR7 KO mice were carried out in SPF environment of Animal Experimental Center of Jinan University with free drinking water and feeding, in temperature-controlled animal facility (temperature: 20 ± 2 °C; humidity: 50%) with 12 h diurnal cycle and individual ventilated cages (IVC). Sixty WT female C57BL/6 mice (6–8 weeks old) were randomly divided into six experimental groups ($n = 10$/group): blank control group, virus control group, oseltamivir group (positive control group), Xinjiaxiangruyin group, Guizhi-and-Mahuang decoction group, and Yinqiao powder group. The same protocol was applied to TLR7 KO mice. Mice were anesthetized by intraperitoneal injection of 130–160 μL 6% chloral hydrate solution, and 50 μL sterile solution of 0.9% NaCl was dropped nasally in blank control group. The rest groups were challenged with 50 μL influenza virus FM1 suspension (dilution 1:640) nasally. None of the mice infected died. The drug dose was calculated based on body-weight differences between humans and mice and the dose for the mice was equivalent to 9.1 times that for human clinical dosage. 24 h after infection, 0.4 mL of Yinqiao powder (560 mg/mL), Xinjiaxiangruyin (230 mg/mL), Guizhi-and-Mahuang decoction (350 mg/mL) and oseltamivir (1.5 mg/mL) were given to mice in treatment groups by gastric gavage once a day for 5 days, respectively. The blank control group and virus control group were treated with the same amount of double distilled water. The mice were placed in an artificial climate incubator (temperature: 18–20 °C; humidity: 50%; light: 3000Lx) and a free diet during the experiment and were observed for 5 days. The mice were sacrificed to collect lung and spleen for examination 6 days after infection.

Table 1 The compositions of Traditional Chinese Medicine

Traditional Chinese Medicine	No.	Herbal drug	Official name	Local name	Batch number	Collection place
Yinqiao powder	1	Fructus Forsythiae	*Forsythia suspensa* (Thunb.) Vahl	Lianqiao	1712002S	Shanxi
	2	Flos Lonicerae	*Lonicera japonica* Thunb.	Jinyinhua	1801002S	Shandong
	3	Radix Platycodonis	*Platycodon grandiflorus* (Jacq.) A.DC.	Jugeng	1712004S	Anhui
	4	Herba Menthae	*Mentha haplocalyx* Briq.	Bohe	1709001S	Jiangsu
	5	Herba Lophatheri	*Lophatherum gracile* Brongn.	Danzhuye	1712002S	Sichuan
	6	Radix Glycyrrhizae	*Glycyrrhiza uralensis* Fisch.	Gancao	1801016S	Gansu
	7	Herba Schizonepetae	*Schizonepeta tenuifolia* Briq	Jingjiesui	1710001S	Hebei
	8	Fermented soybean	*Glycine max* (L.) Merr.	Dandouchi	1704001S	Henan
	9	Fructus arctii	*Arctium lappa* L.	Niubangzi	1801001S	Gansu
	10	Rhizoma Phragmitis	*Phragmites communis* Trin.	Lugen	1709002S	Anhui
Xinjiaxiangruyin	1	Herba Moslae	*Mosla chinensis* Maxim.	Xiangru	1708002S	Jiangxi
	2	Flos Lonicerae	*Lonicera japonica* Thunb.	Jinyinhua	1801002S	Shandong
	3	Dolichos	*Dolichos aciphyllus* R.Wilczek	Biandouhua	161001	Guangdong
	4	Cortex Magnoliae Officinalis	*Magnolia officinalis* Rehder & E.H.Wilson	Houpu	1712003S	Sichuan
	5	Fructus Forsythiae	*Forsythia suspensa* (Thunb.) Vahl	Lianqiao	1712002S	Shanxi
Guizhi-and-Mahuang decoction	1	Herba Ephedrae	*Ephedra intermedia* Schrenk & C.A.Mey.	Mahuang	1706004S	Neimenggu
	2	Ramulus Cinnamomi	*Cinnamomum cassia* (L.) J.Presl	Guizhi	1801003S	Guangxini
	3	Semen Armeniacae Amarum	*Prunus armeniaca* L.	Xingren	1712003S	Hebei
	4	Radix glycyrrhizae preparata	*Glycyrrhiza uralensis* Fisch.	Zhigancao	1712003S	Gansu
	5	Radix Paeoniae Alba	*Paeonia lactiflora* Pall.	Shaoyao	1801001S	Anhui
	6	Radix Glycyrrhizae	*Glycyrrhiza uralensis* Fisch.	Gancao	1801016S	Gansu
	7	Rhizoma Zingiberis Recens	*Zingiber officinale* Roscoe	Shengjiang	–	Guangdong
	8	Jujube	*Ziziphus jujuba* Mill.	Dazao	–	Guangdong

Virus strains

Virus strain: type A influenza virus, FM1 mouse lung adapted strain (FM1), stored at − 80 °C. It was provided by the Department of Microbiology and Immunology, School of Basic Medical Sciences, Jinan University. The hemagglutination titer was 1:40 after two times of routine chick embryo resuscitation. The mortality of mice 14 days after virus infection at different concentrations was determined by double dilution method. The virus concentration causing 20% mouse mortality (blood coagulation titer 1:640) was used and 50 µL of virus solution was given to each mouse.

The changes of body weight, animal condition, survival rate and lung index

Starting at 2 days before infection, the weight of each mouse was recorded at the same time point every day. The changes of symptoms, water and food intake, hair color, activity, survival time, death condition and so on were observed twice a day. The mice were sacrificed

6 days after infection for lung tissue collection. Adipose tissue was removed, and the lung tissue was washed with sterile phosphate buffer saline (PBS). The lungs were then dried with filter paper and weighed. The lung index was calculated using the formula: lung index = lung weight/ body weight × 100%.

Observation of pathological changes in lung tissue

The fresh lungs were fixed in 4% paraformaldehyde, dehydrated, embedded in paraffin wax and serially sectioned at 5 µm. Haematoxylin and eosin (H&E) was employed and the pathological changes of the lung tissue were observed under light microscope.

Detection of the level of Th17 and Treg cells in the spleen of mice

The spleens of mice were rinced with RPMI-1640 medium and continuously grounded. The resultant cell suspension was placed on the upper layer of the lymphocyte separating fluid (Multi Sciences, China). After

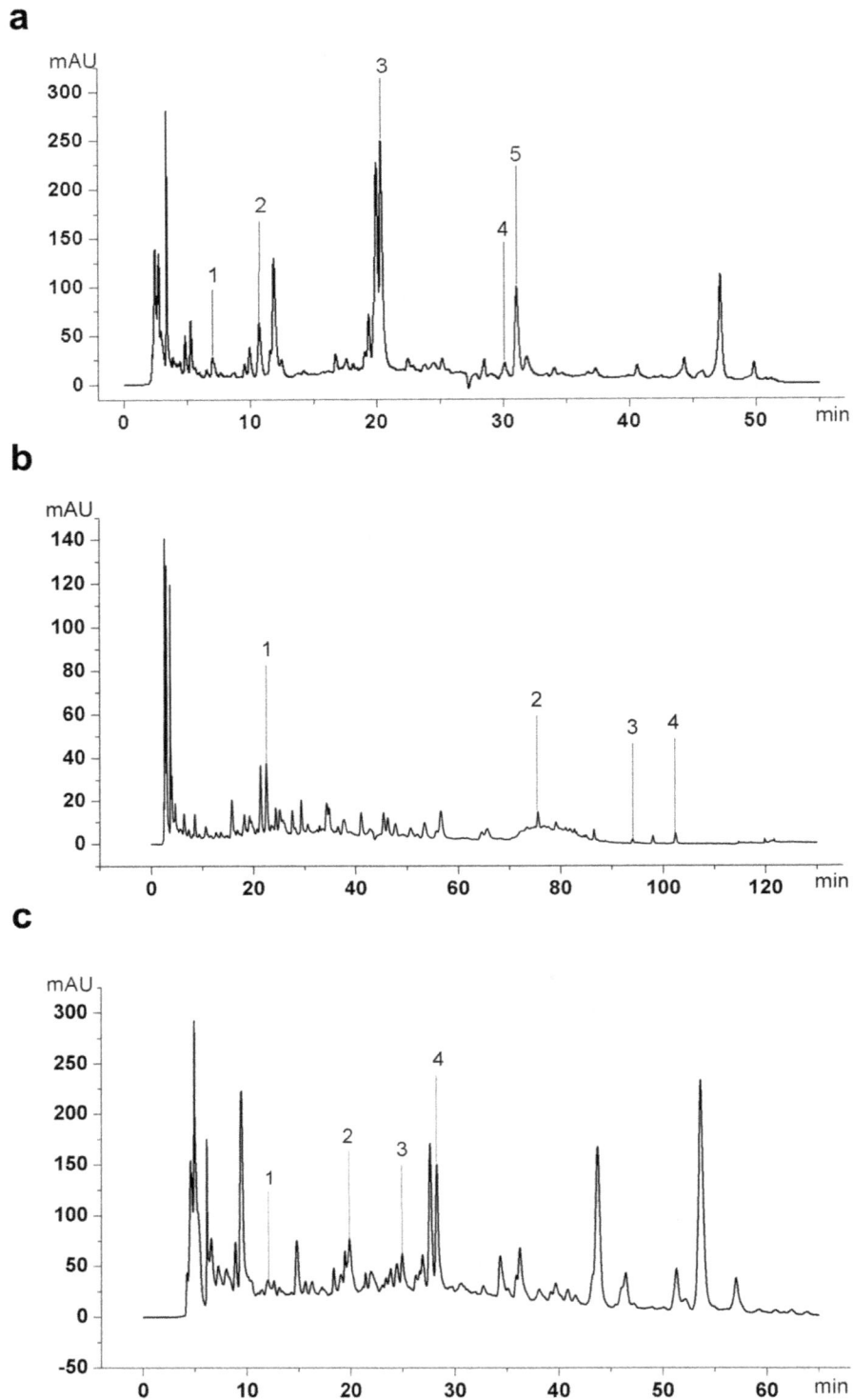

Fig. 1 The fingerprints of TCMs. **a** The fingerprint of Yinqiao powder; peak number and identity, 1: 3,4-dihydroxybenzoic acid; 2: chlorogenic acid; 3: liquiritin; 4: forsythin; 5: arctiin. **b** The fingerprint of Xinjiaxiangruyin; peak number and identity, 1: chlorogenic acid; 2: forsythin; 3: thymol; 4: magnolol. **c** The fingerprint of Guizhi-and-Mahuang decoction; peak number and identity, 1: ephedrine hydrochloride; 2: amygdalin; 3: paeoniflorin; 4: liquiritin

centrifugation, the intermediate white lymphocyte layer was collected and washed with PBS. Lymphocytes were then resuspended in RPMI-1640 medium containing 10% fetal bovine serum (FBS) and adjusted to 1×10^6/mL concentration. To detect Treg cells, 100 μL of cell suspension was incubated with anti-CD4 and anti-CD25 antibodies for 30 min at 4 °C avoiding light, and then washed with precooled PBS. Cells were then resuspended in film breaking working fluid (fixation/permeabilization concentrate: fixation/permeabilization diluent = 1:3) (eBioscience, USA), and incubated for 30 min at 4 °C avoiding light. After washed with 1 × Permeabilization buffer (eBioscience, USA), intracellular antibody Foxp3 was added and incubated for 30 min at 4 °C avoiding light. Finally, cells were washed and resuspended in 200 μL of PBS for analysis on FACSVerse Flow cytometry (Becton–Dickinson Bioscie NCS, Franklin Lakes, NJ, USA). Flowjo7.6.1 (Flow Jo, Ashland, OR, USA) software was used to process and analyze the experimental data. The Antibodies were shown in Table 2.

Detection of mRNA expression levels of TLR7, MyD88, IRAK4 and NF-κB in mouse lung with RT-qPCR

The lung tissue was collected for total RNA extraction using Trizol (TaKaRa, Japan) according to the manufacturer's instructions. First-strand cDNA synthesis and the SYBR® Green qPCR assay were performed using the PrimeScript™ RT Reagent Kit (TaKaRa, Japan). The reverse transcription reactions were performed in the Bio-Rad S1000™ thermocycler (Bio-Rad, USA). qPCR protocol was: 95 °C, 30 s; 95 °C, 5 s; 60 °C, 30 s; with 40 amplification cycle; 95 °C, 10 s using the ABI 7000 Real Time PCR machines. All primers (Table 3) were designed and synthesized by Shanghai Generay Biotech Co. Ltd. Corresponding relative mRNA expression was calculated by the $2^{-\Delta\Delta Ct}$ method [37]. mRNA expression levels of FM1, TLR7, MyD88, IRAK4 and NF-κB were evaluated using GAPDH as an internal standard control.

Table 2 Antibodies used for flow cytometry

Antibody	Clone	Company	Labels used
CD4	RM4-5	eBioscience	PE
IL-17A	eBio17B7	eBioscience	FTIC
CD25	PC61.5	eBioscience	APC
Foxp3	FJK-16 s	eBioscience	PE-cy5.5

PE phyco-erythrin, *FITC* Fluorescein isothiocyanate, *APC* allophycocyanin, *CD4* cluster of differentiation 4, *IL-17A* interleukin-17A, *CD25* cluster of differentiation 25, *Foxp3* forkhead box P3

Table 3 Primers used for RT-qPCR studies

Gene	Forward (5′ to 3′)	Reverse (5′ to 3′)
FM1	GACCAATCCTGTCACCTCTGAC	AGGGCATTNTGGACAAAG CGTCTA
GAPDH	CTGAGCAAGAGAGGCCCT ATCC	CTCCCTAGGCCCCTCCTGTT
TLR7	GGGTCCAAAGCCAATGTG	TGTTAGATTCTCCTTCGTGATG
MyD88	CGATTATCTACAGAGCAAGGA ATG	ATAGTGATGAACCGCAGGATAC
IRAK4	CATCGTGGCGGTGAAGAAG	AGCATACACTAAGCACAGGTTG
NF-κB	ATTCTGACCTTGCCTATCTAC	TCCAGTCTCCGAGTGAAG

GAPDH glyceraldehyde-3-phosphate dehydrogenase, *TLR7* Toll-like receptor 7, *MyD88* Myeloid differentiation primary response 88, *IRAK4* interleukin-1 receptor-associated kinase 4, *NF-κB* nuclear factor kappa-light-chain-enhancer of activated B cells

Determination of protein expression levels of TLR7, MyD88, IRAK4 and NF-κB by Western-blotting

Protein samples were extracted from lung tissue homogenate using a RIPA lysis buffer (Multi Sciences, China) supplemented with protease and phosphatase inhibitors, and the protein concentrations were quantified using BCA assay. Separated with 10% SDS-PAGE, the protein was transferred wetly to the PVDF membrane (Millipore, USA). The PVDF membrane was blocked in TBST containing 5% skimmed milk and incubated with the Rabbit monoclonal antibody (mAb) (CST, USA) of GAPDH, TLR7, MyD88, IRAK4 and NF-κB overnight at 4 °C, respectively, and then incubated for 2 h in the HRP-labeled secondary antibodies against rabbit (Multi Sciences, China). The blots were developed using the ECL color display kit (Multi Sciences, China), and ImageJ image analysis software was used for ALIANCE gel image analyzer and imaging.

Statistical analysis

The experiment data were processed and analyzed with the statistical software SPSS 13.0. All results were presented as mean ± standard deviation (x ± s). Two groups of independent samples were compared by t-test. Multiple experimental groups were analyzed by ANOVA in advance, and SNK was used for comparison of each two groups according to the homogeneity of variance test. $P < 0.05$ indicated that the difference was statistically significant, and $P < 0.01$ means significant difference.

Results

Guizhi-and-Mahuang decoction had a protective effect on virus infection

To evaluate the effects of TCMs on anti-virus and development of lung inflammation, we infected wild-type and

TLR7 KO C57BL/6 mice with Influenza virus FM1 and applied Oseltamivir and three TCMs 24 h post-infection for 5 days, respectively. In wild-type mice, the animals in sham group had good mental state, good hair color, quick action, breathing, normal gait and natural weight growth. Clinical symptoms in virus infected mice were apparent 2 days after infection. In viral control group, mice had typical flu symptoms, including hair discoloring, towering hair, curled up, arch, paralysis, loss of appetite, reduced water drinking, convulsions, faint and breathing difficulties. Meanwhile the body weight was decreased gradually. Compared to virus control, animals in Oseltamivir group, Guizhi-and-Mahuang decoction group were significantly improved with towering hair, convulsions and other symptoms remarkably reduced. Yinqiao powder group only showed slightly improvement. The body weight changes in each group were shown in Fig. 2a. The average body weight of mice on day 6 in virus control group, Xinjiaxiangruyin group and Yinqiao powder group were decreased to 72.08%, 75.16% (NS) and 79.94% ($P < 0.05$) of the original body weight, respectively, while mice in Oseltamivir group and Guizhi-and-Mahuang decoction group were better with 93.29% ($P < 0.01$) and 84.45% ($P < 0.01$) of the original body weight, respectively.

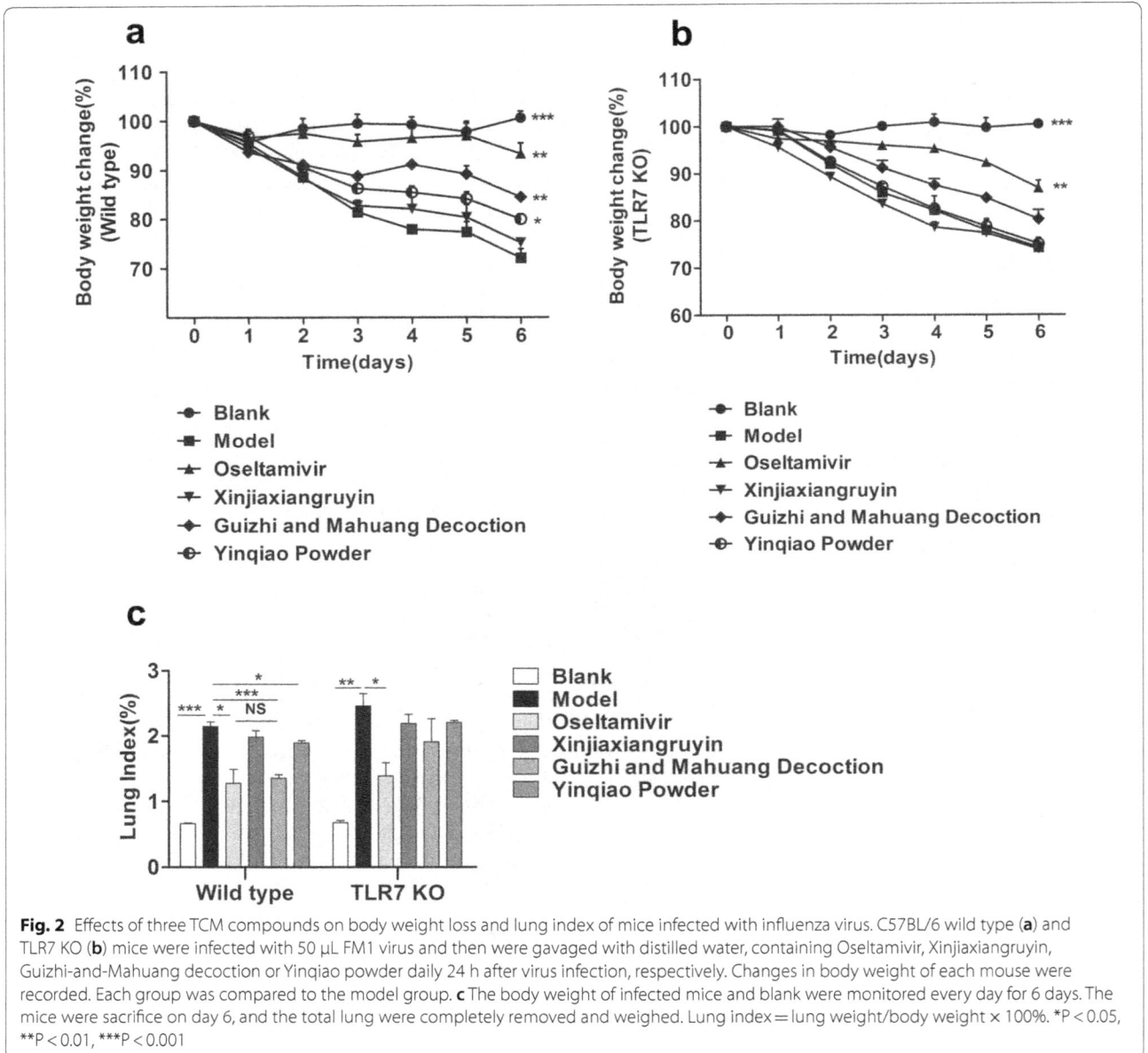

Fig. 2 Effects of three TCM compounds on body weight loss and lung index of mice infected with influenza virus. C57BL/6 wild type (**a**) and TLR7 KO (**b**) mice were infected with 50 μL FM1 virus and then were gavaged with distilled water, containing Oseltamivir, Xinjiaxiangruyin, Guizhi-and-Mahuang decoction or Yinqiao powder daily 24 h after virus infection, respectively. Changes in body weight of each mouse were recorded. Each group was compared to the model group. **c** The body weight of infected mice and blank were monitored every day for 6 days. The mice were sacrifice on day 6, and the total lung were completely removed and weighed. Lung index = lung weight/body weight × 100%. *P < 0.05, **P < 0.01, ***P < 0.001

In TLR7 KO mice, we observed that, except for the blank group and the Oseltamivir group, the body weight of the virus control group and the three TCM groups decreased significantly (Fig. 2b). We further weighed the whole lung of each mouse and calculated the lung index. As shown in Fig. 2c, in both wild type and TLR7 KO mice, there was a significant difference in the lung index between the blank group and the virus control group ($P < 0.01$), indicating that the viral infection was successful. As a positive control drug, Oseltamivir significantly reduced lung index compared to the virus control group ($P < 0.05$). In wild type mice, the lung indexes of animals in Guizhi-and-Mahuang decoction group and Yinqiao powder were significantly decreased compared to the virus control group ($P < 0.05$); and there was no significant difference (NS) between Guizhi-and-Mahuang decoction group and Oseltamivir group. In TLR7 KO mice, the three TCM groups had no significant difference compared to the virus control group or among three groups (NS).

Pathological changes of lung tissue

The amount of replicating virus in the lungs is thought to correlate with the degree of lung pathological changes. Therefore, wild type and TLR7 KO mice were infected with Influenza FM1 virus, and four drugs were used to treat the mice 24 h after infection, respectively. After 5 days of continuous gavage, lungs of the mice were collected. The RNA was extracted from the left lung, and the replication of virus in each group was evaluated. We observed that the virus control group had a significantly higher viral mRNA expression level in lung tissue than blank group in wild type mice ($P < 0.001$), Meanwhile, Oseltamivir, Guizhi-and-Mahuang decoction and Yinqiao powder dramatically decreased the viral load compared to the virus control group ($P < 0.001$). In TLR7 KO mice, the viral load of virus control group was significantly higher than that of blank control group ($P < 0.001$), but only Oseltamivir group reduced the replication of virus ($P < 0.05$). We then performed comparative analysis between wild type and TLR7 KO mice, and found no difference between virus control groups. However, Oseltamivir, Guizhi-and-Mahuang decoction and Yinqiao powder treatment induced significant difference between wild type and TLR7 KO mice, suggesting that TLR7 receptor played a key role in antivirus effects (Fig. 3).

At the same time, the right lungs of mice were fixed in 4% formaldehyde solution and HE staining was performed. In wild type mice (Fig. 4a), blank control group showed clear and intact alveolar structure. The alveolar wall was thin, and there was no inflammatory secretion in alveolar cavity, nor alveolar interstitial infiltration of inflammatory cells. In virus control group, inflammatory

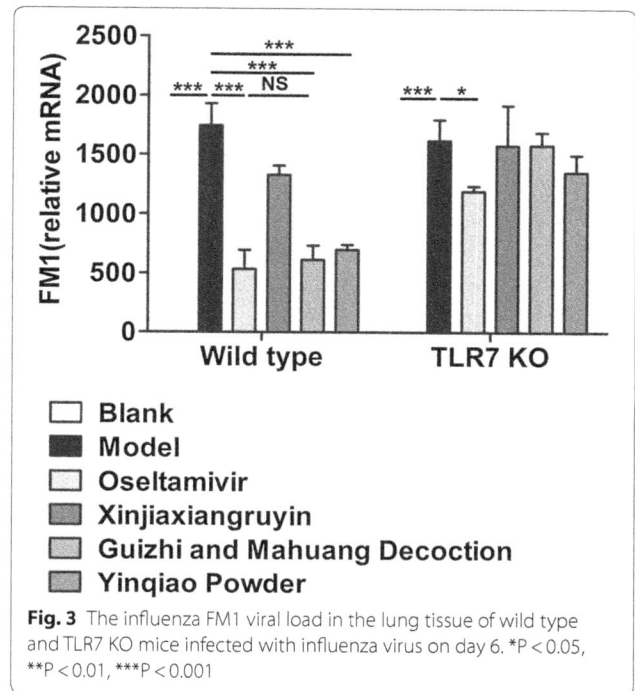

Fig. 3 The influenza FM1 viral load in the lung tissue of wild type and TLR7 KO mice infected with influenza virus on day 6. *$P < 0.05$, **$P < 0.01$, ***$P < 0.001$

damage was observed in lung tissue, including a large number of inflammatory cell infiltration in alveolar cavity, alveolar septum thickening and severe interstitial edema, vascular congestion, bronchial obstruction due to inflammatory exudation. Formation of cavitation was also observed after epithelial cell shedding or necrosis. In the positive control group (oseltamivir group), alveolar inflammatory cells were significantly reduced and peribronchial alveolar wall was thinning with no inflammatory cells, similar to that in the blank control group, and only alveolar wall thickening was observed. In Xinjiaxiangruyin group, alveolar structure destruction was increased. Bronchial wall and alveolar septa were thickened, and there were a large number of infiltrating mononuclear cells, with bronchiole having more infiltrating inflammatory cells. In Guizhi-and-Mahuang decoction group, the inflammatory lesion was more significantly reduced than that in virus control group. The alveolar wall was thin, with less infiltration of mononuclear cells, capillary dilatation and congestion of alveolar wall. The alveolar septum was not obviously thickened, with only a small number of mononuclear cells and lymphocytes. There was no inflammatory exudation in bronchiole, similar to that in the positive control group. In Yinqiao powder group, the alveolar wall was thickened, but alveolar infiltration was not obvious. Compared to the virus control group, the alveolar infiltration and inflammatory reaction was milder and there was no exudate in the bronchiole. In general, the influenza viral

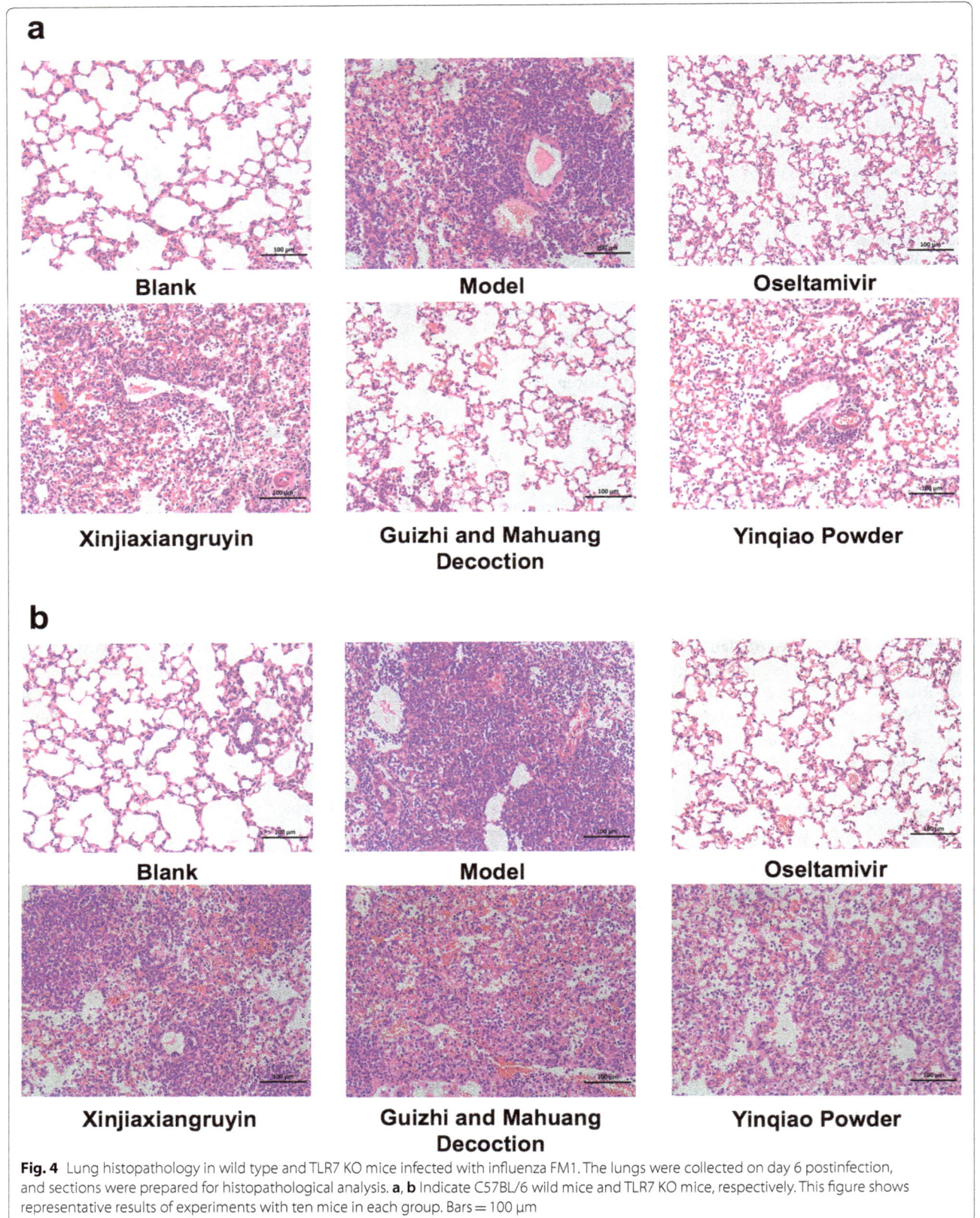

Fig. 4 Lung histopathology in wild type and TLR7 KO mice infected with influenza FM1. The lungs were collected on day 6 postinfection, and sections were prepared for histopathological analysis. **a, b** Indicate C57BL/6 wild mice and TLR7 KO mice, respectively. This figure shows representative results of experiments with ten mice in each group. Bars = 100 μm

infection caused acute inflammatory responses and mononuclear cell infiltration in the respiratory tissue, which contributed to the main pathological basis of the disease. In TLR7 KO mice (Fig. 4b), the Oseltamivir treatment remarkably reduced inflammation compared to virus control. However, neither TCM treatment groups showed any difference compared to the virus control, which indicated that the therapeutic effects of TCM on viral infection induced inflammation needed the participation of TLR7 signaling.

Profiling of Th17 cells and Treg cells in splenocytes

In the process of immuno-regulation, Th17 cells are closely related to Treg cells. IL-17 secreted by Th17 cells can aggravate the inflammatory responses, while Treg cells can reduce the production of inflammatory cytokines and antibody secretion to inhibit immune responses. Th17/Treg balance plays an important role in maintaining the immune homeostasis of the body. In order to further verify the inflammatory response in mice, we used flow cytometry to detect the splenocytes in mice. As shown Fig. 5, in the wild type mice, the ratio of Th17 cells and Treg cells in the virus control group was significantly higher than that in the blank control group ($P < 0.001$). Compared to the virus control, except for Xinjiaxiangruyin group, ratios of Th17 cells and Treg cells in other three groups were significantly decreased (Fig. 5a). In TLR7 KO mice, the ratio of Th17 cells and Treg cells in the virus control group was higher than that in the blank control group. Compared to the virus control group, only the Oseltamivir treatment resulted in significant decrease in the Th17 cell and Treg cell ratio ($P < 0.05$) (Fig. 5b).

Effects of drugs on TLR7/NF-κB signaling pathway

In order to further explore the contribution of Chinese herbal compounds to innate immune response after influenza virus infection, wild type and TLR7 KO mice were infected with influenza virus, respectively. 6 days after infection, the mRNA relative expression and protein levels of components in TLR7 and NF-κB signaling pathways in lung tissue were detected with RT-qPCR and western blotting, respectively. As shown in Fig. 6, virus infection induced significant increase in the mRNA levels of TLR7, MyD88, IRAK4 and NF-κB in wild type mice compared to blank control ($P < 0.001$). Compared to the

virus control group, all treatment, except for Xinjiaxiangzhuyin, resulted in significant decrease in expression levels of TLR7, MyD88, IRAK4 and NF-κB ($P < 0.05$), with Oseltamivir and Guizhi-and-Mahuang decoction treatment having more reduction, followed by Yinqiao powder. These data indicated that influenza virus infection could activate TLR7/NF-κB signaling pathway, while Oseltamivir and Guizhi-and-Mahuang decoction significantly suppressed their expression. We also tested the TLR7 KO mice at the same time. The relative mRNA expression of TLR7 was significantly lower than that in wild type mice, and had no difference among all experimental groups (NS), which confirmed the success of TLR7 KO. Then, we studied the effect of TLR7 gene silencing on the downstream signaling pathway, and found that MyD88 and NF-κB were still activated. We further demonstrated that virus infection increased protein expression levels of TLR7, MyD88, IRAK4 and NF-κB with western blotting, while Oseltamivir, Guizhi-and-Mahuang decoction, Yinqiao powder decreased their expression. The protein levels in each group were in accordance with the expression of mRNA (Fig. 7).

Discussion

Viruses activate immune pathways through three pattern recognition receptors (PRRs), TLRs, RLHs and NLRs (nucleotide-oligomerization domin (NOD) -like receptors) [38–40]. TLR7 recognizes the single-stranded RNA viruses, such as vesicular stomatitis virus and influenza virus [29]. Some studies have shown that TLR7 is mainly expressed in lung, placenta, heart, spleen, bone marrow, lymph nodes and other tissues [34, 41], so we detected mRNA and protein expression levels of TLR7 and its related genes in lung tissue in a mouse model. We infected wild type and TLR7 KO C57BL/6 mice with influenza virus in a normal environment, and applied various TCM treatment to evaluate their anti-virus and anti-inflammation effects. The viral load of the lung tissue in the virus control group was significantly higher than that in the blank control group, indicating that the experimental animal model was successfully established.

The drugs used in our study was selected according to the three main dialectic methods of TCM at the onset of diseases: acrid-warm herbs relieving superficies (Yinqiao powder), cold-pungent diaphoresis (Guizhi-and-Mahuang decoction), and clearing damp

(See figure on next page.)
Fig. 5 Profiling of Th17 cells and Treg cells in splenocytes of mice. C57/6 wild type mice (n = 10/group) and TLR7 KO mice (n = 10/group) were infected with 50 μL of influenza FM1 virus. Splenocytes were isolated from 3 mice out of each group on day 6 post-infection and Th17 cell and Treg cell response were assayed in wild type mice (**a**) and TLR7 KO mice (**b**). Data are presented as the mean ± SEM. Th17 cell response was determined by intracellular CD4, IL-17 staining. Treg cell response was determined by intracellular CD4, CD25 and Foxp3 staining. Data are presented as representative density plots in wild type mice (**c**) and TLR7 KO mice (**d**). *P < 0.05, **P < 0.01, ***P < 0.001

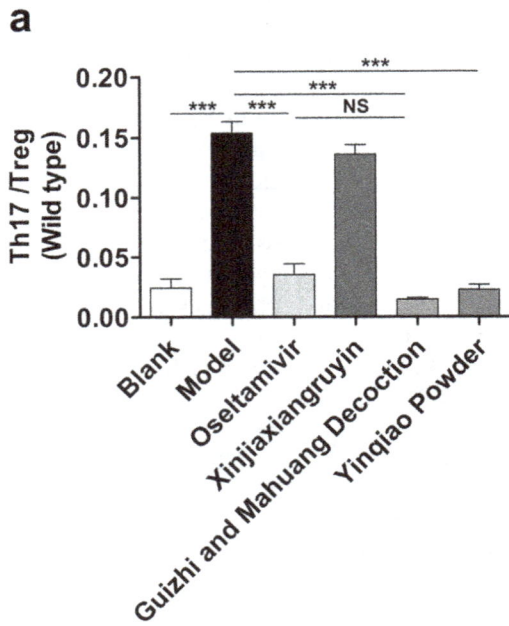

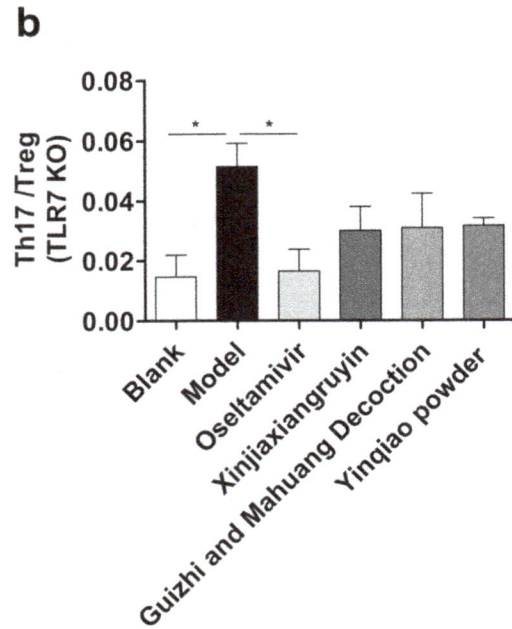

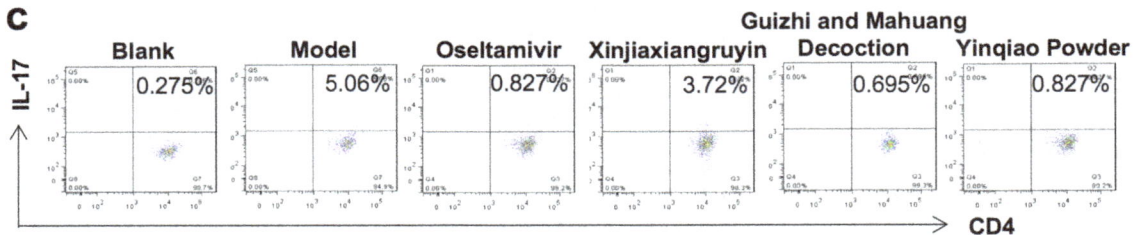

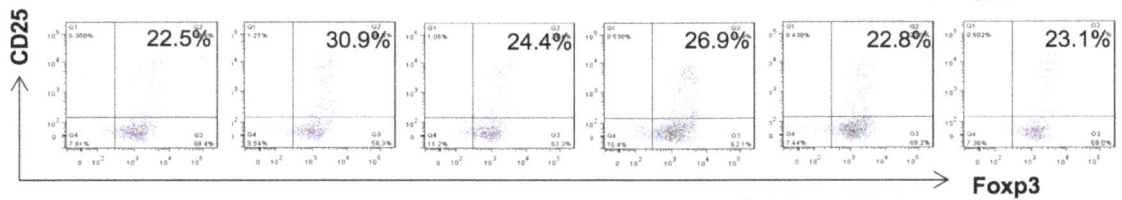

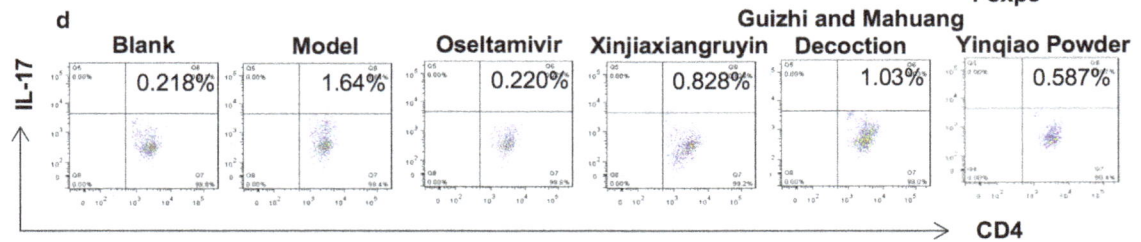

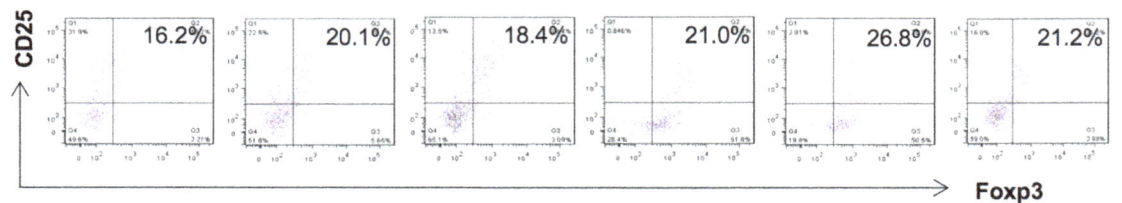

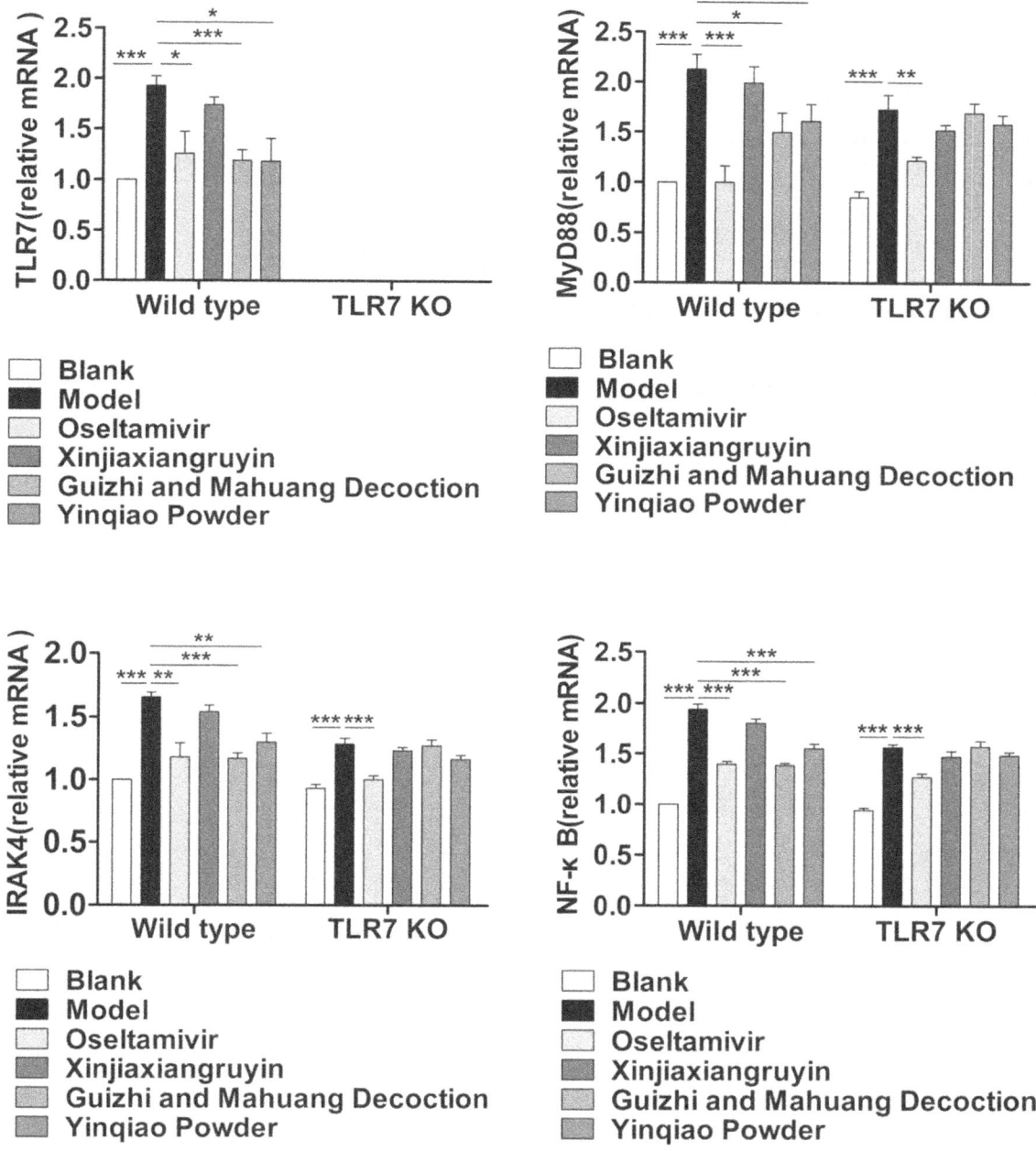

Fig. 6 The effect of different drugs on the mRNA expression of TLR7 and NF-κB signaling pathway in lung tissue of influenza virus infected mice. *P < 0.05, **P < 0.01, ***P < 0.001

(Xinjiaxiangruyin). In different environments, drugs may perform differently against influenza, and our experiment was carried out in the normal environment (temperature: 18–20 °C, humidity 50%, and light: 3000Lx) for the viral infection and drug administration in mice. The experimental results indicated that under normal circumstances, Guizhi-and-Mahuang decoction and Yinqiao powder had defensive effects against influenza virus infection, while the effect of Xinjiaxiangruyin was not obvious in wild type mice. Compared to the positive control oseltamivir, Guizhi-and-Mahuang decoction showed no difference in the lung index, lung pathology change, virus load and the ratio of Th17 cells and Treg cells, demonstrating its efficacy in anti-virus and the potential as

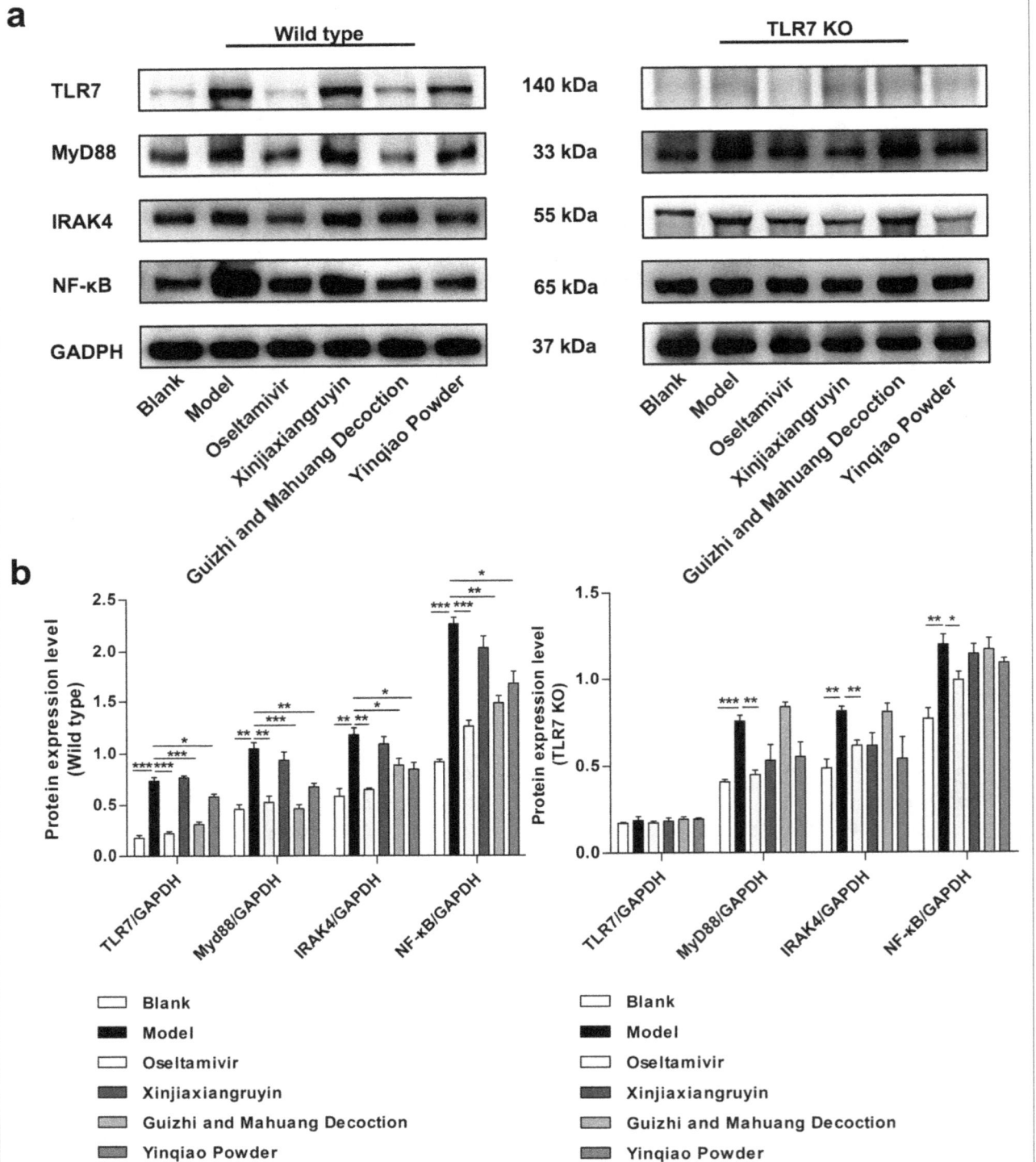

Fig. 7 The effect of different drugs on the protein expression of TLR7 and NF-κB signaling pathway in lung tissue of influenza virus infected mice. **a** Proteins were evaluated by western blotting assay. **b** Quantification of TLR7, MyD88, IRAK4, NF-κB protein was detected by densitometric analysis. *P < 0.05, **P < 0.01, ***P < 0.001

a new anti-influenza drug. Xinjiaxiangruyin may play a good role of anti-influenza in hot and humid environment, which warrants further research and exploration.

In terms of inflammatory response, we further demonstrated the role of Chinese herbal compounds in the anti-influenza process. Th17 cells secrete IL-17 as well as cytokines such as IL-21 and IL-22, and IL-17 can aggravate inflammatory reaction and participate in various autoimmune diseases [42]. Treg is a CD4+ T cell subset with immunosuppressive activity. Treg cells release cytokines IL-10 and TGF- beta to inhibit the function of T cells and antigen presenting cells, and reduce the production of inflammatory cytokines and antibody secretion. Foxp3 is an important transcription factor of Treg, and its continuous expression is the key factor in maintaining the inhibitory activity of Treg. Foxp3+ Treg cells have the function of anti-inflammatory and maintenance of autoimmune tolerance [43]. Foxp3+ Treg cells and Th17 cells inhibit each other in differentiation, development and function [44]. Therefore, Foxp3+ Treg/Th17 balance plays an important role in maintaining immune homeostasis.

Mononuclear cells were isolated from spleen of mice and flow cytometry was used to detect and analyze Th17 cells and Treg cells. The ratio of Th17 to Treg in the virus control group was much greater than that in the blank control group. In wild type mice, Oseltamivir, Guizhi-and-Mahuang decoction, and Yinqiao powder could decrease the ratio of Th17/Treg, which indicated that Treg cells inhibited the release of inflammatory factors and alleviated the inflammatory response in the lungs of mice. In TLR7 KO mice, the deletion of TLR7 gene significantly decreased the antiviral effect of Guizhi-and-Mahuang decoction and Yinqiao powder, which indicated that these two drugs might function through TLR7. The inflammatory response in lung pathology was consistent with the ratio change of Th17/Treg cells.

At both mRNA and protein expression levels, we have demonstrated the effect of TCMs on the TLR7/NF-κB signaling pathway in the process of anti-influenza virus infection. It's found that the TLR7 was up-regulated in the macrophages upon virus infection [45]. Studies have shown that TCMs can play a role in the treatment of influenza by TLR7 mediated MyD88-dependent signaling pathway. In this study, we mainly examined the mRNA and protein expressions of components in TLR7-mediated MyD88-dependent signaling pathway. The results showed that the expression levels of TLR7, MYD88, IRAK4 and NF-κB were remarkably up-regulated upon viral infection, and Guizhi-and-Mahuang decoction and Yinqiao powder could down-regulate their expressions in

wild type mice. In TLR7 KO mice, the mRNA and protein expressions of TLR7 were very low in all groups, indicating that the TLR7 gene was successfully knocked out. However, MyD88 was up-regulated upon viral infection, because all other members of TLRs family, except for TLR3, can be activated by MyD88 dependence [46]. The expression of IRAK4 was low upon viral infection, indicating that the TLR7 knockout might affect IRAK4 expression in the downstream pathway. TLR7 knockout decreased the transcription and translation levels of NF-κB overall, which suggested that TLR7 plays an indispensable role in the pathway. However, there was no significant change in survival rate of TLR7 KO mice, which was probably due to the compensatory role of the RLH signaling pathway. RIG-I (RIG-like receptors) is also a type of pattern recognition receptor [47] and involves in the recognition of influenza virus [48]. NF-κB is the common nuclear factor of TLR7 and RIG-I, so when TLR7 gene is knocked out, RIG-I may play a compensatory role, and ultimately activate NF-κB to maintain stable expression.

Oseltamivir is a neuraminidase inhibitor [49], which blocks the activity of neuraminidase, inhibiting the replication and toxicity of virus so as to effectively prevent and even alleviate the symptoms of influenza. It can be combined with the flu vaccine without affecting the antibody production. However, oseltamivir resistant influenza A and influenza B virus strains have continuously emerged in recent years [5], and many side effects have been reported, such as vomiting, nausea, headache, and rash [50]. TCM has a lot of advantages. It not only has the functions of inhibiting virus replication, preventing cytopathic effect, improving host immunity and blood circulation, but also greatly reduces the drug resistance due to its compatibility, which makes TCM a unique and effective option in the prevention and treatment of influenza.

Conclusion

The results of this study show that, under normal circumstances, Guizhi-and-Mahuang decoction and Yinqiao powder play a more significant role in the process of anti-influenza virus. After influenza virus infection, transcription and translation levels of components in the TLR7/NF-κB pathway were increased in mouse lungs, and Guizhi-and-Mahuang decoction and Yinqiao powder effectively reduced those changes to achieve viral clearance and inflammation recovery. Although different from oseltamivir in antiviral mechanisms, Guizhi-and-Mahuang decoction showed similar effects on therapeutic effects.

Authors' contributions
JZY, TXL and CXY conceived and designed the experiments. FYJ, YYQ, QHQ and ZX performed the experiments. FYJ and YYQ analyzed the data. WS, SSS and WPC provided reagents and advice. Wrote the paper: FYJ. All authors read and approved the final manuscript.

Acknowledgements
Not applicable.

Competing interests
The authors declare that they have no competing interests.

Consent for publication
The manuscript is approved by all authors for publication.

Funding
This work was supported by the National Natural Science Foundation of China [Grant Numbers 81473454, 81473557, 81774164] and the Natural Science Foundation of Guangdong, China [Grant Numbers 2015A030313331].

References
1. Nogales A, Martínez-Sobrido L. Reverse genetics approaches for the development of influenza vaccines. Int J Mol Sci. 2016;18:20.
2. Ozawa M, Kawaoka Y. Crosstalk between animal and human influenza viruses. Annu Rev Anim Biosci. 2013;1:21–42.
3. Kumar A, Zarychanski R, Pinto R, Cook D, Marshall J. Critically Ill patients with 2009 influenza A(H1N1) infection in Canada. JAMA. 2009;302:1872–9.
4. Tomoko N, Kazufumi S, Torahiko T, Kazumichi K. Bacterial neuraminidase rescues influenza virus replication from inhibition by a neuraminidase inhibitor. PLoS ONE. 2012;7:e45371.
5. Poland GA, Jacobson RM, Ovsyannikova IG. Influenza virus resistance to antiviral agents: a plea for rational use. Clin Infect Dis. 2009;48:1254–6.
6. Moscon A. Neuraminidase inhibitors for influenza. New Engl J Med. 2005;353:1363.
7. Gubareva L, Okomo-Adhiambo M, Deyde V, Sheu TG, Garten R. Update: drug susceptibility of swine-origin influenza A (H1N1) viruses, april 2009. MMWR Morb Mortal Wkly Rep. 2009;58:433–5.
8. Zhang ZY, Zhang HM, Zhou Z, Wang SQ. Protective effect of Yin Qiao San on H1N1 viral infection in the mice. World J Integr Trad West Med. 2015;10:771–87.
9. Ding Y, Cao Z, Cao L, Ding G, Wang Z, Xiao W. Antiviral activity of chlorogenic acid against influenza A (H1N1/H3N2) virus and its inhibition of neuraminidase. Sci Rep. 2017;7:45723.
10. Qu XY, Li QJ, Zhang HM, Zhang XJ, Shi PH, Zhang XJ, Yang J, Zhou Z, Wang SQ. Protective effects of phillyrin against influenza A virus in vivo. Arch Pharm Res. 2016;39:998–1005.
11. Wang Z, Xia Q, Li X, Liu W, Huang W, Mei X, Luo J, Shan M, Lin R, Zou D, Ma Z. Phytochemistry, pharmacology, quality control and future research of *Forsythia suspensa* (Thunb.) Vahl: a review. J Ethnopharmacol. 2018;210:318–39.
12. Kobayashi M, Davis SM, Utsunomiya T, Pollard RB, Suzuki F. Antivrial effect of Gingyo-san, a traditional Chinese medicine herbal medicine, on influenza A2 virus in mice. Am J Med. 1999;27:53–62.
13. Hayashi K, Narutaki K, Nagaoka Y, Hayashi T, Uesato S. Therapeutic effect of arctiin and arctigenin in immunocompetent and immuno-compromised mice infected with influenza A virus. Biol Pharm Bull. 2010;33:1199–205.
14. Deng L, Nie J, Pang P, Chen XY. Comparative study on the effects of Xinjiaxiangruyin in influenza viral pneumonia mice in a damp and hot environment. J New Chin Med. 2016;48:235–8.
15. Ding CX, Ju JL. Research advance of the chemical componentand pharmacological action of elsholtzia. Shanghai J Trad Chin Med. 2005;39:64.
16. Bao Z, Yang X, Ding Z, Cao Q, Zou Y. Simultaneous determination of magnolol and honokiol by UV spectrophotometry and study on free radical scavenger activity. Nat Prod Res Devel. 2004;16:435–8.
17. Schuhly W, Hufner A, Pferschy-Wenzig EM, Prettner E, Adams M, Bodensieck A, Kunert O, Oluwemimo A, Haslinger E, Bauer R. Design and synthesis of ten biphenyl-neolignan derivatives and their in vitro inhibitory potency against cyclooxygenase-1/2 activity and 5-lipoxygenase-mediated LTB4-formation. Bioorg Med Chem. 2009;17:4459–65.
18. Shen P, Zhang Z, He Y, Gu C, Zhu K, Li S, Li Y, Lu X, Liu J, Zhang N, Cao Y. Magnolol treatment attenuates dextran sulphate sodium-induced murine experimental colitis by regulating inflammation and mucosal damage. Life Sci. 2018;196:69–76.
19. Li M, Zhang F, Wang X, Wu X, Zhang B, Zhang N, Wu W, Wang Z, Weng H, Liu S, Gao G, Mu J, Shu Y, Bao R, Cao Y, Lu J, Gu J, Zhu J, Liu Y. Magnolol inhibits growth of gallbladder cancer cells through the p53 pathway. Cancer Sci. 2015;106:1341.
20. Fang CY, Chen SJ, Wu HN, Ping YH, Lin CY, Shiuan D, Chen CL, Lee YR, Huang KJ. Honokiol, a lignan biphenol derived from the magnolia tree, inhibits dengue virus type 2 infection. Viruses. 2015;7:4894–910.
21. Lan KH, Wang YW, Lee WP, Lan KL, Tseng SH, Hung LR, Yen SH, Lin HC, Lee SD. Multiple effects of Honokiol on the life cycle of hepatitis C virus. Liver Int. 2012;32:989–97.
22. Ma L, Li JB, Sheng D, Liu Y. Effect of three therapies on interleukin 2 and t lymphocyte subgroups in mice infected with influenza a virus of type 1 or type 3. Chin J Exp Trad Med Formulae. 2010;16:108–11.
23. Jia CH, Pang ZR, Yang HM, Wei XF, Liu BS, Zhao TH, Yang HS. Pharmacodynamic study on the antipyretic and analgesic effect of GUI Ma He Fang. Chin J Basic Med Trad Chin Med. 2004;10:32–4.
24. Liu XG, Jia CH, Guo YC, Li JH, Li XJ, Pang ZR. Effects of GUI Ma He Fang on asthma latent period and pathological changes of lung tissue in asthmatic guinea pigs. J Chengde Med Coll. 2006;23:3–6.
25. Dai GD, Zheng P, Li HQ. Action of pseudo-ephedrine and ephedrine on the rings of isolated rabbit's and rat's aorta. J Ningxia Med Coll. 2001;23:318–9.
26. Hayashi K, Imanishi N, Kashiwayama Y, Kawano A, Terasawa K, Shimada Y, Ochiai H. Inhibitory effect of cinnamaldehyde, derived from Cinnamomi cortex, on the growth of influenza A/PR/8 virus in vitro and in vivo. Antiviral Res. 2007;74:1–8.
27. Ding Y, Qiu L, Zhao G, Xu J, Wang S. Influence of cinnamaldehyde on viral myocarditis in mice. Am J Med Sci. 2010;340:114–20.
28. Lin YC, Huang DY, Chu CL, Lin WW. The tyrosine kinase Syk differentially regulates toll-like receptor signaling downstream of the adaptor molecules TRAF6 and TRAF3. Sci Signal. 2013;6:71.
29. Lund JM, Alexopoulou L, Sato A, Karow M, Adams NC, Gale NW, Iwasaki A, Flavell RA. Recognition of single-stranded RNA viruses by Toll-like receptor 7. P Natl Acad Sci. 2004;101:5598–603.
30. Blasius AL, Beutler B. Intracellular toll-like receptors. Immunity. 2010;32:305–15.
31. Diebold SS, Kaisho T, Hemmi H, Akira S. Reis CeS. innate antiviral responses by means of TLR7-mediated recognition of single-stranded RNA. Science. 2004;303:1529.
32. Iwasaki A, Medzhitov R. Toll-like receptor control of the adaptive immune responses. Nat Immunol. 2004;5:987.
33. Takeda K, Akira S. TLR signaling pathways. Semin Immunol. 2004;16:3–9.
34. Du X, Poltorak A, Wei Y, Beutler B. Three novel mammalian Toll-like receptors: gene structure, expression, and evolution. Eur Cytokine Netw. 2000;11:362–71.
35. Lee J, Chuang TH, Redecke V, She L, Pitha PM, Carson DA, Raz E, Cottam HB. Molecular basis for the immunostimulatory activity of guanine nucleoside analogs: activation of Toll-like receptor 7. Proc Natl Acad Sci. 2003;100:6646–51.
36. Heil F, Ahmad-Nejad P, Hemmi H, Bauer S. The Toll-like receptor 7 (TLR7)-specific stimulus loxoribine uncovers a strong relationship within the TLR7, 8 and 9 subfamily. Eur J Immunol. 2010;33:2987–97.
37. Livak KJ, Schmittgen TD. Analysis of relative gene expression data using real-time quantitative PCR and the $2^{-\Delta\Delta Cq}$ method. Methods. 2001;25:402–8.
38. Dovedi SJ, Melis MH, Wilkinson RW, Adlard AL, Stratford IJ, Honeychurch J, Illidge TM. Systemic delivery of a TLR7 agonist in combination with radiation primes durable antitumor immune responses in mouse models of lymphoma. Blood. 2013;121:251–9.

39. Walter A, Schafer M, Cecconi V, Matter C, Urosevic-Maiwald M, Belloni B, Schonewolf N, Dummer R, Bloch W, Werner S, Beer HD, Knuth A, van den Broek M. Aldara activates TLR7-independent immune defence. Nat Commun. 2013;4:1560.

40. Greiff L, Cervin A, Ahlstrom-Emanuelsson C, Almqvist G, Andersson M, Dolata J, Eriksson L, Hogertatt E, Kallen A, Norle P, Sjolin IL, Widegren H. Repeated intranasal TLR7 stimulation reduces allergen responsiveness in allergic rhinitis. Respir Res. 2012;13:53.

41. Hemmi H, Kaisho T, Takeuchi O, Akira S. Small anti-viral compounds activate immune cells via the TLR7 MyD88-dependent signaling pathway. Nat Immunol. 2002;3:196–200.

42. Yang JN, Liu XG, Li T, Chen H, Zhang YY. Function of Th17/Treg balance in rheumatoid arthritis. Chin Pharmacol Bull. 2013;29:1045–8.

43. Ray A, Khare A, Krishnamoorthy N, Qi Z, Ray P. Regulatory T cells in many flavors control asthma. Mucosal Immunol. 2010;3:216–29.

44. Ivanov II, Zhou L, Littman DR. Transcriptional regulation of Th17 cell differentiation. Semin Immunol. 2007;19:409–17.

45. Chen C, Jiang ZY, Yu B, Wu XL, Dai CQ, Zhao CL, Ju DH, Chen XY. Study on the anti-H1N1 virus effects of quercetin and oseltamivir and their mechanism related to TLR7 pathway. J Asian Nat Prod Res. 2012;14:877–85.

46. Kawai T, Akira S. Toll-like receptors and their crosstalk with other innate receptors in infection and immunity. Immunity. 2011;34:637–50.

47. Kutikhin AG, Yuzhalin AE. C-type lectin receptors and RIG-I-like receptors: new points on the oncogenomics map. Cancer Manag Res. 2012;4:39–53.

48. Yoneyama M, Kikuchi M, Natsukawa T, Shinobu N, Imaizumi T, Miyagishi M, Taira K, Akira S, Fujita T. The RNA helicase RIG-I has an essential function in double-stranded RNA-induced innate antiviral responses. Nat Immunol. 2004;5:730–7.

49. Stephenson I, Democratis J, Lackenby A, Mcnally T, Smith J, Pareek M, Ellis J, Bermingham A, Nicholson K, Zambon M. Neuraminidase inhibitor resistance after oseltamivir treatment of acute influenza A and B in children. Clin Infect Dis. 2009;48:389–96.

50. Strong M, Burrows J, Stedman E, Redgrave P. Adverse drug effects following oseltamivir mass treatment and prophylaxis in a school outbreak of 2009 pandemic influenza A(H1N1) in June 2009, Sheffield, United Kingdom. Euro Surveill. 2010;15:19565.

8

Effective authentication of Placenta Hominis

Yat-Tung Lo, Mavis Hong-Yu Yik and Pang-Chui Shaw[*]

Abstract

Background: Human placenta is used to make the medicinal product Placenta Hominis in Asian countries. With its therapeutic benefits and limited supply, intentional or inadvertent adulteration is found in the market. In order to enforce the implementation of product description laws and protect customer rights, we established a hierarchical protocol involving morphological, chemical, biochemical and molecular diagnosis to authenticate this medicinal product.

Methods: Ten samples claimed as Placenta Hominis were collected from herbal shops in China, Hong Kong and Taiwan. Species-specific diagnostic primers for human, cow, deer and sheep were designed for PCR amplification and subsequent DNA sequencing for species identification. Commercially available pregnancy test strip was used to detect human chorionic gonadotropin (hCG), and progesterone competitive ELISA kit was used to detect the presence of progesterone in samples. The presence of starch in samples was tested by adding small amount of iodine solution onto the samples.

Results: Among the ten samples studied, results showed that no cow, deer and sheep DNA sequence was found in all samples. Five samples were genuine with the presence of human DNA, hCG and progesterone accompanied with the absence of starch fillers. On the other hand, four samples were adulterants which may be made from starch products. In addition, a sample was found as a mixture of Placenta Hominis and starch fillers, and it did not conform to the product requirement of Placenta Hominis.

Conclusions: The comprehensive protocol developed involving morphological, chemical, biochemical and molecular diagnosis provides an accurate method to regulatory bodies and testing laboratories for the quality control of Placenta Hominis.

Keywords: Competitive ELISA, Diagnostic PCR, Human chorionic gonadotropin, Iodine test, Molecular authentication, Placenta Hominis, Pregnancy test strips, Progesterone

Background

Placenta Hominis is a medicinal material made from human placenta. It is listed in Compendium of Materia Medica written by LI Shi-zhen in the sixteenth century. In this reference, Placenta Hominis has the action to warm the *kidney* and replenish *vital essence*, *qi* and blood. It is used to treat various diseases such as emaciation, hectic fever, night sweating, cough, anorexia, impotence,

*Correspondence: pcshaw@cuhk.edu.hk
Li Dak Sum Yip Yio Chin R & D Centre for Chinese Medicine, State Key Laboratory of Phytochemistry and Plant Resources in West China (CUHK) and School of Life Sciences, The Chinese University of Hong Kong, Shatin, N.T., Hong Kong, China

shortness of infertility and lack of lactation [1]. Nowadays, Placenta Hominis has been found to increase cell proliferation and metabolism [2], boost immune system [3] and it is used to treat bronchitis, asthma [4] and gastric ulcer [5]. Since human placenta is normally not available for trading, the material supply for making Placenta Hominis is limited and intentional or inadvertent adulteration is often found in the market. For instant, some dishonest merchants may use placenta from other mammals such as cow, deer and sheep, or even use starch products as adulterants [6].

Traditional methods to authenticate Placenta Hominis involve morphological and chemical approaches.

However, variation in morphological appearance due to different preparation treatment and product form like powder [7] makes the morphological authentication difficult. Chemical authentication investigates the characteristic chemical markers in the medicinal materials. Thin layer chromatography (TLC) [8] and high-performance liquid chromatography (HPLC) [9] are the commonly used methods for identifying placenta, but they are not able to distinguish adulterants derived from placenta of other mammals as they share similar chemical components [10]. High-performance capillary electrophoresis (HPCE) has also been developed for authentication of Placenta Hominis from sheep's placenta [11]. However, chemical constituents in individual placenta samples may vary [12] due to difference in physiological conditions, storage and processing methods.

Molecular authentication is especially suitable for animal-derived material since only few characteristic chemical compounds are present for chemical authentication when compared with plant-derived material. In addition, DNA markers are abundant, tissue independent with high resolution power [13]. For instance, DNA techniques have been employed to authenticate crocodile [14], snake species [15] and processed animal-derived concentrated Chinese medicine granules [16]. However, molecular techniques sometimes may not be applicable on processed products which have the DNA highly degraded or absent.

Therefore, it is beneficial to employ a battery of independent methods to increase the accuracy of authentication. In this study, we have established a comprehensive protocol involving morphological, chemical, biochemical and molecular diagnosis (Fig. 1) for accurate and quick authentication of Placenta Hominis samples obtained from different places. A comprehensive protocol is needed for better implementation of Trade Descriptions Ordinance (Chapter 362) of Hong Kong and similar laws in other jurisdictions.

Methods

The Minimum Standards of Reporting Checklist contains details of the experimental design, and statistics, and resources used in this study (Additional file 1).

Sample studied

Ten samples claimed as Placenta Hominis were collected from herbal shops in China, Hong Kong and Taiwan. All specimens were deposited in the Institute of Chinese Medicine, The Chinese University of Hong Kong (Table 1). Images of the samples studied are shown in Fig. 2.

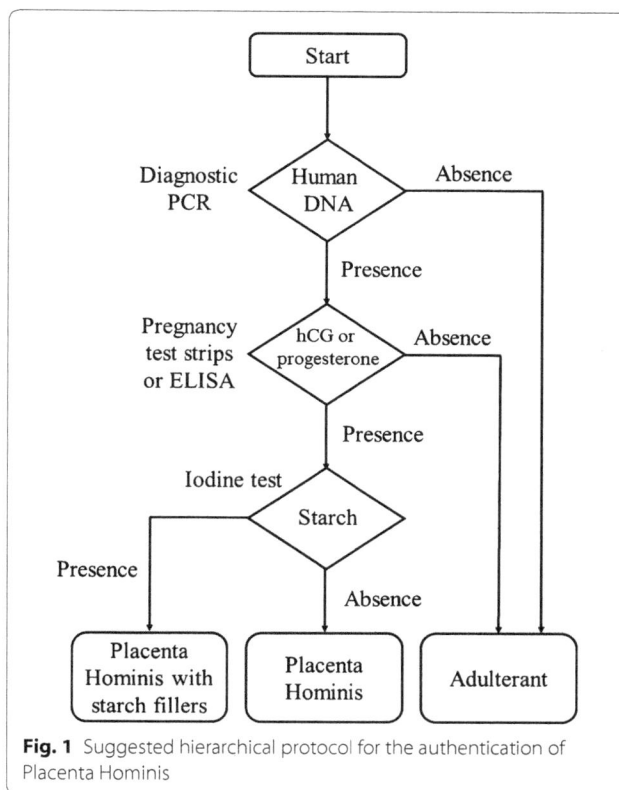

Fig. 1 Suggested hierarchical protocol for the authentication of Placenta Hominis

Extraction of DNA and hormones

Each sample was washed with 70% ethanol and water to remove dusts and soils on the surface, followed by grinding into powder. For DNA extraction, 20 mg of the ground samples were extracted by following the manufacturer's instruction in cell/tissue genomic DNA extraction kit (Biomed, Beijing, China) to obtain 50 µl DNA extract. For human chorionic gonadotropin (hCG) extraction, 300 mg of ground samples was first incubated in 1 ml of 10 mM phosphate-buffered saline (PBS) [137 mM NaCl, 2.7 mM KCl, 4.3 mM Na_2HPO_4, 1.47 mM KH_2PO_4, pH 7.4] for 3 h at 30 °C, followed by centrifugation at $604 \times g$ for 20 min to obtain the supernatant. For progesterone extraction, 300 mg of desiccated ground sample was shaken vigorously with 3 ml ethanol for 1 h in room temperature, followed by centrifugation at $1677 \times g$ for 15 min. The ethanol portion in the supernatant was then evaporated in a SpeedVac™ concentrator (Thermo Fisher Scientific, Waltham, MA, USA) and finally re-dissolved the extracted sample in 100 µl ethanol.

Polymerase chain reaction (PCR) amplification and molecular analysis

DNA sequences of cytochrome c oxidase subunit I (COI) gene from human (*Homo sapiens*), cow (*Bos*

Table 1 Samples of Placenta Hominis studied

Sample code	Place of collection
PH01	Nanjing
PH02	Yunnan
PH03	Guangzhou
PH04	Guangzhou
PH05	Guangzhou
PH06	Taipei
PH07	Hong Kong
PH08	Yunnan
PH09	Guangzhou
PH10	Guangzhou

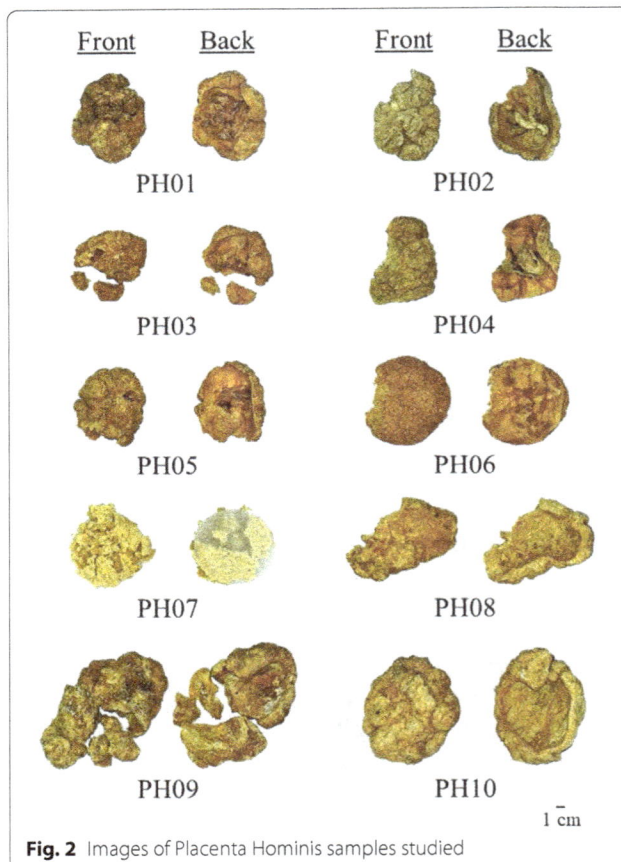

Fig. 2 Images of Placenta Hominis samples studied

PCR amplification was performed in a 25 µl of reaction mixture with 2.5 µl of 10X PCR buffer [75 mM Tris, pH 8.8, 20 mM $(NH_4)_2SO_4$, 1.5 mM $MgCl_2$, 0.01% Tween 20], 2 µl of 2.5 mM dNTP mixture (Biomed), 1 µl of each 10 µM species-specific diagnostic primers, 1 µl of DNA sample and 0.4 µl of 5 U/µl *Taq* polymerase. PCR was conducted using Veriti™ Thermal Cycler (Thermo Fisher Scientific). The PCR programme included 35 cycles of 94 °C for 30 s, indicated annealing temperature (Table 2) for 30 s and 72 °C for 1 min. The amplification product was analyzed on 1.5% TAE gel electrophoresis stained with SYBR Safe DNA Gel Stain (Thermo Fisher Scientific), purified by DNA gel purification kit (Biomed) and performed DNA sequencing (BGI, Hong Kong). The obtained sequences were performed Basic Local Alignment Search Tool (BLAST) against GenBank nucleotide database. Query sequences were identified to species level with top hit of similarity.

Detection of hCG by pregnancy test strips
Home pregnancy test strip (Mannings, Hong Kong) was purchased from a local pharmaceutical store. Each of the 100 µl extracted sample in PBS was added to the adsorbent tip of the test strip. The solution was then absorbed across the whole test strip until pink band appeared at the C (Control) section which indicated the test strip was working properly. For positive results with hCG concentration more than or equal to 20 mlU/ml, pink bands should be appeared for both C and T (Test) sections. For negative results, only a single pink band appeared at the C section.

Detection of progesterone by enzyme-linked immunosorbent assay (ELISA)
Progesterone competitive ELISA kit (Thermo Fisher Scientific) was used to detect the presence of progesterone in samples. 400 µl of 1X Assay Buffer in the ELISA kit was added to 100 µl of each extracted sample in ethanol. The solution was then diluted into 1000 times using the same 1X Assay Buffer and transferred in 50 µl aliquots to the antibody coated wells. Competitive ELISA was then performed followed the manufacturer's instruction. Results were measured at 450 nm with microtiter plate reader (BioTek Instruments, Inc., Winooski, VT, USA).

Iodine test
The presence of starch in samples was tested by adding small amount of iodine solution onto the samples. Samples with color changed from brown to blue indicated the presence of starch and were labelled as positive, while samples remained unchanged in brown color indicated the absence of starch and were labelled as negative.

taurus), deer (*Cervus elaphus* and *Cervus nippon*) and sheep (*Ovis aries*) were obtained from the GenBank database in National Center for Biotechnology Information (NCBI) and aligned using BioEdit 7 software. Species-specific diagnostic primers to differentiate each species were designed according to the polymorphic sites (Additional file 2) and shown in Table 2.

Table 2 Primers for amplification and sequencing

Species specificity	Primer name	Sequence (5′–3′)	Amplicon size (bp)	Annealing temp. (°C)
Homo sapiens	COI_human_F	GCAACCTTCTAGGTAACGACCAC	120	63
	COI_human_R	GGGGAACTAGTCAGTTGCCAAAG		
Bos taurus	COI_cow_F	CGACCAAATCTACAACGTAG	102	61
	COI_cow_R	GGAACAAGTCAGTTACCG		
Cervus elaphus and *Cervus nippon*	COI_deer_F	CTGCTTGGAGATGACCAAATT	125	59
	COI_deer_R	CCAATTATTAGGGGAACTAGTCAA		
Ovis aries	COI_sheep_F	GGCAACTGACTAGTTCCT	117	59
	COI_sheep_R	CATAGAGGATGCTAGGAGTAAC		

Results

Morphological characterization

Morphologies of the samples are shown in Fig. 2. They were majorly divided into three groups. For samples PH01–PH05, the irregular round or oval shape of samples had diameter around 10 cm. The color was yellow-white or yellow-purple. The outer surface was rough and uneven with grooves. The inner surface was relatively smooth with the remnant of umbilical cord-like structure in the center. The texture was crispy and there was a smell of blood. For samples PH06–PH07, they were pale yellow in color with a sheet of paper at the bottom. Their texture was biscuit-like and brittle. For samples PH08–PH10, the color was yellow-white and the sizes were ranged from 13 to 18 cm, which were much larger than other samples.

The texture was very hard and without the presence of umbilical cord-like structure.

Authentication by diagnostic PCR

For effective differentiation between *Homo sapiens* and other mammals which were commonly used as adulterants of Placenta Hominis, species-specific diagnostic primers were employed. With polymorphic sites at the primer 3' end sequences (Additional file 2), only the concerned species could be amplified without non-specific PCR amplification for controls (Fig. 3). Using the human diagnostic PCR developed, PCR products with 120 bp were amplified from samples PH01–PH06 (Fig. 3a) with identity matched *Homo sapiens* perfectly (Additional

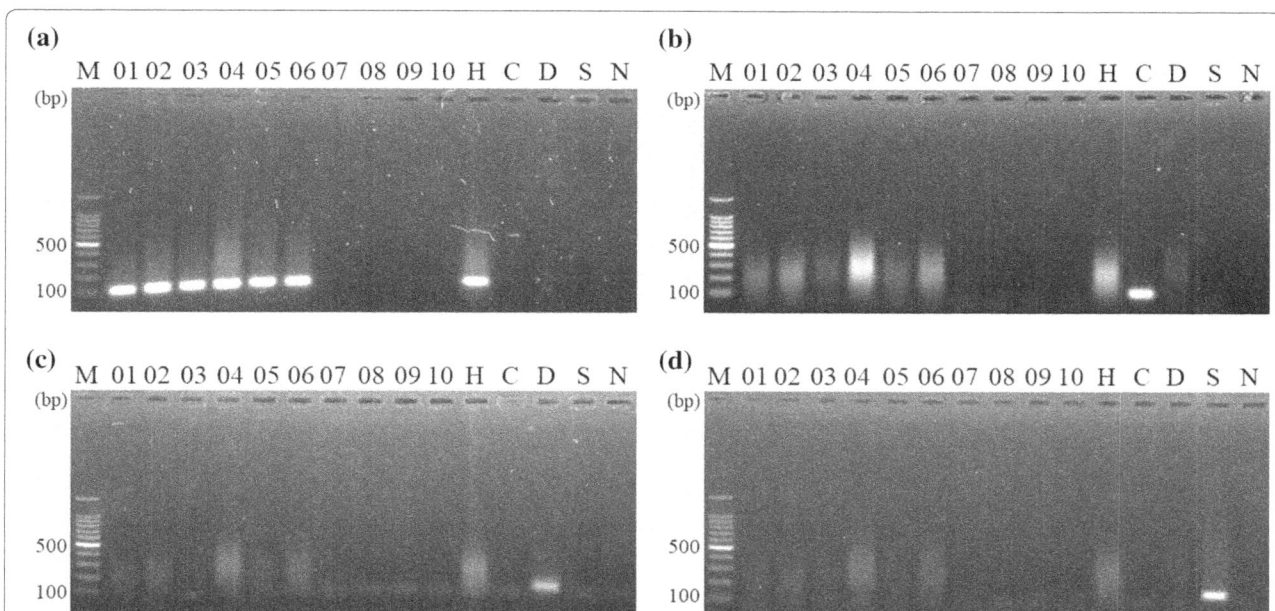

Fig. 3 Diagnostic PCR using species-specific diagnostic primers for **a** human (*Homo sapiens*), **b** cow (*Bos taurus*), **c** deer (*Cervus elaphus* and *Cervus nippon*) and **d** sheep (*Ovis aries*). Lanes 01–10 represent PH01-PH10 samples, lanes H, C, D and S are positive controls with DNA from human, cow, deer and sheep, respectively. Lane M and N represent the DNA size ladder and negative control, respectively

file 3). In addition, no cow, deer and sheep DNA sequence was found in all samples (Fig. 3 and Table 3).

Authentication by hormone assays

Commercially available pregnancy test strip was a rapid chromatographic immunoassay device for qualitative determination of hCG in samples with more than 99% accuracy of detection according to the manufacturer's claim. The presence of two pink bands in the result window indicated the presence of hCG while one pink band in the C section indicated the absence of it. Results with no band in the C section should be regarded as invalid. In this study, hCG was detected in samples PH01–PH06 with two pink bands, while only one pink band appeared in the C section for samples PH07–PH10 (Fig. 4 and Table 3).

Placenta-derived progesterone in samples were detected by progesterone competitive ELISA kit. Progesterone level can also be quantified by comparing the absorbance reading at 450 nm with external standard curve. In this study, progesterone was found in samples PH01–PH06 with concentration ranged from 265 to 843 ng/ml. On the other hand, no progesterone above the detection limit of 47.9 pg/ml was detected in samples PH07–PH10 (Table 3).

Authentication by iodine test

Presence of starch in sample was revealed by adding small amount of iodine solution onto the sample. The aqueous solution of the triiodide anion (I_3^-) from the iodine solution bound with starch molecule to form a very dark blue-black complex for visual determination. Results showed the presence of starch with dark

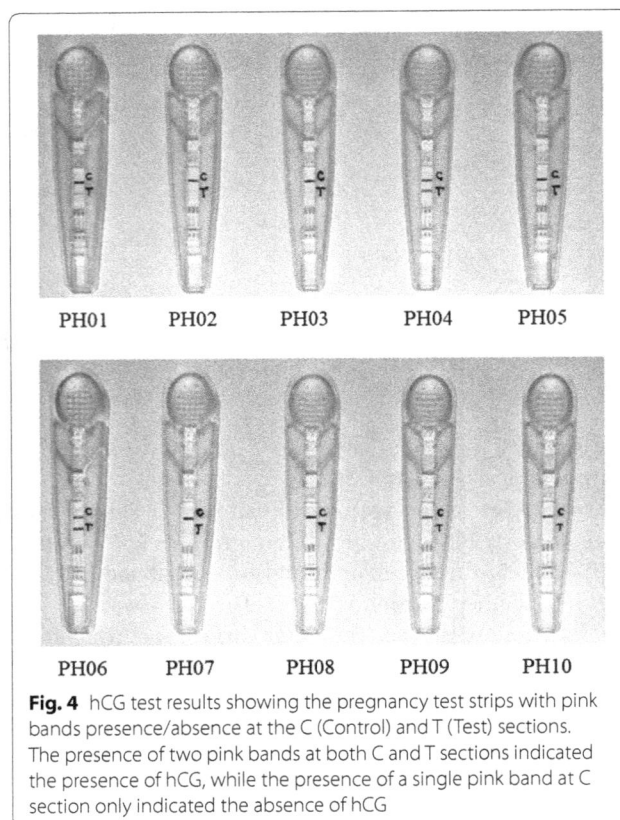

Fig. 4 hCG test results showing the pregnancy test strips with pink bands presence/absence at the C (Control) and T (Test) sections. The presence of two pink bands at both C and T sections indicated the presence of hCG, while the presence of a single pink band at C section only indicated the absence of hCG

blue-black color upon addition of iodine solution for samples PH06–PH10. On the other hand, the brown color of the iodine solution remained for samples PH01–PH05 which indicated the absence of starch in samples (Fig. 5 and Table 3).

Table 3 Summary of iodine test, detection of hCG and progesterone hormones and diagnostic PCR results

Sample code	Iodine test[a]	HCG detection[b]	Progesterone conc.[c] (ng/ml)	Diagnostic PCR[d]			
				Human	Cow	Deer	Sheep
PH01	N	Y	544.19±120.76	Y	N	N	N
PH02	N	Y	435.17±86.80	Y	N	N	N
PH03	N	Y	265.34±49.59	Y	N	N	N
PH04	N	Y	461.48±78.98	Y	N	N	N
PH05	N	Y	316.37±52.92	Y	N	N	N
PH06	Y	Y	843.43±93.75	Y	N	N	N
PH07	Y	N	Not detected	N	N	N	N
PH08	Y	N	Not detected	N	N	N	N
PH09	Y	N	Not detected	N	N	N	N
PH10	Y	N	Not detected	N	N	N	N

[a] In iodine test, Y and N indicate positive result with observable color change from brown to blue, and negative result without color change (i.e. brown), respectively

[b] In hCG detection, Y represents the presence of two pink bands at the Test (T) and Control (C) sections of pregnancy test strip, while N represents the presence of a single pink band at the C section only

[c] Assay buffer was set as blank and the data represent mean±standard deviation (n = 3)

[d] In diagnostic PCR, Y and N represent the presence and absence of amplified products, respectively

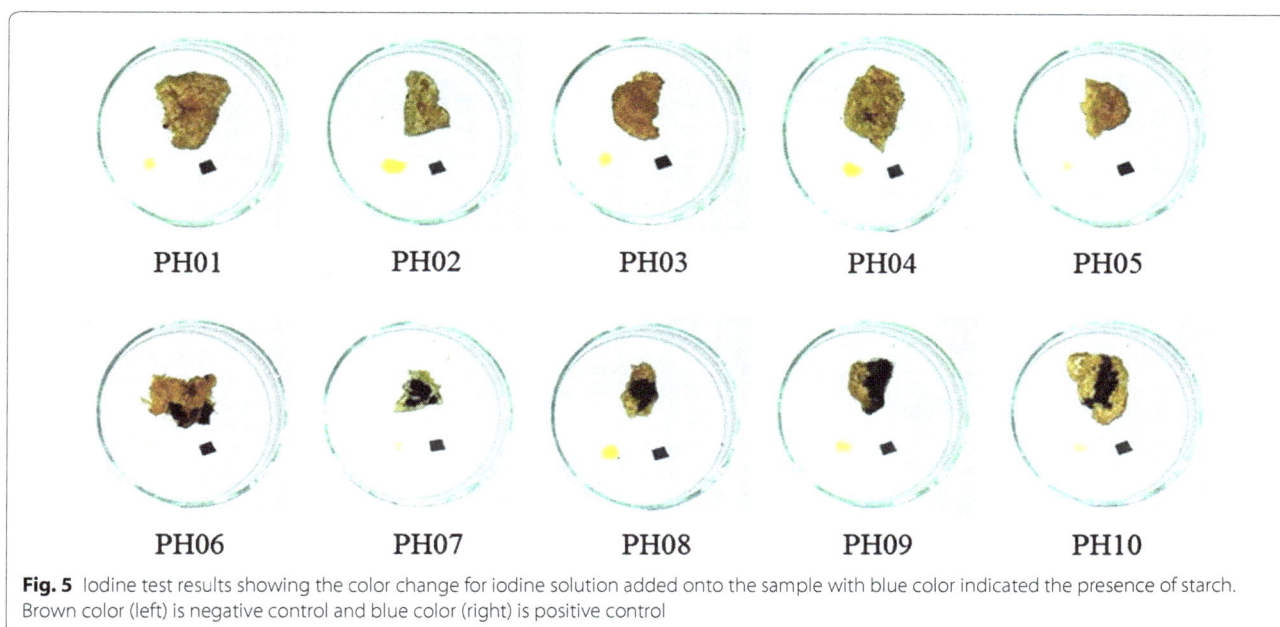

Fig. 5 Iodine test results showing the color change for iodine solution added onto the sample with blue color indicated the presence of starch. Brown color (left) is negative control and blue color (right) is positive control

Discussion

In the present study, a comprehensive protocol was established to reveal the authenticity and quality of Placenta Hominis sold in market. According to the 2010 edition of Chinese Pharmacopoeia, genuine Placenta Hominis should be rounded or dish-shaped with 9–15 cm in diameter, yellow or yellowish-brown in color. One side of the material is uneven with irregular strips while another side is relatively smooth with remnant of umbilical cord in often. In this study, morphological appearance of samples PH01–PH05 match the above description.

The presence of human or other mammalian tissue was determined by using species-specific diagnostic primers for PCR amplification. In the preparation of Placenta Hominis, human placenta was steamed or boiled in water for a period of time, DNA in the samples was thus somewhat degraded. When designing the primers for diagnostic PCR, the amplicon to be amplified should keep as small as possible, while not compromising the differentiation power at species level, so as to reduce false negative results due to DNA fragmentation [16–19].

hCG is a glycoprotein produced by the human placenta after implantation [20, 21]. Progesterone is a steroid hormone involved in the female menstrual cycle, gestation and embryogenesis, and it is present in placenta [22, 23]. The presence of hCG and progesterone in the tested samples were indicated by commercially available pregnancy test strip and progesterone competitive ELISA kit, respectively. The positive results of pregnancy test strip indicated the hCG concentration was equal to or more than 20 mIU/ml. For sample PH03, the band intensity on

the T section of the result window was lighter than others (Fig. 4). Nevertheless, it was still regarded as positive according to the manufacturer's instruction. This sample also had a lower progesterone concentration (Table 3). These show that the quality of PH03 is inferior to other genuine samples.

In Placenta Hominis, starch should not be found. Samples PH07–PH10 had starch while without human DNA, hCG and progesterone (Table 3), implied that they were adulterants of Placenta Hominis and they may be made from starch products. An interesting finding is that for sample PH06, starch as well as human DNA, hCG and progesterone were found (Table 3). It is concluded that sample PH06 may be a mixture of Placenta Hominis and starch fillers. Traditionally, Placenta Hominis is produced from the whole human placenta only and thus the presence of starch in PH06 does not conform to the product requirement.

Establishing an objective method to identify Placenta Hominis is critical for the effective implementation of product description laws and safeguarding the consumer rights. In this study, a hierarchical protocol combining morphological, chemical, biochemical and molecular approach has been proposed to identify Placenta Hominis and assess its quality (Fig. 1). It is suggested that for Chinese medicine practitioners and customers without laboratory facilities, the authenticity of Placenta Hominis can be preliminary tested by observing morphological traits and using commercially available pregnancy test strips plus iodine test (Fig. 6). Diagnostic PCR and ELISA may be used for further

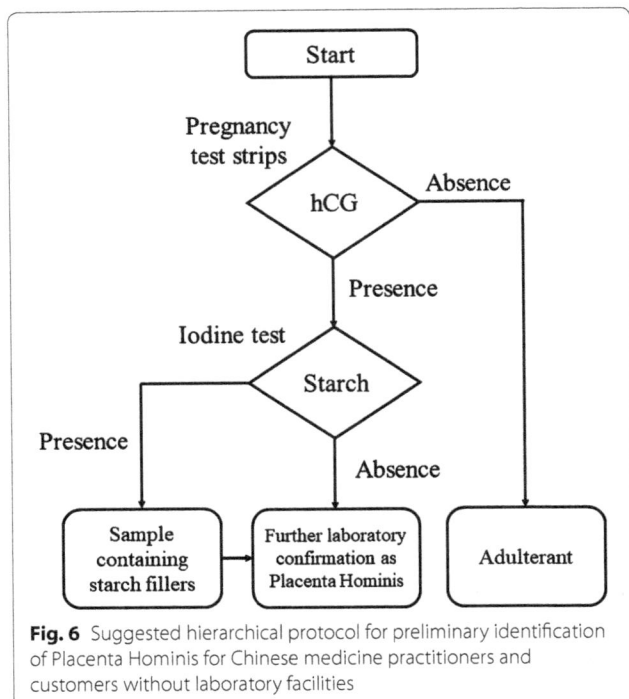

Fig. 6 Suggested hierarchical protocol for preliminary identification of Placenta Hominis for Chinese medicine practitioners and customers without laboratory facilities

confirmation. Our work showed that samples PH01–PH05 were genuine, with samples PH01, PH02, PH04 and PH05 of higher quality. On the other hand, samples PH07–PH10 were adulterants and sample PH06 was manufactured unconventionally.

Conclusion

Our work has established a multi-disciplinary approach (morphological inspection, molecular identification, hormone assays and iodine test) for the authentication of Placenta Hominis and revealed that a substantial amount of this medicinal material in the market are adulterated.

Abbreviations

COI: Cytochrome c oxidase subunit I; DNA: Deoxyribonucleic acid; ELISA: Enzyme-linked immunosorbent assay; hCG: Human chorionic gonadotropin; HPCE: High-performance capillary electrophoresis; HPLC: High-performance liquid chromatography; NCBI: National Center for Biotechnology Information; PBS: Phosphate-buffered saline; PCR: Polymerase chain reaction; TLC: Thin layer chromatography.

Authors' contributions

YTL and MHYY performed experiments. YTL designed the study, performed

data analyses and wrote the manuscript. PCS coordinated the study. All authors read and approved the final manuscript.

Acknowledgements

Not applicable.

Competing interests

The authors declare no potential conflict of interest.

Consent for publication

Not applicable.

Funding

Not applicable.

References

1. Li SZ, Luo XW. Compendium of Materia Medica: Bencao Gangmu. Beijing: Foreign Languages Press; 2003.
2. Wang L. The culture of the new small rat epidermal cells: the evaluation of effect for the human placental tissue extract on the cell's physiological function. Chin Surfactant Deterg Cosmet. 2001;1:61–2.
3. Cui YD, Cai YJ, Jin HK, Jin XJ, Jin SZ, Li YJ. Study on immunological function of placental powder. Chin J Basic Med Trad Chin Med. 2001;7:29–31.
4. Wu L, Li JX, Wang GL, Sun B, Xia C. The evolution on pharmacological effect and clinic application of domestic animals and human placenta. Heilongjiang Bayi Nongken Daxue Xuebao. 2001;13:68–71.
5. Zhuang JX. Analysis of 40 cases in ulcer-curing of Placenta Hominis. Jiangxi J Trad Chin Med. 2002;33:56.
6. Lu WC, Li YQ. Beware of adulterants in Placenta Hominis powder. J Chin Med Med. 2000;20:270.
7. Ou Yang CG. The study on quality control of Placenta Hominis and its capsules. Chin J Info Trad Chin Med. 2004;11:888–9.
8. Zhu ZX. Authentication of Placenta Hominis and its adulterants by thin layer chromatography (TLC). Zhong Yao Cai. 1996;19:27–8.
9. Zhu ZX. Authentication of Placenta Hominis and its adulterants by UV light. Chin Trad Patent Med. 1996;18:16–7.
10. Shi JY, Lü PY, Cheng JY, Liu YQ. Studies of identification and quality to pangolin scales, Placenta Homins and their adulterants. J Shandong Univ Trad Chin Med. 1998;22:379–83.
11. Gu J, Liu P, Li W. Study on identification of Placenta Hominis and pseudo-placenta with high performance capillary electrophoresis. Acad J PLA Postgrad Med Sch. 2006;27:46–7.
12. Zhang LB, Qiao CZ. Comparison of progesterone, HCG and HPL contents in Placenta Hominis, other mammalian placentas and its processed products. Ti Erh Chun i Ta Hsueh Hsueh Pao. 1994;15:187–9.
13. Mafra I, Ferreira IMPLVO, Oliveira MBPP. Food authentication by PCR-based methods. Eur Food Res Technol. 2008;277:649–65.
14. Yau FC, Wong KL, Wang J, But PP, Shaw PC. Generation of a sequence characterized amplified region probe for authentication of crocodilian species. J Exp Zool. 2002;294:382–6.
15. Wong KL, Wang J, But PP, Shaw PC. Application of cytochrome b DNA sequences for the authentication of endangered snake species. Forensic Sci Int. 2004;139:49–55.
16. Jiang LL, Lo YT, Chen WT, Shaw PC. DNA authentication of animal-derived concentrated Chinese medicine granules. J Pharm Biomed Anal. 2016;129:398–404.
17. Aslan O, Hamill RM, Sweeney T, Reardon W, Mullen AM. Integrity of nuclear genomic deoxyribonucleic acid in cooked meat: implications for food traceability. J Anim Sci. 2009;87:57–61.
18. Zimmermann J, Hajibabaei M, Blackburn DC, Hanken J, Cantin E, Posfai J, Evans TC Jr. DNA damage in preserved specimens and tissue samples: a molecular assessment. Front Zool. 2008;5:18.
19. Lo YT, Li M, Shaw PC. Identification of constituent herbs in ginseng decoctions by DNA markers. Chin Med. 2015;10:1.

20. Gregory JJ Jr, Finlay JL. Alpha-fetoprotein and beta-human chorionic gonadotropin: their clinical significance as tumour markers. Drugs. 1999;57:463–7.

21. Cole LA. New discoveries on the biology and detection of human chorionic gonadotropin. Reprod Biol Endocrinol. 2009;7:8.

22. Conti M, Chang RJ. Folliculogenesis, ovulation, and luteogenesis. In: Jameson JL, De Groot LJ, editors. Endocrinology: adult and pediatric. 7th ed. Philadelphia: Elsevier Health Sciences; 2015. p. 2179–91.

23. Brucker MC, Likis FE. Steroid hormones. In: King TL, Brucker MC, editors. Pharmacology for women's health. Sudbury: Jones and Bartlett Publishers; 2010. p. 362–80.

9

Metabonomic study of the protective effect of Fukeqianjin formula on multi-pathogen induced pelvic inflammatory disease in rats

Yan Zhang[1†], Wei Li[1†], Liang Zou[1*], Yun Gong[2], Peng Zhang[2], Shasha Xing[3] and Hang Yang[1]

Abstract

Background: Fukeqianjin formula has been effectively used in the treatment of pelvic inflammatory disease (PID) and the related complications in clinic. Although there have been some studies about the underlying mechanism that focus on its anti-inflammatory and immunoregulatory activities. But the mechanism is still not fully understood. The aim of this study was to investigate the alteration of plasma metabolic profiles in PID rats and the regulatory effect of Fukeqianjin formula on potential biomarkers.

Methods: Pelvic inflammatory model was established by intrauterine inoculation of multiple pathogens combined with mechanical injury of endometrium. Rats were randomly divided into normal group, model group, azithromycin group, high-and low-dose of Fukeqianjin formula treatment group (FF-H, and FF-L, respectively). After 14 days of intragastric administration, the plasm levels of interleukin-1β (IL-1β) and nitric oxide (NO) were measured. To further recognize and identify potential biomarkers and metabolic pathways, an ultra-performance liquid chromatography-quadrupole-Exactive Orbitrap-mass spectrometry (UPLC-Q-Exactive Orbitrap-MS) metabonomic method combined with multivariate analyses including principal component analysis (PCA), partial least squares discriminant analysis (PLS-DA) and orthogonal partial least squares discriminant analysis (OPLS-DA), was employed to analyze the metabolic profiling.

Results: Compared with normal group, the plasma levels of IL-1β and NO were significantly increased in the PID model group ($P < 0.05$), and obviously decreased after high-dose intervention of Fukeqianjin formula ($P < 0.01$). The PCA, PLS-DA and OPLS-DA analysis showed that PID rats were clearly separated from normal rats. Compared with the PID model group, the metabolite profiles of Fukeqianjin formula treatment group was gradually restored to normal. Meanwhile, 14 potential metabolite biomarkers, which were mainly related to the metabolic pathways of intervening glycerophospholipid metabolism, linoleic acid metabolism/alpha-linolenic acid metabolism, amino acid metabolism, arachidonic acid metabolism, and unsaturated fatty acids biosynthesis, have been identified. Fukeqianjin formula exerts good regulatory effect on the abnormal metabolism of PID rats.

Conclusions: Intrauterine inoculation of multiple pathogens combined with mechanical injury of endometrium could significantly disturb the plasma metabolic profiles of rats. Fukeqianjin formula has potential therapeutic effect on multi-pathogen-induced PID by ameliorating metabolism disorders and alleviating the inflammatory response.

Keywords: Fukeqianjin formula, Anti-inflammatory, UPLC-Q-Exactive Orbitrap-MS, Metabonomic, Pelvic inflammatory disease

*Correspondence: zouliangcdu@126.com
†Yan Zhang and Wei Li contribute equally as co-first authors
[1] School of Medicine, Chengdu University, No. 2025, Cheng Luo Road,
Chengdu 610106, Sichuan, People's Republic of China

Background

Pelvic inflammatory disease (PID) is a multiple bacterial infection and inflammatory disorder on the upper female genital tract, typically involving the uterus, fallopian tubes, and ovaries [1]. The widespread gynecologic disease, which can lead to serious sequelae, such as tubal infertility, ectopic pregnancy, and chronic pelvic pain, is considered to be a major threat to reproductive age women [2]. Studies based on the updated meta-analysis have also demonstrated that PID might be a potential risk factor of ovarian cancer, especially among Asian women [3]. The most common pathogens cause to PID were *Neisseria gonorrhoeae*, *Chlamydia trachomatis*, *Mycoplasma genitalium*, and gram-negative bacilli [4]. In addition, studies confirm that *Staphylococcus aureus*, *Escherichia coli*, and *S. sanguinegens* were also associated with PID [5, 6]. Currently, PID is commonly treated with broad spectrum antibiotics. A randomized clinical trial confirmed that azithromycin monotherapy or azithromycin monotherapy in combination with metronidazole has an excellent therapeutic effect [7]. Moreover, several antibiotics including ceftriaxone, cefoxitin, doxycycline, and metronidazole also provide a good antibacterial efficacy and high clinical cure rate on pelvic inflammation [8, 9].

In recent years, accumulating evidence suggests that Chinese medicine has a remarkable curative effect in the treatment of PID. Research confirms that apart from the infection caused by pathogenic microorganisms, long-term chronic inflammation can also result in the decline of the immune system or pelvic microcirculation disturbance [10], while traditional Chinese medicine has various functions including anti-bacterial, anti-inflammatory, regulating immunity, or promoting blood circulation. An experimental study has demonstrated that *Patrinia villosa* can provide a good therapeutic effect on pelvic inflammatory rats by significantly reduce the levels of pro-inflammatory cytokines such as IL-6, IL-8 and TNF-α in serum [11]. Studies have shown that Danzhi Decoction not only has a positive anti-inflammatory effect, but also can relieve chronic pelvic pain and ameliorate the pelvic microcirculation disorders in PID mice [12]. The laboratory study confirms that *Cortex phellodendri* and *Humulus japonicus* exert good therapeutic effect on mice with chronic PID by inhibiting the expression of inflammatory cytokines and neutrophil infiltration [13]. Furthermore, Feiyangchangweiyan is reported to suppress infiltration and apoptosis of inflammatory cells in uterine tissues by preventing NF-κB nuclear translocation in pathogen-induced PID rats [14]. Fukeqianjin formula, consisting of *Moghania macrophylla*, *Radix Rosa laevigata*, *Andrographis paniculata*, *Mahonia fortunei*, *Zanthoxylum dissitum hemsl*,

Angelica sinensis, *Spatholobus suberectus*, and *Codonopsis pilosula*, is a traditional Chinese medicine prescription which has been widely applied to treat various gynecological inflammation disease clinically in China. Previous studies have verified that Fukeqianjin tablet could improve the immune function by promoting the production of IgA, IgG, and IgM in acute PID rats [15]. Furthermore, the experimental study confirmed that the anti-inflammation mechanism of Fukeqianjin tablets might be associated with reducing level of inflammatory cytokines IL-1β, IL-8 and TNF-α, and down-regulating of the expression of TNF-α, IL-10, and IL-2 mRNA [16, 17]. Additionally, Fukeqianjin tablets can improve the expression of caspases-3 and caspases-8, mediate inflammatory cells apoptosis, and ultimately alleviate pathological damage of ovarian tissue [18].

As an important branch of systematic biology, metabolomics is mainly used to evaluate the effects of environment, disease status, or drug intervention on endogenous small molecular metabolites like fatty acids, amino acids, peptides, and lipids [19]. Recently, metabolomic investigation has been widely used in the evaluation of biological efficacy and possible mechanism of traditional Chinese medicine. An GC/MS-based metabolomics research revealed that the metabolic disorders of citric acid circulation, glucose metabolism, unsaturated fatty acids and amino acids in acute liver injury mouse can be regulated by *Hedyotis diffusa* [20]. A recent metabolomic study suggested that 12 biomarkers were identified in carbon tetrachloride (CCl4)-induced liver fibrosis in rats, and Shu Gan Jian Pi formula could ameliorate the energy, amino acid, sphingolipid, cytochrome P450, glucose and water–electrolyte metabolism [21]. Meanwhile, PID-associated metabolomic study in the urine of PID rats based on GC–MS has yet been reported, eighteen potential biomarkers of PID were found, and *Patrinia scabiosaefolia Fisch* showed a holistic interventional effect on disease-associated metabolomic changes [22, 23].

In the present study, the effect of Fukeqianjin formula on inflammatory cytokines was investigated in PID rats induced by intrauterine inoculation of multiple pathogens combined with mechanical injury of endometrium. Moreover, an UPLC-Q-Exactive Orbitrap-MS-based metabonomic method combined with multivariate analyses including principal component analysis (PCA), partial least squares discriminant analysis (PLS-DA) and orthogonal partial least squares discriminant analysis (OPLS-DA), were used to analyze the metabolic profiling and to recognize and identify potential biomarkers and the metabolic pathways.

Methods

Information of experimental design and resources

The information regarding the experimental design, statistics, and resources used in this study are attached in the minimum standards of reporting checklist (Additional file 1).

Chemicals and reagents

Ferulic acid (Batch No. 110773-200611) was obtained from the National Institutes for Food and Drug Control (Beijing, China). Chlorogenic acid (Batch No. MUST-17030620) was obtained from Chengdu Manchester biotech Co., Ltd. (Chengdu, China). Lobetyolin (Batch No. 16022204), Andrographolide (Batch No. 16073103), and dehydrated andrographolide (Batch No. 16022501) were obtained from Chengdu Zhuo Pu Instrument Co., Ltd (Chengdu, China). Fukeqianjin tablets were obtained from Zhuzhou Qianjin pharmaceutical Co., Ltd. (Hunan, China). Azithromycin (Batch No. R37977) was purchased from Pfizer pharmaceutical Co., Ltd. (NY, USA). *Staphylococcus aureus* (ATCC25923) and *E. coli* were purchased from Chinese national fungus storehouse. Methanol and acetonitrile with HPLC-grade were purchased from Thermo Fisher Scientific Inc. (Iowa, USA). Formic acid was purchased from Sigma Chemical Co. (St. Louis, MO, USA). Water used in this study was prepared by ULUP Ultrapure Water System (Chengdu, China).

Animals

Healthy female Sprague–Dawley rats (specific pathogen-free, 220 ± 20 g) were supplied by DaShuo Biotechnology Co., Ltd [Approval Number: SCXK (Sichuan) 2015-030, Chengdu, China]. This study was strictly in accordance with the Guidelines for the Care and Use of Laboratory Animals. The animal protocol was approved by the Animal Ethics Committee of Chengdu University.

Preparation and quality control of Fukeqianjin formula

Fukeqianjin formula powder (4 g) was extracted with 20 mL 70% ethanol by ultrasonic extraction for 60 min. Then the supernatant was concentrated and dissolved with 5 mL methanol after centrifugation for 10 min at 12,000 rpm. Samples for High Performance Liquid Chromatography (HPLC) detection were obtained by filtration through a 0.22 μm membrane filter.

A HPLC method was established for the identification of the major compounds in Fukeqianjin formula (LC-20AT HPLC system, Shimadzu, Japan). A ZORBAX SB-C18 analytical column (4.6×250 mm, 5 μm, Agilent, USA) was used with the column temperature maintained at 35 °C. Acetonitrile and 0.1% phosphoric acid in water were treated as mobile phase A and B, respectively. The gradient elution was programmed as follows: 10% A–20% (0–15 min), 20–47.5% A (15.1–45 min), 47.5–68.5% A (45.1–50 min). The detection wavelength is 220 nm. The flow rate was set at 1.0 mL/min, and the sample injection volume was set at 5 μL.

Induction of PID model rats

The preparation of PID model was based on the methods described in the previous literature with some revisions [23]. Rats were anesthetized with 20% urethane (5 mL/kg) by intraperitoneal injection. Endometrial tissue was injured by a blunt needle-tip syringe that entered the uterine cavity and pulls back and forth twice along the uterine wall. At the same time, 0.1 mL of the prepared multi-pathogen solution which was composed of *S. aureus* and *E. coli* (1×10^8 ccu/mL, respectively) was injected into the ovary, and the rats were positioned upside down for 5 min. Rats in control group were treated identically with saline solution without endometrial tissue injured.

Histopathological analysis of PID model rats

Ten days after establishment of PID model, the uterine tissue samples of model and normal rats (n = 6 per group) were randomly collected and fixed in 4% paraformaldehyde, followed by embedded in paraffin, cut into 5-μm sections (RM2235, Leica, Germany). Furthermore, paraffin sections were deparaffinized in xylene, then stained with hematoxylin and eosin (H&E) and the pathological changes were evaluated randomly, nonconsecutive chosen fields at a magnification of 200× using optical microscopy (CX21FS1, Olmpus, Japan).

Drug administration and sample collection

After histological analysis, PID rats were randomly divided into model group, azithromycin group (AZM, 10 mg/kg), high-dose of Fukeqianjin formula group (FF-H, 1.6 g/kg) and low-dose of Fukeqianjin formula group (FF-L, 0.8 g/kg). All drugs were dissolved in distilled water. Normal control group were given equal volume of distilled water. Each group was consisted of 10 rats. After 14 days of intragastric administration, blood samples were collected from abdominal aorta. The plasma samples were centrifuged at 3500 rpm for 10 min at 4 °C and immediately stored at − 80 °C until analysis.

Measurement of inflammatory cytokines

Concentrations of interleukin-1β (IL-1β) was measured by enzyme linked immunosorbent assay (ELISA) kits (Batch Number: 2301B61242, MultiSciences Biotech Co., Ltd. Hangzhou, China). The concentration of nitric oxide (NO) was quantified based on the nitric reductase method (Batch Number: 20161114, Nanjing Jiancheng Institute of Biotechnology, Nanjing, China). All date was carried out by Varioskan Multifunctional full wave-length microplate reader (Thermo Fisher Scientific, USA) according to the manufacturers.

Plasm sample preparation

A total of 300 μL acetonitrile was added into 100 μL of plasm sample for protein precipitation, and then the mixture was vortexed for 3 min, centrifuged at 12,000 rpm for 10 min at 4 °C. The supernatant was transferred to an auto-sampler vial for UPLC-Q-Exactive Orbitrap-MS analysis.

UPLC-Q-Exactive Orbitrap-MS analysis

Chromatographic separation was carried out on an Ultimate-3000 RS LC system (Dionex, USA) using an Acquity UPLC BEH C18 column (2.1 mm × 100 mm, 1.7 μm, Waters, USA) with the column temperature maintained at 35 °C. The mobile phase consisted of 0.1% formic acid in water (A) and 0.1% formic acid in acetonitrile (B). The gradient elution was modified as follows: 0–25 min, 5–95% B; 25–30 min, 95% B; 30–31 min, 95–5% B; and 31–35 min, 5% B. The sample injection volume was set at 10 μL for analysis with a flow rate of 0.4 mL/min.

Mass spectrometry was performed on a Q-Exactive Orbitrap-MS system (Thermo Fisher Scientific, USA) equipped with an electrospray ionization source operating in the positive ion mode with the following parameters: scan type, full MS; scan range, 80 to 1000 m/z; scan resolution, 7000 m/z/s; sheath gas flow rate, 30 arb; aux gas flow rate, 10 arb; spray voltage, 3.5 kV, capillary temperature, 320 °C; aux gas heater temperature, 150 °C.

The quality control (QC) samples mixed by 100 μL of 10 experimental samples were determined by duplicate analysis of six injections before analysis to evaluate the precision and repeatability of the instrument. In addition, QC samples were measured every 10 samples during the testing process in order to investigate the stability of analytical method by determining relative standard deviations (RSD) of intensity and retention time of 10 randomly selected characteristic ion peaks of QC samples.

Data analysis

The raw MS data were exported to MZ mine for normalization treatment before multivariate analysis. The principal component analysis (PCA), partial least-squares discriminant analysis (PLS-DA) and orthogonal partial least-squares discriminant analysis (OPLS-DA) were performed with Metabolomics Univariate and Multivariate Analysis (MUMA) of R software (URL: http://www.R-project.org/). For potential biomarker identifications, the information was obtained from the following databases: http://www.genome.jp/kegg/, http://metlin.scripps.edu/, http://www.lipidmaps.org/. Potential metabolic pathways

were analyzed by Metabo Analyst 2.0. All results were expressed as the mean ± standard deviation (SD). One-way analysis of variance (ANOVA) was applied to the statistical analysis and P values less than 0.05 were considered significantly different between groups.

Results

Quality control of Fukeqianjin formula

Five major characteristic chemical constituents from Fukeqianjin formula were determined. A typical HPLC chromatogram was shown in Fig. 1. As a result, the concentration of chlorogenic acid, ferulic acid, lobetyolin, andrographolide and dehydrated andrographolide was 0.46 mg/g, 0.33 mg/g, 0.25 mg/g, 2.06 mg/g, and 1.67 mg/g, respectively. Fukeqianjin formula conform to the relevant quality standards.

Histopathological examination of PID model

In PID group, the uterus of rats were characterized by obvious congestion and edema, epithelial cell proliferation and degeneration, and chronic inflammatory cell infiltration was observed in the endometrium and myometrium. It indicated that the multi-pathogen treatment with endometrial tissue injure could result in the inflammation reaction in the upper genital tract (Fig. 2).

Anti-inflammation activity

As illustrated in Fig. 3, compared with normal control group, the inflammatory cytokines including IL-1β and NO were significantly increased in PID rats. Treatment with either AZM or FF-H could remarkably decrease the level of IL-1β and NO in plasma, which can be inferred that AZM and FF-H can alleviate genital inflammatory response in rats with pelvic inflammation.

Validation of UPLC-Q-Exactive Orbitrap-MS conditions

The representative UPLC-Q-Exactive Orbitrap-MS total ion chromatogram (TIC) of the plasma samples were shown in Fig. 4. By calculating the peak area, m/z data, and retention time of the selected ions, the precision, repeatability of the instrument, and stability of analytical method were evaluated. All of the relative standard deviation (RSD%) values were less than 6%, which indicated that this established rat plasma metabolomics analysis method was reliable and accurate.

Pattern recognition and potential biomarkers identification

First, PCA analysis was used for unsupervised pattern recognition in all groups. Additionally, two supervised pattern recognition methods, PLS-DA and OPLS-DA, were employed to provide better discrimination and to carry out metabolites differences between groups in this

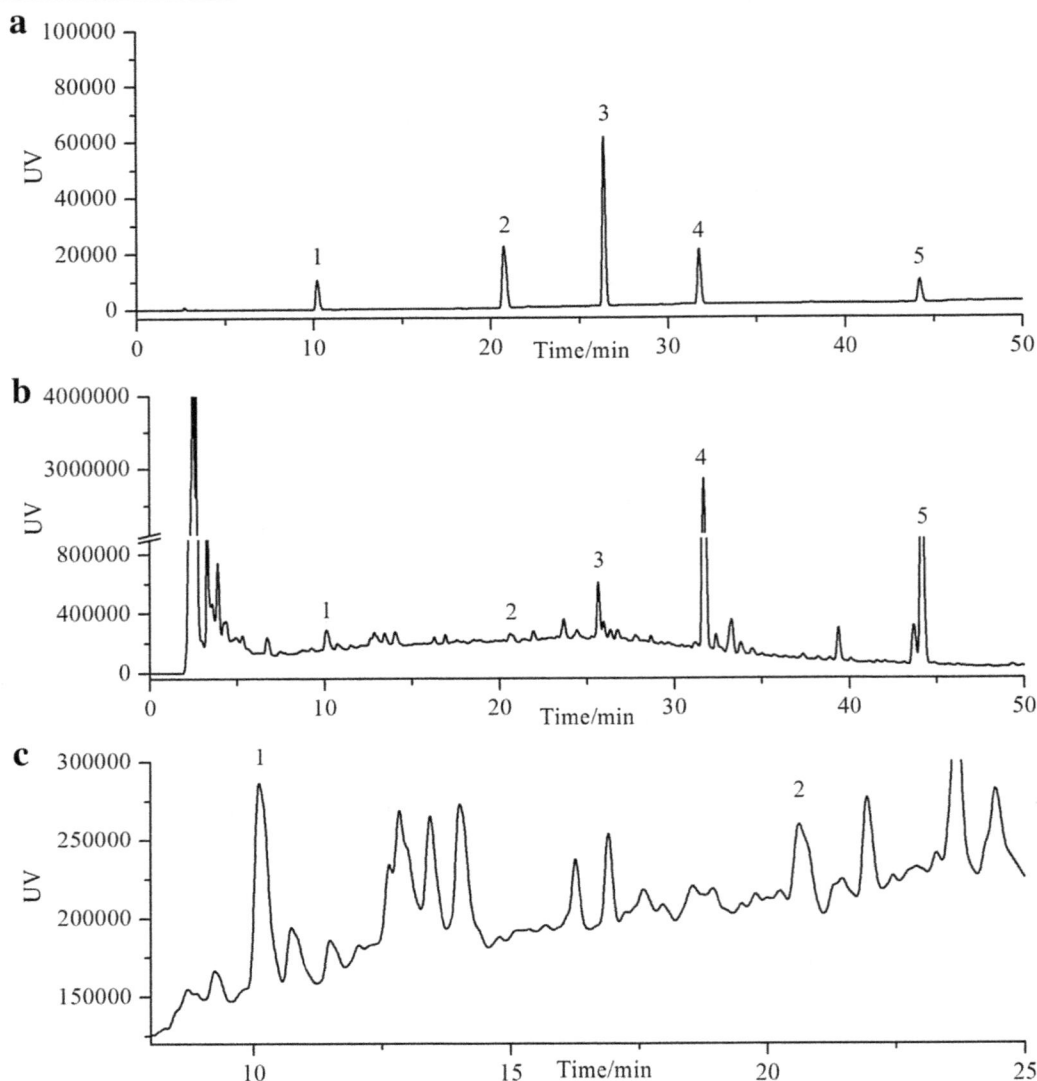

Fig. 1 The typical HPLC chromatogram of Fukeqianjin formula. **a** Mixed standard reference substance. 1: chlorogenic acid (10.163 min); 2: ferulic acid (20.775 min); 3: lobetyolin (26.385 min); 4: andrographolide (31.671 min); 5: dehydrated andrographolide (44.164 min). **b** Fukeqianjin formula extract (0–50 min). **c** Fukeqianjin formula extract (8–25 min)

study. As shown in Fig. 5, the corresponding scores plots from PCA, PLS-DA and OPLS-DA showed that PID rats were clearly separated from normal rats, which suggested that intrauterine inoculation of multiple pathogens combined with mechanical injury of endometrium could significantly disturb the plasma metabolic profiles of rats. Meanwhile, compared with the PID model group, the metabolite profiles of Fukeqianjin formula treatment group was gradually restored to normal, indicating that the treatment of Fukeqianjin formula can significantly alleviate the metabolic disorders caused by pelvic inflammation in rats.

A total of 14 potential metabolite biomarkers, including L-alanine, Ser-Lys-Lys-Ile, taurodeoxycholic acid, tridecyl phloretate, 12-ketodeoxycholic acid, diaminomethylidene-L-ornithine, adrenic acid, docosatrienoic acid, Arg-Met-Arg-Thr, Ergine, PC(20:3(8Z,11Z,14Z)/0:0), LysoPC(15:0), LysoPC(16:0), and stearoylcarnitine, which are mainly related to the metabolic pathways of intervening glycerophospholipid metabolism, linoleic acid metabolism/alpha-linolenic acid metabolism, amino acid metabolism, arachidonic acid metabolism, and unsaturated fatty acids biosynthesis were

Metabonomic study of the protective effect of Fukeqianjin formula on multi-pathogen induced pelvic...

89

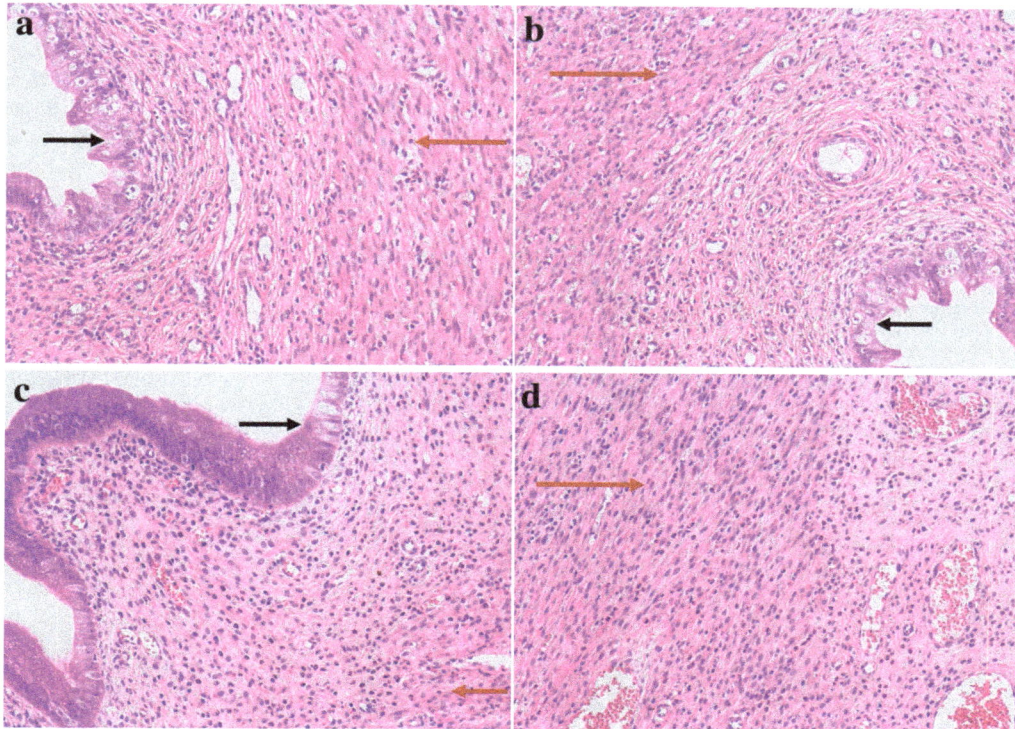

Fig. 2 Representative histopathological micrographs of uterus. **a, b** Saline solution treatment. **c, d** Multi-pathogen solution treatment. H&E stain, ×200. Black arrow stands for endometrium, red arrow stands for myometrium

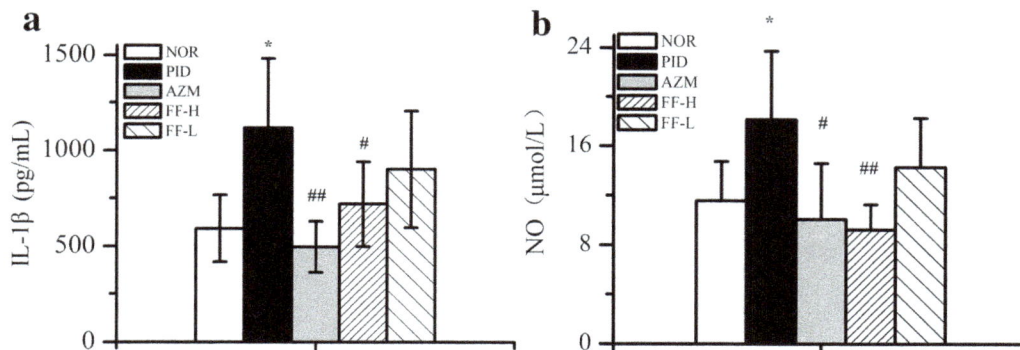

Fig. 3 Effect of Fukeqianjin formula on the inflammatory response in PID rats. **a** Level of IL-1β. **b** Level of NO. *$P < 0.05$ compared to the control group; #$P < 0.05$ and ##$P < 0.01$ compared to the PID model group

identified (shown in Table 1). The different intensity of these biomarkers was shown in Fig. 6. The results also suggested that the plasma biomarkers of rats with pelvic inflammation have obvious changes compared with normal rats, and Fukeqianjin formula has potential therapeutic effect on PID rats.

Discussion

Nitric oxide (NO), an important endogenous bioinformatic molecule produced from L-arginine by constitutive and inducible nitric oxide synthases, plays a key role in inflammatory cascade reaction and immune regulation [24, 25]. Inhibiting the excessive production of NO

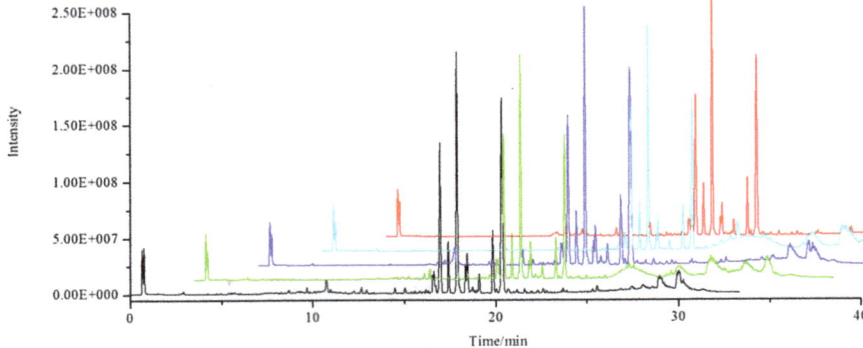

Fig. 4 Representative UPLC-Q-Exactive Orbitrap-MS TIC chromatograms of the plasma samples. Black line: NOR group, Green line: AZM group, Blue line: FF-H group, Light blue line: FF-L group, Red line: PID group

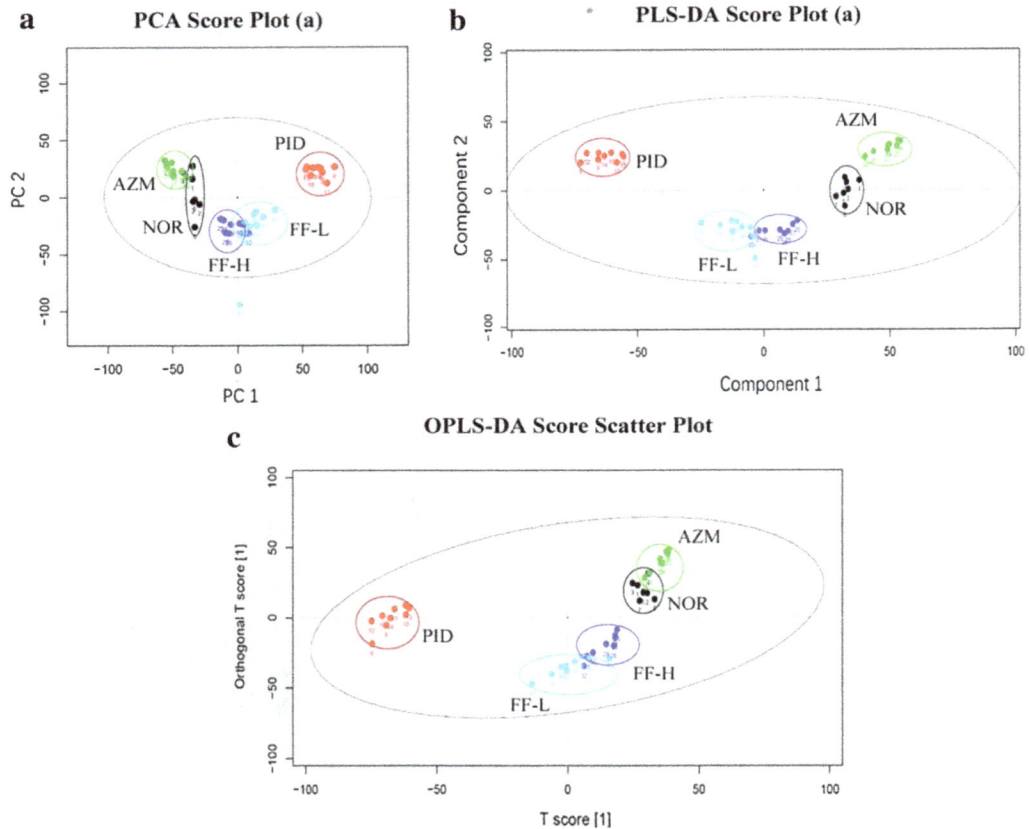

Fig. 5 Scores plots of PCA (**a**), PLS-DA (**b**) and OPLS-DA (**c**) analysis on the PID rat plasm metabolic profiles of normal control (NOR), model (PID), azithromycin treatment (AZM) and Fukeqianjin formula treatment (FF-H, FF-L) group

has been regarded as an effective strategy for the treatment of inflammation-related diseases due to its harmful consequences such as tissue damage in the process of chronic inflammation [26]. It was previously reported

that stimulating IL-1β would increase the expression of iNOS, which may further cause an increased production of NO [27]. Study indicated the amount of NO in endometrial tissues was comparatively higher in patients with

Table 1 The potential metabolite biomarkers

No.	RT (min)	Mass (m/z)	Formula	Identity names	Trend
1	0.74	90.0544	$C_3H_7NO_2$	L-Alanine	↓
2	5.67	475.3232	$C_{21}H_{42}N_6O_6$	Ser-Lys-Lys-Ile	↓
3	10.06	500.3023	$C_{26}H_{45}NO_6S$	Taurodeoxycholic acid	↓
4	11.37	357.2775	$C_{22}H_{36}O_3$	Tridecyl phloretate	↓
5	11.39	391.2826	$C_{24}H_{38}O_4$	12-Ketodeoxycholic acid	↓
6	11.54	750.3722	$C_{28}H_{51}N_{11}O_{13}$	Diaminomethylidene-L-ornithine	↓
7	12.61	355.2618	$C_{22}H_{36}O_2$	Adrenic acid	↓
8	15.34	357.2775	$C_{22}H_{38}O_2$	Docosatrienoic acid	↓
9	16.99	563.3104	$C_{21}H_{42}N_{10}O_6S$	Arg-Met-Arg-Thr	↓
10	17.13	496.3379	$C_{24}H_{50}NO_7P$	LysoPC (16:0)	↑
11	17.41	268.1477	$C_{16}H_{17}N_3O$	Ergine	↓
12	17.78	546.3533	$C_{28}H_{52}NO_7P$	PC (20:3(8Z,11Z,14Z)/0:0)	↓
13	20.18	482.3223	$C_{23}H_{48}NO_7P$	LysoPC (15:0)	↓
14	22.91	428.3715	$C_{25}H_{49}NO_4$	Stearoylcarnitine	↑

endometriosis [28]. Rocha et al. reported that NO levels appeared to be elevated in women with chronic pelvic pain diagnosed as secondary stage to endometriosis, and was directly associated with reduction in pain intensity and increase in pain threshold after treatment [29]. Meanwhile, recent experiments have shown that the productions of inflammatory cytokines including IL-1β, IL-6, and TNF-α were significantly increased in upper genital tract of PID rats [16, 17]. In patients with upper genital tract inflammatory diseases, the level of interleukins IL-1β were prominently elevated [30]. In this study, NO and IL-1β level in PID rat plasma was detected to evaluate the anti-inflammatory function of Fukeqianjin formula. Results show that the level of NO and IL-1β were significantly increased (Fig. 3), indicating inflammatory response has been induced in PID rats. Moreover, treatment with FF-H remarkably decrease these cytokines levels, suggesting a potent anti-inflammatory effect of FF-H.

A systematic review and meta-analysis drew a conclusion that A. paniculata, an important drug in Fukeqianjin formula, was safe and effective in the treatment of acute respiratory tract infections [31]. Andrographolide is the main chemical constituent of A. paniculata and is also considered to be a major contributor to the therapeutic activity [32, 33]. It has been reported that andrographolide has a broad-spectrum antimicrobial activity against both Gram (+) and Gram (−), especially to S. aureus, Bacillus subtilis, E. coli, Pseudomonas aeruginosa, and Klebsiella pneumoniae [34]. In addition, andrographolide was able to inhibit Chlamydia trachomatis-induced human cervical epithelial cell infection and reduce the level of inflammatory factors such

as IFNγ-induced protein10, CXCL8, and IL-6 [35]. Study also confirmed that andrographolide administration in both LPS-activated RAW264.7 cells and peritoneal macrophages could decrease IFN-β, iNOS, TNF-α, and COX-2 expression as well as the downstream NO and PGE2 productions [36]. Andrographis paniculata has also been proved to have potent therapeutic effect on pathogen-induced PID rats by significantly reduce the excessive secretion of cytokines and chemokines including IL-1β, IL-6, CXCL-1, and MCP-1 through blocking the NF-κB signal pathway transduction [37]. Based on our experimental results and previous studies, we speculate that A. paniculata may be one of the main anti-inflammatory drugs in Fukeqianjin formula.

Besides, it was previously reported that the total flavonoids from R. laevigata Michx fruit markedly downregulated the expression levels of IL-1β, IL-6, TNF-α by inhibiting NF-κB and AP-1 transcriptional activities during inflammatory courses, and thus has protective effect on pathological processes including renal and hepatic ischemia–reperfusion damage [38, 39]. Berberine, as the main ingredient of Mahonia fortunei, was widely recognized for its considerable anti-inflammatory effects. Study has demonstrated that berberine has a protective effect on adenomyosis, a complication of PID, by inhibiting the expression of IL-6, IL-8, TGF-β, VEGF and MMP-2 [40]. Its anti-inflammatory mechanism mainly involves signaling pathways such as NF-κB, AMPK, and caspase-1/IL-1β inflammatory signal transduction axis [41, 42]. Combination of the above herbal medicine can enhance the anti-inflammatory effect of the compound, and produce a good therapeutic effect on pelvic inflammation.

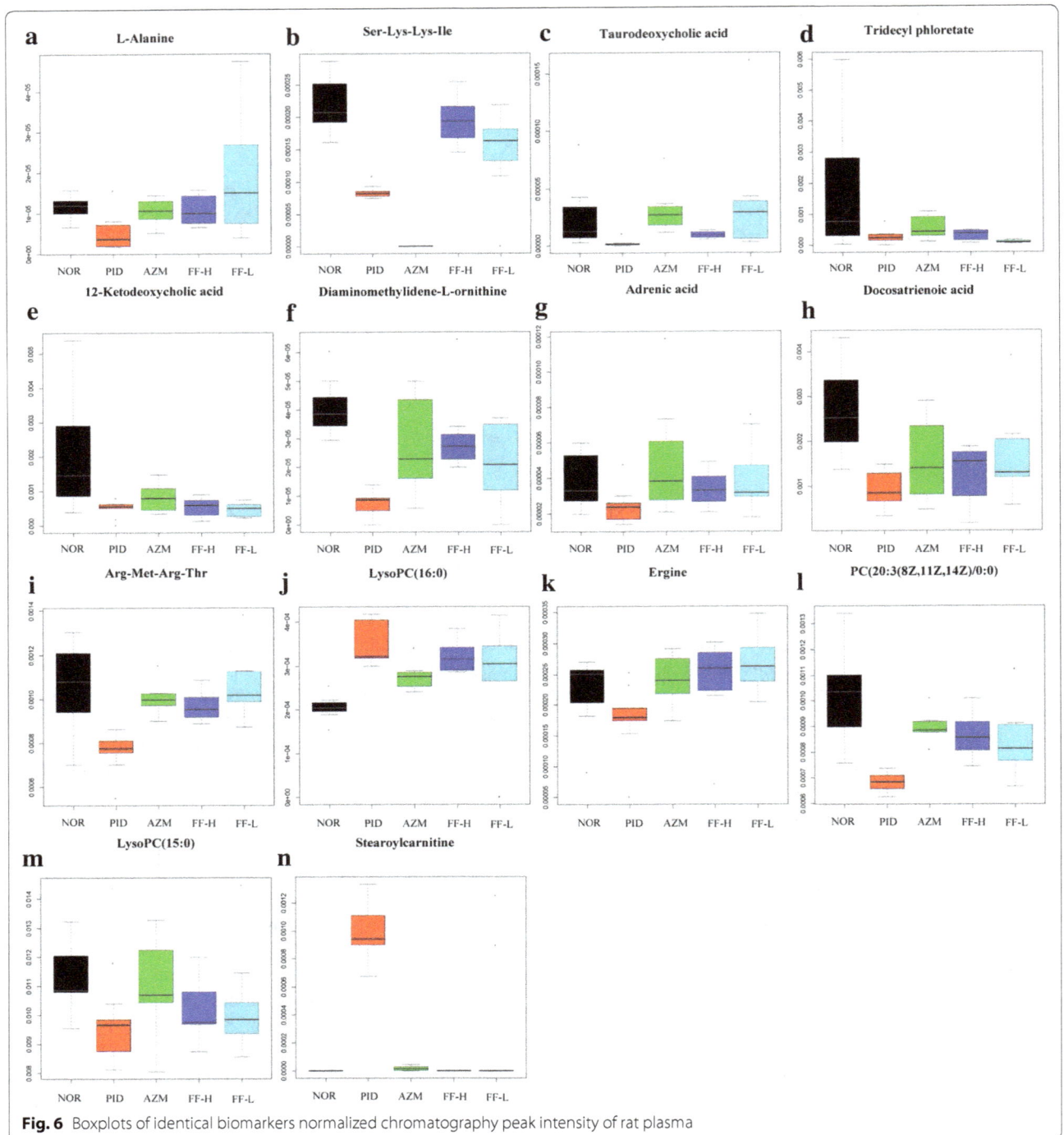

Fig. 6 Boxplots of identical biomarkers normalized chromatography peak intensity of rat plasma

At the same time, although PID is recognized as a multiple bacterial infectious disease, chronic inflammation and correlative complications also participate in its progression. So, in addition to short-term antimicrobial targets, long-term sequelae prevention and treatment is also an important therapeutic goal [43]. Some studies indicates that chronic PID are often under a situation of microcirculation disorder and immune deficiency. *Angelica sinensis* is commonly used in Chinese medicine to promote hematopoietic function, improve microcirculation and regulate the immune system [44]. Ferulic acid, Z-ligustilide and polysaccharides are the main chemical constituents of *Angelica sinensis* [45]. Liu et al. reported polysaccharides may promote the recovery of platelets and other blood cells and the formation of hematopoiesis in rat by regulating the PI3K/Akt pathway [46]. *Spatholobus suberectus* contains various types of polyphenolic compounds mainly including flavonoids, isoflavones, flavonols, and flavanones [47]. Among them, total flavonoids of *S. suberectus* have been proved to inhibit oxidative stress and regulate immune function, and it can also play an anti-viral role [48]. Through reasonable compatibility, the whole compound can not only achieve good anti-inflammatory effect, but also improve microcirculation and immunity. It has significant advantages in the treatment of pelvic inflammatory disease and its complications.

In addition, since the complex composition of Chinese herbal compound, it is difficult to elucidate its mechanism of action. Metabonomics methodology covers a wide range of substances, focusing on holistic and dynamic evaluation, which was in coincidence with the holistic theory of traditional Chinese medicine. In recent years, metabonomics has been widely used in the study of inflammatory diseases. Previous studies have shown that collagen-induced arthritis was characterized by metabolic disorders of lipid, tricarboxylic acid cycle, tryptophan and phenylalanine metabolism [49]. According to Ahn et al. the mechanism of curcumin in the treatment of rheumatoid arthritis may be related to the abnormal regulation of glycine, citrulline, arachidonic acid and saturated fatty acid levels [50]. In this study, the plasma metabolomics method based on UPLC-Q-Exactive Orbitrap-MS was used to investigate the underlying mechanism of Fukeqianjin formula on pelvic inflammation. Our results demonstrate that 14 endogenous compounds can be considered as potential metabolite biomarkers of PID (Table 1). Studies have confirmed that the metabolites including amino acids, fatty acids, organic acids, and sugars in urine could considered to be the potential biomarkers of PID [22]. In addition, *Patrinia scabiosaefolia Fisch* is believed to play a therapeutic role in pelvic inflammation by regulating tricarboxylic acid circulation, glucose metabolism, and amino acid metabolism [23]. However, the above studies were based on the urine metabolomics of gas chromatography–mass spectrometry and our study can be used as complementary biological information for PID.

Previous studies suggested that the lipids metabolism, including bile acids and unsaturated fatty acids, is involved in the occurrence and development of inflammatory reaction [51]. Taurine deoxycholic acid has been shown to ameliorate insulin resistance in mice by inhibiting the increase of phospholipid, myelin sheath and neuramide [52]. Moreover, taurine deoxycholic acid

can significantly up-regulate the expression of MUC4 (a membrane-bound mucin) by activating phosphatidylinositol 3-kinase, thereby affecting cell proliferation and tumor progression [53, 54]. As a long chain polyunsaturated fatty acids, docosatrienoic acid is of great benefit to health. As a metabolite of arachidonic acid, adrenic acid can be converted into a variety of oxygenated metabolites, and plays an important role in cardiovascular system and immune system [55]. In this study, a variety of bile acids and unsaturated fatty acids, including taurodeoxycholic acid, 12-ketodeoxycholic acid, docosatrienoic acid and adrenic acid, were identified (Table 1). After treatment with Fukeqianjin formula for 14 days can significantly correct the abnormal changes of these substances (Fig. 6).

Studies have shown that some kinds of phosphatidylcholine (PC) were important biomarkers of inflammation. Glycerophospholipids metabolism profiles can characterize the progress of inflammation and provide valuable evidence for the diagnosis and prognosis of inflammation [56]. It has been confirmed that various drugs in Fukeqianjin formula can affect lipid metabolism. For instance, the total flavonoids of *R. laevigata* Michx can regulate lipid metabolism in LPS-induced liver injury mice by mainly reducing the expression levels of fatty acid synthase, acetyl coenzyme A carboxylase-1, and stearoyl coenzyme A desaturase-1, and improving the level of carnitine palmitoyltransferase 1 [57]. Besides, some new polyynes from *Codonopsis pilosula* may affect lipid metabolism by inhibiting the expression of squalene monooxygenase gene in HepG2 cells [58]. Our data suggested that there were significant changes in biomarkers, including LysoPC (16:0), PC (20:3(8Z,11Z,14Z)/0:0), and LysoPC (15:0), in PID rats, which could be regulated by Fukeqianjin formula intervention (Fig. 6).

Amino acids are not only essential substances of proteins, but also as signal molecules regulate various physiological functions of the organism, such as precursors of many neurotransmitters and hormones, and intermediates of TCA circulation and glyconeogenesis [59]. Previous reports have demonstrated that branched-chain amino acids can increase the expression of eNOS and nitrotyrosine, and induce inflammatory response by activating the transcription factor NF-κB in endothelial cells [60]. Four potential biomarkers related to amino acid metabolism, including L-alanine, Ser-Lys-Lys-Ile, diaminomethylidene-L-ornithine, and Arg-Met-Arg-Thr, have been shown in Table 1. Fukeqianjin formula was observed to have an obvious regulatory effect on the abnormal changes of these substances (Fig. 6). To summarize, the results illustrated that the metabolic pathways were mainly related to glycerophospholipid metabolism, linoleic acid metabolism/alpha-linolenic acid metabolism, amino acid metabolism, arachidonic acid metabolism, and unsaturated fatty acids biosynthesis. Fukeqianjin formula has potential therapeutic effect on multi-pathogen-induced PID rats by ameliorating metabolism disorders.

Conclusions

In summary, these results indicate that intrauterine inoculation of multiple pathogens combined with mechanical injury of endometrium could significantly disturb the plasma metabolic profiles of rats. Fukeqianjin formula has potential therapeutic effect on multi-pathogen-induced PID rats by ameliorating metabolism disorders and alleviating the inflammatory response.

Abbreviations

PID: pelvic inflammatory disease; FF: Fukeqianjin formula; AZM: azithromycin; IL-1β: interleukin-1β; IL-8: interleukin-8; IL-10: interleukin-10; IL-2: interleukin-2; NO: nitric oxide; TNF-α: tumor necrosis factor-α; NF-κB: nuclear factor-κb; IgA: immunoglobulin A; IgG: immunoglobulin G; IgM: immunoglobulin M; UPLC-Q-Exactive Orbitrap-MS: ultra-performance liquid chromatography-quadrupole-Exactive Orbitrap-mass spectrometry; NMR: nuclear magnetic resonance; GC–MS: gas chromatography–mass spectrometer; HPLC: high performance liquid chromatography; PCA: principal component analysis; PLS-DA: partial least squares discriminant analysis; OPLS-DA: orthogonal partial least squares discriminant analysis; CCl4: carbon tetrachloride; H&E: hematoxylin and eosin; QC: quality control; RSD: relative standard deviations; MUMA: Metabolomics Univariate and Multivariate Analysis; SD: standard deviation; ANOVA: one-way analysis of variance; TIC: total ion chromatogram; IFNγ: interferon γ; LPS: lipopolysaccharide; iNOS: inducible nitric oxide synthase; COX-2: cyclooxygenase-2; PGE2: prostaglandin E2; TFs: total flavonoids; VEGF: vascular endothelial growth factor; TGF-β: transforming growth factor-β; AMPK: adenosine 5′-monophosphate (AMP)-activated protein kinase; MMP-2: matrix metalloproteinases-2.

Authors' contributions

LZ and YG designed the research. YZ, WL, HY and PZ performed this study. WL, YZ and SSX analyzed the data. YZ and WL wrote the paper. YZ was responsible for the critical revision of the paper. All authors read and approved the final manuscript.

Author details

[1] School of Medicine, Chengdu University, No. 2025, Cheng Luo Road, Chengdu 610106, Sichuan, People's Republic of China. [2] Zhuzhou Qianjin Pharmaceutical Ltd. Co., No. 801 Zhuzhou Avenue, Tianyuan District, Zhuzhou 412000, Hunan, People's Republic of China. [3] Drug Clinical Trial Center, Affiliated Hospital of Chengdu University, 2nd Ring Road, Jinniu District, Chengdu 610081, Sichuan, People's Republic of China.

Acknowledgements
Not applicable.

Competing interests
The authors declare that they have no competing interests.

Consent for publication
All authors have provided consent for publication in the journal of Chinese Medicine.

Funding
This work was supported by Chengdu science and Technology Bureau (2016-HM01-00096-SF), Sichuan Provincial Department of Education (17TD0010), Health and Family Planning Commission of Chengdu-Key disciplines of clinical pharmacy.

References
1. Mitchell C, Prabhu M. Pelvic inflammatory disease: current concepts in pathogenesis, diagnosis and treatment. Infect Dis Clin N Am. 2013;27(4):793–809.
2. Haggerty CL, Schulz R, Ness RB. Lower quality of life among women with chronic pelvic pain after pelvic inflammatory disease. Obstet Gynecol. 2003;102(5 Pt 1):934–9.
3. Zhou Z, Zeng F, Yuan J, Tang J, Colditz GA, Tworoger SS, et al. Pelvic inflammatory disease and the risk of ovarian cancer: a meta-analysis. Cancer Causes Control. 2017;28(5):415–28.
4. Sharma H, Tal R, Clark NA, Segars JH. Microbiota and pelvic inflammatory disease. Semin Reprod Med. 2014;32(1):43–9.
5. Haggerty CL, Totten PA, Tang G, Astete SG, Ferris MJ, Norori J, et al. Identification of novel microbes associated with pelvic inflammatory disease and infertility. Sex Transm Infect. 2016;92(6):441–6.
6. Spencer TH, Umeh PO, Irokanulo E, Baba MM, Spencer BB, Umar AI, et al. Bacterial isolates associated with pelvic inflammatory disease among female patients attending some hospitals in Abuja, Nigeria. Afr J Infect Dis. 2014;8(1):9–13.
7. Bevan CD, Ridgway GL, Rothermel CD. Efficacy and safety of azithromycin as monotherapy or combined with metronidazole compared with two standard multidrug regimens for the treatment of acute pelvic inflammatory disease. J Int Med Res. 2003;31(1):45–54.
8. Piyadigamage A, Wilson J. Improvement in the clinical cure rate of outpatient management of pelvic inflammatory disease following a change in therapy. Sex Transm Infect. 2005;81(3):233–5.
9. Ness RB, Soper DE, Holley RL, Peipert J, Randall H, Sweet RL, et al. Effectiveness of inpatient and outpatient treatment strategies for women with pelvic inflammatory disease: results from the pelvic inflammatory disease evaluation and clinical health (peach) randomized trial. Am J Obstet Gynecol. 2002;186(5):929–37.
10. Zhou J, Qu F. Treating gynaecological disorders with traditional Chinese medicine: a review. Afr J Tradit Complement Altern Med. 2009;6(4):494–517.
11. Zheng Y, Jin Y, Zhu HB, Xu ST, Xia YX, Huang Y. The anti-inflammatory and anti-nociceptive activities of Patrinia villosa and its mechanism on the proinflammatory cytokines of rats with pelvic inflammation. Afr J Tradit Complement Altern Med. 2012;9(3):295–302.
12. Bu X, Liu Y, Lu Q, Jin Z. Effects of "danzhi decoction" on chronic pelvic pain, hemodynamics, and proinflammatory factors in the murine model of sequelae of pelvic inflammatory disease. Evid Based Complement Altern Med. 2015;2015:547251.
13. Oh Y, Kwon YS, Jung BD. Anti-inflammatory effects of the natural compounds cortex Phellodendri and Humulus japonicus on pelvic inflammatory disease in mice. Int J Med Sci. 2017;14(8):729–34.
14. Li Y, Liu Y, Yang Q, Shi Z, Xie Y, Wang S. Anti-inflammatory effect of Feiyangchangweiyan capsule on rat pelvic inflammatory disease through JNK/NF-κB pathway. Evid Based Complement Altern Med. 2018;2018:8476147.

15. Yuan J, Guo J, Wu C, Yue Z, Zeng G. Effect of Qianjin tablets on serum IgA, IgG and IgM in acute pelvic inflammation in rats. J TCM Univ Hunan. 2010;30(9):87–9 **(In Chinese)**.

16. Lu Y, Qu J, Guo J, Zuo Z, Shi Z, Wang X, Gui L. Effect of Fuke Qianjin tablet on TNF-α and IL-2 mRNA transcription in the uteri and ovary tissues of acute pelvic inflammatory disease in rats. Chin Tradit Patent Med. 2012;34(1):29–33 **(In Chinese)**.

17. Li X, Guo J, Shi Z, Nie J. Effect of Fuke Qianjin tablets on inflammatory cytokines in blood serum in rats with chronic pelvic inflammatory disease. Chin J Exp Tradit Med Formulae. 2013;19(10):226–8 **(In Chinese)**.

18. Nie J, Li X, Shi Z, Guo J. Influence of FukeQianjin tablets to rat's caspase-3 and caspase-8 expression of ovary with chronic pelvic inflammatory disease. Northwest Pharm J. 2014;29(4):385–7 **(In Chinese)**.

19. Wang X, Sun H, Zhang A, Sun W, Wang P, Wang Z. Potential role of metabolomics apporoaches in the area of traditional Chinese medicine: as pillars of the bridge between Chinese and Western medicine. J Pharm Biomed Anal. 2011;55(5):859–68.

20. Dai M, Wang F, Zou Z, Xiao G, Chen H, Yang H. Metabolic regulations of a decoction of *Hedyotis diffusa* in acute liver injury of mouse models. Chin Med. 2017;12:35.

21. Jiang H, Qin XJ, Li WP, Ma R, Wang T, Li ZQ. Effects of Shu Gan Jian Pi formula on rats with carbon tetrachloride-induced liver fibrosis using serum metabonomics based on gas chromatography-time of flight mass spectrometry. Mol Med Rep. 2017;16(4):3901–9.

22. Zou W, Wen X, Sheng X, Zheng YI, Xiao Z, Luo J, et al. Gas chromatography-mass spectrometric method-based urine metabolomic profile of rats with pelvic inflammatory disease. Exp Ther Med. 2016;11(5):1653–60.

23. Zou W, Wen X, Zheng Y, Xiao Z, Luo J, Chen S, et al. Metabolomic study on the preventive effect of *Patrinia scabiosaefolia* Fisch on multipathogen induced pelvic inflammatory disease in rats. Evid Based Complement Altern Med. 2015;2015:170792.

24. Niedbala W, Alves-Filho JC, Fukada SY, Vieira SM, Mitani A, Sonego F, et al. Regulation of type 17 helper T-cell function by nitric oxide during inflammation. Proc Natl Acad Sci USA. 2011;108(22):9220–5.

25. Xu L, Zhu J, Yin W, Ding X. Astaxanthin improves cognitive deficits from oxidative stress, nitric oxide synthase and inflammation through upregulation of PI3K/Akt in diabetes rat. Int J Clin Exp Pathol. 2015;8(6):6083–94.

26. Zhou MX, Wei X, Li AL, Wang AM, Lu LZ, Yang Y, et al. Screening of traditional Chinese medicines with therapeutic potential on chronic obstructive pulmonary disease through inhibiting oxidative stress and inflammatory response. BMC Complement Altern Med. 2016;16:360.

27. Ying X, Chen X, Cheng S, Shen Y, Peng L, Xu HZ. Piperine inhibits IL-β induced expression of inflammatory mediators in human osteoarthritis chondrocyte. Int Immunopharmacol. 2013;17(2):293–9.

28. Wu MY, Chao KH, Yang JH, Lee TH, Yang YS, Ho HN. Nitric oxide synthesis is increased in the endometrial tissue of women with endometriosis. Hum Reprod. 2003;18(12):2668–71.

29. Rocha MG, Gomes VA, Tanus-Santos JE, Rosa-e-Silva JC, Candido-dos-Reis FJ, Nogueira AA, et al. Reduction of blood nitric oxide levels is associated with clinical improvement of the chronic pelvic pain related to endometriosis. Braz J Med Biol Res. 2015;48(4):363–9.

30. Cheng W, Shivshankar P, Li Z, Chen L, Yeh IT, Zhong G. Caspase-1 contributes to *Chlamydia trachomatis*-induced upper urogenital tract inflammatory pathologies without affecting the course of infection. Infect Immun. 2008;76(2):515–22.

31. Hu XY, Wu RH, Logue M, Blondel C, Lai LYW, Stuart B, et al. *Andrographis paniculata* (Chuān Xīn Lián) for symptomatic relief of acute respiratory tract infections in adults and children: a systematic review and meta-analysis. PLoS ONE. 2017;12(8):e0181780.

32. Jayakumar T, Hsieh CY, Lee JJ, Sheu JR. Experimental and clinical pharmacology of *Andrographis paniculata* and its major bioactive phytoconstituent andrographolide. Evid Based Complement Altern Med. 2013;2013:846740.

33. Pholphana N, Rangkadilok N, Saehun J, Ritruechai S, Satayavivad J. Changes in the contents of four active diterpenoids at different growth stages in *Andrographis paniculata* (Burm.f.) Nees (Chuanxinlian). Chin Med. 2013;8(1):2.

34. Arifullah M, Namsa ND, Mandal M, Chiruvella KK, Vikrama P, Gopal GR. Evaluation of anti-bacterial and anti-oxidant potential of andrographolide and echiodinin isolated from callus culture of *Andrographis paniculata* Nees. Asian Pac J Trop Biomed. 2013;3(8):604–10.

35. Hua Z, Frohlich KM, Zhang Y, Feng X, Zhang J, Shen L. Andrographolide inhibits intracellular *Chlamydia trachomatis* multiplication and reduces secretion of proinflammatory mediators produced by human epithelial cells. Pathog Dis. 2015;73(1):1–11.

36. Shen T, Yang WS, Yi YS, Sung GH, Rhee MH, Poo H, et al. AP-1/IRF-3 targeted anti-inflammatory activity of andrographolide isolated from *Andrographis paniculata*. Evid Based Complement Altern Med. 2013;2013:210736.

37. Zou W, Xiao Z, Wen X, Luo J, Chen S, Cheng Z, et al. The anti-inflammatory effect of *Andrographis paniculata* (Burm. f.) Nees on pelvic inflammatory disease in rats through down-regulation of the NF-κB pathway. BMC Complement Altern Med. 2016;16(1):483.

38. Tao X, Sun X, Xu L, Yin L, Han X, Qi Y, et al. Total flavonoids from *Rosa laevigata* Michx fruit ameliorates hepatic ischemia/reperfusion injury through inhibition of oxidative stress and inflammation in rats. Nutrients. 2016;8(7):E418.

39. Zhao L, Xu L, Tao X, Han X, Yin L, Qi Y, Peng J. Protective effect of the total flavonoids from *Rosa laevigata* Michx fruit on renal ischemia-reperfusion injury through suppression of oxidative stress and inflammation. Molecules. 2016;21(7):E952.

40. Liu L, Chen L, Jiang C, Guo J, Xie Y, Kang L, et al. Berberine inhibits the LPS-induced proliferation and inflammatory response of stromal cells of adenomyosis tissues mediated by the LPS/TLR4 signaling pathway. Exp Ther Med. 2017;14(6):6125–30.

41. Ma X, Chen Z, Wang L, Wang G, Wang Z, Dong X, et al. The pathogenesis of diabetes mellitus by oxidative stress and inflammation: its inhibition by berberine. Front Pharmacol. 2018;9:782.

42. Jin H, Jin X, Cao B, Wang W. Berberine affects osteosarcoma via downregulating the caspase-1/IL-1β signaling axis. Oncol Rep. 2017;37(2):729–36.

43. Sweet RL. Treatment of acute pelvic inflammatory disease. Infect Dis Obstet Gynecol. 2011;2011:561909.

44. Wu YC, Hsieh CL. Pharmacological effects of Radix *Angelica sinensis* (Danggui) on cerebral infarction. Chin Med. 2011;6:32.

45. Chao WW, Lin BF. Bioactivities of major constituents isolated from *Angelica sinensis* (Danggui). Chin Med. 2011;6:29.

46. Liu C, Li J, Meng FY, Liang SX, Deng R, Li CK, et al. Polysaccharides from the root of *Angelica sinensis* promotes hematopoiesis and thrombopoiesis through the PI3K/AKT pathway. BMC Complement Altern Med. 2010;10:79.

47. Huang Y, Chen L, Feng L, Guo F, Li Y. Characterization of total phenolic constituents from the stems of *Spatholobus suberectus* using LC-DAD-MS(n) and their inhibitory effect on human neutrophil elastase activity. Molecules. 2013;18(7):7549–56.

48. Fu YF, Jiang LH, Zhao WD, Xi-Nan M, Huang SQ, Yang J, et al. Immunomodulatory and antioxidant effects of total flavonoids of *Spatholobus suberectus* Dunn on PCV2 infected mice. Sci Rep. 2017;7(1):8676.

49. Yue R, Zhao L, Hu Y, Jiang P, Wang S, Xiang L, et al. Rapid-resolution liquid chromatography TOF-MS for urine metabolomic analysis of collagen-induced arthritis in rats and its applications. J Ethnopharmacol. 2013;145(2):465–75.

50. Ahn JK, Kim S, Hwang J, Kim J, Lee YS, Koh EM, et al. Metabolomic elucidation of the effects of curcumin on fibroblast-like synoviocytes in rheumatoid arthritis. PLoS ONE. 2015;10(12):e0145539.

51. Dai D, Gao Y, Chen J, Huang Y, Zhang Z, Xu F. Time-resolved metabolomics analysis of individual differences during the early stage of lipopolysaccharide-treated rats. Sci Rep. 2016;6:34136.

52. Qi Y, Jiang C, Cheng J, Krausz KW, Li T, Ferrell JM, et al. Bile acid signaling in lipid metabolism: metabolomic and lipidomic analysis of lipid and bile acid markers linked to anti-obesity and anti-diabetes in mice. Biochim Biophys Acta. 2015;1851(1):19–29.

53. Mariette C, Perrais M, Leteurtre E, Jonckheere N, Hémon B, Pigny P, et al. Transcriptional regulation of human mucin MUC4 by bile acids in oesophageal cancer cells is promoter-dependent and involves activation of the phosphatidylinositol 3-kinase signalling pathway. Biochem J. 2004;377(Pt 3):701–8.

54. Carraway KL, Ramsauer VP, Haq B, Carothers Carraway CA. Cell signaling through membrane mucins. BioEssays. 2003;25(1):66–71.

55. Guijas C, Astudillo AM, Gil-de-Gómez L, Rubio JM, Balboa MA, Balsinde J. Phospholipid sources for adrenic acid mobilization in RAW 264.7 macrophages. Comparison with arachidonic acid. Biochim Biophys Acta. 2012;1821(11):1386–93.

56. Wu X, Cao H, Zhao L, Song J, She Y, Feng Y. Metabolomic analysis of glycerophospholipid signatures of inflammation treated with non-steroidal anti-inflammatory drugs-induced-RAW264.7 cells using (1)H NMR and U-HPLC/Q-TOF-MS. J Chromatogr B Analyt Technol Biomed Life Sci. 2016;1028:199–215.

57. Dong L, Han X, Tao X, Xu L, Xu Y, Fang L, et al. Protection by the total flavonoids from *Rosa laevigata* Michx fruit against lipopolysaccharide-induced liver injury in mice via modulation of FXR signaling. Foods. 2018;7(6):E88.

58. Hu XY, Qin FY, Lu XF, Zhang LS, Cheng YX. Three new polyynes from *Codonopsis pilosula* and their activities on lipid metabolism. Molecules. 2018;23(4):E887.

59. Bröer S, Bröer A. Amino acid homeostasis and signalling in mammalian cells and organisms. Biochem J. 2017;474(12):1935–63.

60. Zhenyukh O, González-Amor M, Rodrigues-Diez RR, Esteban V, Ruiz-Ortega M, Salaices M, et al. Branched-chain amino acids promote endothelial dysfunction through increased reactive oxygen species generation and inflammation. J Cell Mol Med. 2018. https://doi.org/10.1111/jcmm.13759.

10

Paeoniflorin exerts neuroprotective effects by modulating the M1/M2 subset polarization of microglia/macrophages in the hippocampal CA1 region of vascular dementia rats via cannabinoid receptor 2

Xian-Qin Luo[1], Ao Li[2], Xue Yang[3], Xiao Xiao[2], Rong Hu[4], Tian-Wen Wang[3], Xiao-Yun Dou[5], Da-Jian Yang[3] and Zhi Dong[1*]

Abstract

Background: Cerebral hypoperfusion is a pivotal risk factor for vascular dementia (VD), for which effective therapy remains inadequate. Persistent inflammatory responses and excessive chemotaxis of microglia/macrophages in the brain may accelerate the progression of VD. Endocannabinoids are involved in neuronal protection against inflammation-induced neuronal injury. Cannabinoids acting at cannabinoid receptor 2 (CB_2R) can decrease inflammation. Based on the identification of paeoniflorin (PF) as a CB_2R agonist, we investigated the neuroprotective and microglia/macrophages M1 to M2 polarization promoting effects of PF in a permanent four-vessel occlusion rat model.

Methods: One week after surgery, PF was intraperitoneally administered at a dose of 40 mg/kg once a day for 28 successive days. The effects of PF on memory deficit were investigated by a Morris water maze test, and the effects of PF on hippocampal neuronal damage were evaluated by light microscope and electron microscope. The mRNA and protein expression levels of key molecules related to the M1/M2 polarization of microglia/macrophages were assessed by RT-qPCR and Western blotting, respectively.

Results: Administration of PF could significantly attenuate cerebral hypoperfusion-induced impairment of learning and memory and reduce the morphological and ultrastructural changes in the hippocampal CA1 region of rats. Moreover, PF promoted an M1 to M2 phenotype transition in microglia/macrophages in the hippocampus of rats. In addition to its inhibitory property against proinflammatory M1 mediator expression, such as IL-1β, IL-6, TNF-α and NO, PF dramatically up-regulated expression of anti-inflammatory cytokines IL-10 and TGF-β1. Importantly, CB_2R antagonist AM630 abolished these beneficial effects produced by PF on learning, memory and hippocampus structure in rats, as well as the polarization of microglia/macrophages to the M2 phenotype. Additionally, PF treatment significantly inhibited cerebral hypoperfusion-induced mTOR/NF-κB proinflammatory pathway and enhanced PI3K/Akt anti-inflammatory pathway. Effects of PF on these signaling pathways were effectively attenuated when rats were co-treated with PF and AM630, indicating that the mTOR/NF-κB and PI3K/Akt signaling pathways were involved in the PF effects through CB_2R activation.

*Correspondence: dongzhidyx@163.com
[1] Chongqing Key Laboratory of Biochemistry and Molecular Pharmacology, School of Pharmacy, Chongqing Medical University, Chongqing 400016, China

Conclusion: These findings demonstrated PF exerts its neuroprotective effect and shifts the inflammatory milieu toward resolution by modulation of microglia/macrophage polarization via CB_2R activation.

Keywords: Paeoniflorin, Cannabinoid receptor 2, Vascular dementia, Neuroprotection

Background

Vascular dementia (VD) is a cognitive impairment syndrome caused by cerebral hemorrhage, ischemia or acute/chronic cerebral hypoxia, and other cerebrovascular diseases. VD often presents as an impairment in memory, speech, calculation, and visuospatial functions, and severely affects the patient's daily life [1, 2]. Dementia due to VD accounts for 20% of all cases of dementia, with an incidence secondary only to dementia caused by Alzheimer's disease [3]. With an increasing human lifespan and an increase in the incidence of cerebrovascular diseases, the population of people affected by VD is increasing year-by-year, leading to huge burdens on families and society [2].

The pathogenesis of VD is still not completely clear. Neurological imaging and pathological studies have shown that pathological changes due to cerebrovascular obstruction or injury results in insufficient cerebral perfusion and are the main cause of VD-induced cognitive impairments [4]. In addition, inflammatory responses are an important factor of secondary brain injury caused by cerebral ischemia. Studies have found that after ischemic brain damage, microglial cells in the brain and macrophages that infiltrated the central nervous system (CNS) due to damage to the blood–brain barrier will rapidly migrate to the site of inflammation. In the damaged environment, these cells are activated through the classical pathway to undergo M1 polarization and secrete large amounts of reactive oxygen species and inflammatory mediators, such as IL-1β, tumor necrosis factor-α (TNF-α), and nitric oxide (NO), which promote inflammatory responses in the CNS and accelerate neuronal death. In the later stage of neuroinflammation, microglia/macrophages that are polarized into the M2 phenotype by the alternative activation pathway can secrete arginase-1, IL-10, and other anti-inflammatory factors. This will inhibit synaptic damage due to excessive inflammation and promote the regeneration of axons. Therefore, regulating the activation status of microglia/macrophages can be a new treatment strategy for VD.

In the CNS, neurotransmission and neuroinflammation are mediated by the cannabinoid signaling system. Cannabinoid receptors include cannabinoid receptor 1 (CB_1R) and cannabinoid receptor 2 (CB_2R). CB_1R is primarily expressed in the CNS and peripheral neuronal tissues and mainly regulates neuropsychological functions, while CB_2R belongs to the Gi/Go G-protein-coupled receptor. CB_2R is mainly expressed in cells associated with innate immunity, such as microglial cells, dendritic cells, and cerebrovascular endothelial cells, and participates in immunoregulation in the brain. In VD animal models, selective agonists of CB_2R can decrease memory impairments and infarction areas in rats caused by insufficient cerebral perfusion and vascular dementia [5]. Similarly, for microglial cells and neurons that are cultured in vitro, endocannabinoids or the CB_2R agonist JWH-015 can decrease lipopolysaccharide (LPS)-induced synthesis of IL-1β, TNF-α and NO [6, 7]. In cultures of mouse cortical microglial cells, activated CB_2R can induce the synthesis of the anti-inflammatory cytokine IL-10, inhibiting the activation of microglial cells and suppressing neuroinflammation [8]. These study results mentioned above suggest that CB_2R activation can aid in converting M1 microglia/macrophages during the recovery phase of cerebral ischemia into the M2 phenotype, thereby decreasing inflammatory responses after cerebral ischemia and promoting the recovery of neurobehavioral functions.

Besides IFN-γ, IL-4, and other classical induction factors, more regulatory factors that induce conversion of microglia/macrophage polarization have been identified recently. As an example, it has been shown that increasing mammalian target of rapamycin (mTOR) activity could significantly increase the survival of microglial cells in an in vitro ischemia/hypoxia model that is deprived of oxygen and glucose. In addition, inducible nitric oxide synthase (iNOS) expression was induced, and this promoted NO synthesis [9]. In contrast, inhibition of mTOR activity can significantly decrease microglia activation in the glucose and oxygen deprivation model, inducing its conversion from the M1 phenotype to an M2 phenotype [10]. At the same time, this ameliorates learning and memory impairments in mice caused by insufficient cerebral perfusion. Furthermore, in microglial cells that have been transfected with interferon regulatory factor 3-overexpressing gene via adenoviruses, up-regulation of the phosphatidylinositol-3-kinase (PI3K)/protein kinase B (PKB/Akt) signaling pathway can similarly mediate the conversion of microglial cells from an M1 phenotype into an M2 phenotype [11]. In mouse microglial cells, β-amyloid can activate nuclear factor-κB (NF-κB) signaling and at the same time reduce PI3K/Akt signaling, leading to down-regulation of mRNA expression of M2 phenotype marker genes [12]. In summary, the results presented above suggest that the mTOR, NF-κB and PI3K/Akt signaling pathways may participate in the conversion of the M1/M2 polarization of microglia/macrophages after CB_2R activation.

Previously, we have established a CB_2R agonist screening system using a combination of PIRES2-EGFP-CB_2R eukaryotic expression plasmid and the luc2P/CRE/Hygro reporter gene [13, 14]. Using this system, we screened more than 100 ingredients and extracts used in the traditional Chinese medicine and found that paeoniflorin (PF) shows the strongest CB_2R stimulation activity. PF, a monoterpene glycoside, is one of the main active ingredients of the traditional Chinese medicine *Paeonia lactiflora* Pall and *Paeonia veitchii* Lynch. Studies in recent years have found that PF can activate the muscarinic acetylcholine receptors [15] and adrenaline receptors [16] to improve spatial recognition as well as learning and memory functions. PF can also elicit analgesic effects by acting on opioid receptors [17]. Several studies have implicated that PF acting through adenosine A_1 receptors decreases infarction caused by acute or chronic cerebral ischemia and alleviates neurobehavioral impairments [18]. Recent studies have also found that PF can significantly improve cognitive impairments in VD rat models by increasing cerebral blood flow and inhibiting the hippocampal neuronal apoptosis and NF-κB-mediated inflammatory signaling pathway [19, 20]. Our previous data also showed that PF could protect hippocampal neurons in rats subjected to cerebral ischemia–reperfusion through activating CB_2R [21]. However, there are no reports so far on whether PF can activate CB_2R to inhibit cerebral ischemia-induced polarization of microglia/macrophages in the hippocampal regions and thus protect adjacent neurons and restore spatial memory and cognitive functions. Therefore, we studied here a four-vessel occlusion (4-VO) rat model to delineate the potential molecular mechanisms by which PF inhibits neuroinflammation and elicits its neuroprotective effects in a CB_2R dependent manner.

Methods

Information of experimental design and resources

The Minimum Standards of Reporting Checklist (Additional file 1) contains details of the experimental design, and statistics, and resources used in this study.

Reagents

Paeoniflorin (> 98% purity) was obtained from Shanghai Daibo Chemical Technology Co., Ltd (Shanghai, China); HU308 (a selective CB_2R agonist) and AM630 (a selective CB_2R antagonist) were obtained from Cayman Chemicals (Ann Arbor, MI, USA). CB_2R antibody was obtained from Thermo Fisher Scientific Inc. (Waltham, MA, USA), NF-κB p65 antibody was obtained from Abcam

Inc (Cambridge, MA, UK), Phospho-Akt (Ser473), Akt, mTOR, Phospho-mTOR (Ser2448) and Phospho-IκBα (Ser32) antibodies were obtained from Cell Signaling Technology Inc. (Beverly, MA, USA), iNOS, CD206, IκBα and lamin B1 antibodies were obtained from Santa Cruz Biotechnology Inc. (Santa Cruz, CA, USA), CD68 antibody was obtained from AbD Serotec (Kidlington, Oxford, UK), Iba1 was from Wako Pure Chemical (Osaka, Tokyo, Japan), and phospho-PI3K p85α (Tyr467)/ phospho-PI3K p55γ (Tyr199), PI3K and β-actin antibodies were obtained from Bioworld Technology Inc. (Minneapolis, MN, USA). An NO assay kit was obtained from Beyotime Institute of Biotechnology (Jiangsu, China).

Animals

Male Sprague–Dawley (SD) rats, weighing 300–400 g, SPF grade, were obtained from the Experimental Animal Research Center of Chongqing Academy of Chinese Materia Medica; Approval No. SCXK (Yu) 2012-0006. All rats were housed in the experimental animal room of the Chongqing Academy of Chinese Materia Medica with free access to food and water, under a 12:12 h light–dark cycle, at a constant environmental temperature of 22–25 °C and a relative humidity of 50–60%. The animals were allowed to acclimatize for 1 week before the experiments. All protocols in this study conformed to the National Institutes of Health guidelines for the Care and Use of Laboratory Animals (8th Edition, 2011), and the use of animals was approved by the animal ethics committee of the Chongqing Academy of Chinese Materia Medica.

Surgery

Rats were subjected to the Morris water maze test, and rats that failed to find the platform within 90 s were excluded. Four-vessel occlusion was carried out in qualified rats according to the method described by Pulsinelli et al. [22, 23]. After the rats were fasted for 24 h, intraperitoneal injections of 45 mg/kg pentobarbital sodium were used to anesthetize the rats. The rats were fixed on the operating station in a prone position and routine skin preparation was carried out. An incision was made in the middle of the neck, and the latissimus dorsi and trapezius muscles were gradually separated. The transverse foramen on the left and right sides of the 1st cervical vertebra was exposed and a 0.5-mm diameter electrocoagulation needle was inserted 1–2 mm into the transverse foramen from the tail end, to cause permanent occlusion of the vertebral arteries. Twenty-four hours later, the rats were re-anesthetized by intraperitoneal injections of 40 mg/kg pentobarbital sodium. The rats were kept at the supine position, and an incision was made in the middle of the neck. Blunt separation was carried out on the common carotid arteries on both sides, and non-invasive microvascular clips were used to clip both common carotid arteries to induce cerebral ischemia. Ten minutes later, the vascular clips were removed to restore the blood flow to the carotid arteries. In order to decrease inter-animal differences, the following conditions had to be strictly met during the 10-min ischemia period and the subsequent 20 ± 5-min comatose stage: loss of righting reflex and dilation of both pupils. During the 6 h after ischemia, the anal temperature of the rats was maintained at 37 ± 0.5 °C. Besides no vertebral artery cauterization on the first day and ischemic treatment of bilateral common carotid arteries on the second day in the sham treatment group, the remaining procedures were identical to those performed in the treatment group.

Animal grouping and drug treatment

One week after surgery, 120 rats of dementia were selected, based on the results from the Morris water maze with the following success criterion: using the mean value of the time taken by sham-operated rats to escape from the maze as a reference value, rats with a ratio of the difference between the escape latency period and the reference value greater than 20% were defined as dementia rats [24, 25]. In addition to the sham-operated group ($n = 24$), successful models were randomly assigned to five groups ($n = 24$): the model group, the PF (40 mg/kg) group (Additional file 2: Figure S1), the PF (40 mg/kg) + AM630 (3 mg/kg) group, the AM630 (3 mg/kg) group, and the HU308 (3 mg/kg) group. All drugs were dissolved in Tween 80 and dimethyl sulfoxide (DMSO), and then was diluted by saline (Tween 80:DMSO:saline = 1:1:18), which was administered intraperitoneally to rats at a volume of 5 ml/kg 15 min after permanent four-vessel occlusion and then with the same dose once a day for 27 successive days. In order to study the role of CB_2R in the neuroprotection and anti-neuroinflammation of PF, a specific CB_2R antagonist AM630 was administered intraperitoneally 15 min prior to the PF administration each time.

Morris water maze

The Morris water maze was provided by Beijing Zhongshidichuang Science and Technology Development Co., Ltd (Beijing, China), and different combinations of experimental apparatus were used to test positioning and navigation as well as spatial exploration abilities. Ten rats were randomly selected from each group for the water maze test. The water maze consisted of a circular pool of a diameter of 130 cm and a height of 50 cm, with a water depth of 30 cm and a water temperature of 26 ± 1 °C. At the walls of the maze, there were four labeled entry spots,

dividing the maze into four quadrants. At the 4th quadrant, a platform with a diameter of 12 cm and a height of 29 cm was placed 1 cm below the water surface. The positioning and navigation experiment mainly tested the learning ability of the rats. On day 24 after drug administration, the rats in each group were placed into the pool at the four different entry points. The time the rats took to find and climb the platform ("escape latency time") within 90 s was recorded, and the rats were continuously observed for 5 days. If the rats were unable to find the platform within 90 s, they were placed on the platform for 15 s and their escape latency period was recorded as 90 s. In addition, spatial exploration experiments were used to test the ability of the rats to remember the location of the platform. On day 5 when the positioning and navigation experiment ended, the platform was removed and the rats were placed into the 4th quadrant, into the water, facing the wall. The number of times that the rats crossed the original location of the platform within 120 s and the percentage of swimming routes within the 4th quadrant (relative to the total route) were recorded.

Histopathological analysis

On the day after the water maze experiment ended, six rats were selected from each group and 45 mg/kg pentobarbital sodium was administered for anesthesia by intraperitoneal injection. Cardiac perfusion of 150 ml physiological saline was administered and 100 ml of 4% paraformaldehyde was used for fixation before the brains were extracted. A 3-mm-thick tissue block behind the optic chiasm was extracted and routine paraffin embedding was carried out. Continuous coronal sections (4 μm thick) were cut using a microtome (Leica Microsystems, Wetzlar, Germany) and stained with conventional hematoxylin and eosin (HE) staining. An Olympus BX51 light microscope was used to observe morphological and structural changes in the hippocampal CA1 region. The extent of the neuronal damage was quantified by counting the number of intact pyramidal neurons in the hippocampal CA1 area, which was expressed as a neuronal cell density.

Electron microscopy observations

After rats in each group were anesthetized by intraperitoneal injection of 45 mg/kg pentobarbital sodium, 100 ml physiological saline was rapidly perfused into the left ventricular aorta. Then ice-cold fixing solution (4% paraformaldehyde in phosphate buffered saline; PBS) was perfused for 30 min. A sharp blade was used to rapidly resect the left hippocampal CA1 region and slice it into $1 \times 1 \times 1$ mm^3 hippocampal blocks. The blocks were immersed in 2.5% glutaraldehyde solution for 24 h. After that, 0.1 M PBS was used to wash the tissue blocks, and then 1% osmic acid was used for 1 h of fixation. An alcohol gradient was used for dehydration and the block was embedded in epoxy resin 618. After positioning and embedding of semithin sections, an ultramicrotome was used to process the slices into 60-nm ultrathin sections. The sections were collected in a polyvinyl formal-coated copper grid. Double staining with uranyl acetate and lead citrate was carried out. The ultrastructure of the hippocampal CA1 region of rats was observed under an H-7500 transmission electron microscopy (Hitachi, Tokyo, Japan) at 15,000× magnification.

Enzyme-linked immunoassay (ELISA)

Six rats were selected from each group and rapidly decapitated for brain extraction. The hippocampus was rapidly isolated in an ice bath and blood was washed off the tissue surface using a 4 °C pre-cooled physiological saline. After blotting dry, the hippocampus was weighed and 4 °C pre-cooled physiological saline was added. An electric homogenizer was used to generate hippocampal homogenates with a 10% mass fraction. The homogenates were centrifuged at 3000 rpm for 10 min, and the supernatant was collected for assay. IL-1β, IL-6 and TNF-α concentrations in rat hippocampal tissues were measured using ELISA test kits (Shanghai JiJin Chemistry Technology Co. Ltd., Shanghai, China) following the manufacturer's instructions. The detection limits for IL-1β, IL-6, and TNF-α were 0.1, 1 and 1 pg/ml, respectively. The concentration of each sample was calculated according to the corresponding standard curve and normalized to the protein concentration of the sample. The final unit used was pg/mg protein. Protein concentrations of the tissues were quantitated according to the bicinchoninic acid (BCA) assay kit (Beyotime). This method was used for subsequent protein concentration determination.

Quantitation of nitrite concentrations

The NO concentration of rat hippocampal homogenates was indirectly measured by using the Griess reagent to measure the NO metabolite, nitrite (NO_2^-). The specific steps were as follows: 50 μl hippocampal homogenate and 50 μl Griess reagent (1% sulfanilamide, 0.1% N-[1-naphthyl-ethylenediamine dihydrochloride] and 0.1 M HCl) were allowed to react. Subsequently, a microplate reader (Thermo Electron Co., Waltham, MA, USA) was used to measure the optical density (OD) at 540 nm wavelength. The NO_2^- concentration of the sample was calculated by plotting a standard $NaNO_2$ curve (1–100 μM), and the unit used was nmol/g tissue.

Western blotting analysis

Hippocampal specimens (30–50 mg) were removed from the −80 °C freezer and 150–250 μl protein lysis buffer (Beyotime) and protease inhibitors (Roche Applied Science, Indianapolis, IN, USA) were added. The specimens were homogenized on ice and lysed for 30 min. In addition, nuclear lysates from tissues were obtained using the nuclear extraction kit (Pierce Biotechnology, Rockford, IL, USA). Equivalent amounts of protein samples (30 μg) were loaded on a 10–15% (w/v) SDS-PAGE for electrophoretic separation. The proteins in the gel were then transferred onto a polyvinylidene difluoride (PVDF; Millipore, Bedford, MA, USA) membrane and the membrane was blocked with 5% skim milk in Tris-buffered saline (TBS) containing 0.1% Tween 20 (TBS-T) at room temperature for 1 h. Subsequently, corresponding primary antibodies were added for incubation overnight at 4 °C. After washing thrice with TBS-T, the membranes were incubated at room temperature with anti-rabbit or anti-mouse secondary antibodies (Bioworld Technology) that were conjugated to horseradish peroxidase at a dilution of 1:10,000. The membranes were washed four times with TBS-T and visualized using enhanced chemiluminescence (ECL; Millipore). Images were obtained using the Amersham Imager 600 (GE Healthcare Biosciences, Little Chalfont, UK). The Quantity One software (Bio-Rad, Hercules, CA, USA) was used to analyze the integrated absorbance value of every band, with β-actin and lamin B1 being used as reference proteins for loading control in total cell lysates and nuclear extracts, respectively. The ratio of the integrated absorbance value of the target band in the sham-operated group and the reference protein band was set as 1. The ratio of the integrated absorbance value of target band in the different treatment groups and the reference protein band were compared to obtain the relative expression level of target proteins in each group.

RNA reverse transcription and quantitative polymerase chain reaction (RT-qPCR)

Six rats were selected from each group and rapidly decapitated, and their hippocampi were rapidly isolated in an ice bath. Total RNA from the rat hippocampus was extracted using the RNApure high-purity total RNA rapid extraction kit (spin-column, BioTeke, Beijing, China) following the manufacturer's instructions. Of the total RNA, 2 μg was used as a template, and Oligo (dT) was used as a primer with M-MuLV reverse transcriptase (BioTeke) in a 20 μl reaction system for reverse transcription to obtain cDNA. The cDNA was added into the SYBR FAST qPCR Master Mix (Kapa Biosystems, Woburn, MA, USA), together with primers for real-time quantitative PCR. Table 1 shows the primer sequences for rat CB_2R, IL-1β, IL-6, TNF-α, IL-10, arginase-1, Ym1, TGF-β1 and β-actin. Representative cDNAs for various groups were mixed and a 5-fold dilution method

Table 1 Primer sequences used for quantitative real-time PCR amplification

Gene	Forward primer (5'–3')	Reverse primer (5'–3')	Product length (bp)
CB$_2$R	ACCTATGTCTGTGCTACCCACC	CCAGCCCAGGAGGTAGTCG	188
iNOS	AGTGGCAACATCAGGTCGG	CGATGCACAACTGGGTGAAC	166
IL-1β	ATGACCTGTTCTTTGAGGCTGAC	CGAGATGCTGCTGTGAGATTTG	114
TNF-α	GCCACCACGCTCTTCTGTC	GCTACGGGCTTGTCACTCG	149
IL-6	GTTGCCTTCTTGGGACTGATG	GCCATTGCACAACTCTTTTCTC	183
IL-10	GTTTTACCTGGTAGAAGTGATGCC	CCACTGCCTTGCTTTTATTCTC	155
Arginase-1	GGGAAAAGCCAATGAACAGC	CCAAATGACGCATAGGTCAGG	148
Ym1	TTGGAGGCTGGAAGTTTGG	AGGAGGGCTTCCACGAGAC	161
TGF-β1	GGCGGTGCTCGCTTTGTA	ATTGCGTTGTTGCGGTCC	135
β-Actin	CCCATCTATGAGGGTTACGC	TTTAATGTCACGCACGATTTC	150

was used to plot a standard curve to examine the qPCR amplification efficiency. The threshold cycle (Ct) is the number of the cycle in which the fluorescence signal becomes detectable above background. The Ct value is inversely proportional to the original template number. The comparative Ct method ($2^{-\Delta\Delta Ct}$) was used for comparison of relative mRNA levels in different groups. Here, the ΔCt value represents the difference in Ct between the target genes in different groups and that of the internal reference gene β-actin. Subsequently, the ΔCt values in each treatment group were subtracted from those in the sham-operated group to obtain ΔΔCt.

Immunofluorescence

After rats were decapitated, their brains were extracted and fixed in 4% paraformaldehyde at 4 °C for 24 h. The brains were then immersed in 30% sucrose solution overnight. Three-mm-thick tissue blocks in front of and behind the optic chiasm were extracted and cut into 14 μm thick cryosections. Subsequently, the sections were rinsed with PBS four times for 5 min each time. Then 10% goat serum was added for blocking at 37 °C for 1 h. In order to carry out staining with double fluorescence markers, the sections were co-incubated with mouse anti-CD68 monoclonal antibody and goat anti-CD206 polyclonal antibody (both 1:100 dilution) at 4 °C overnight. Subsequently, sections were further incubated with FITC-labeled goat anti-mouse and TRITC-labeled rabbit anti-goat IgG (both at a 1:100 dilution; Beijing Zhongshan Golden Bridge Biotechnology Co., Ltd., Beijing, China) at 37 °C for 1.5 h. After sufficient washing, in order to visualize cell nucleus, DAPI (Sigma Chemical Company, St. Louis, MO, USA) was added for nuclear staining for 10 min. Finally, stained sections were scanned and photographed with an A$_1$R confocal laser scanning microscope (Nikon Instruments, Melville, Japan).

Statistical analysis

Experimental data were collected and presented as mean ± standard deviation (SD). Two-way analysis of variance (ANOVA) was applied to compare the length of the escape latency period of rats. One-way ANOVA was used for intergroup comparisons of continuous variables. If the statistical analysis showed that differences between multiple groups were significant, Fisher's least significant difference (LSD) post hoc analysis was employed for comparison of differences between two groups. All statistical analyses were carried out with SPSS version 19.0 software (IBM, Chicago, IL, USA), and a $P < 0.05$ was considered to be statistically significant.

Results

Influence of PF on behavior of the VD rat model

Learning and memory deficits constitute some of the most injurious symptoms of VD. In behavioral research, the Morris water maze task is widely used for testing spatial learning and memory abilities in a VD rat model [26]. In the present study, rats in each group were subjected to the spatial navigation task at 24–28 days after 4-VO (Fig. 1A) and showed decreased escape latencies over time, indicating that spatial learning and memory abilities improved with the prolong of training time. The escape latency of rats in the 4-VO model group was significantly longer than that in the sham operation group at each point during the training, indicating that the spatial learning ability of rats in the model group was severely impaired. However, compared with the model group, after the administration of PF or CB$_2$R selective agonist HU308, the escape latency of rats in the model group was significantly shortened, and the reduction was most prominent from the 3rd to the 5th day of the training, demonstrating that PF and HU308 can significantly improve learning and memory abilities in rats following 4-VO. Compared with the PF group, the CB$_2$R

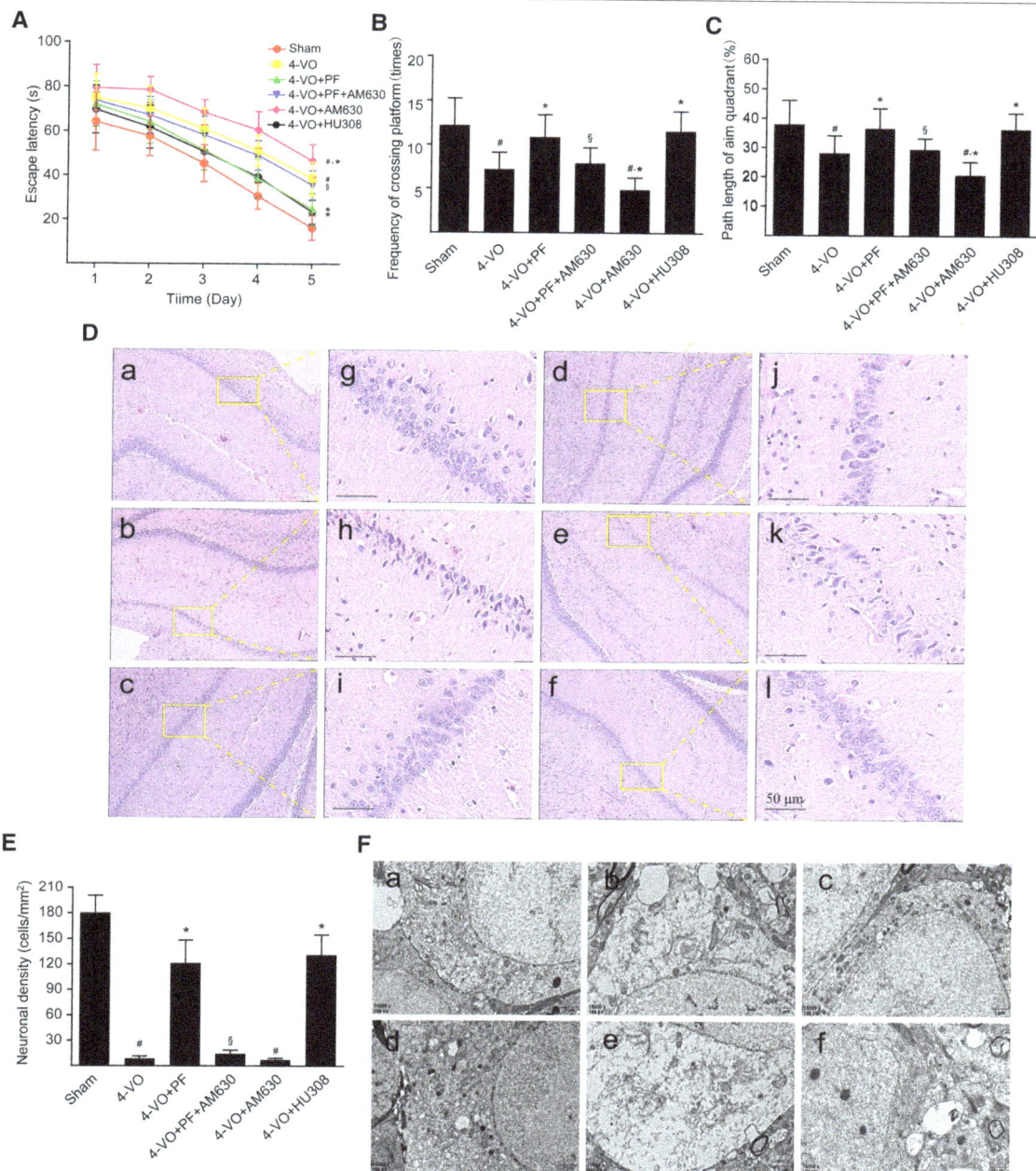

Fig. 1 Effects of paeoniflorin on learning and memory abilities, histopathology and ultrastructure of the hippocampal CA1 area of rats after cerebral ischemia. One week after four-vessel occlusion (4-VO) surgery, rats were intraperitoneally administered saline (4-VO), paeoniflorin (4-VO+PF; 40 mg/kg/day), paeoniflorin+AM630 (4-VO+PF+AM630; 40 + 3 mg/kg/day), AM630 (4-VO+AM630; 3 mg/kg/day) or HU308 (4-VO+HU308; 3 mg/kg/day) for consecutive 28 days. Sham-operated group (Sham) was performed using the same surgical procedures, except that vertebral artery and bilateral common carotid arteries were not occluded. **A** Mean escape latency of rats in the water maze task was recorded during the last 5 days (23–28 days) of treatment. The spatial probe trial was performed on the last day (day 28) of water maze training, and the parameters measured included (**B**) the number of times rats crossed the platform and (**C**) relative path length in the target quadrant/path length in the whole pool within 120 s. **D** Rats were sacrificed after 28 days consecutive drug treatment. Representative photomicrographs of hematoxylin–eosin-stained hippocampal regions of rats are shown in different groups: (**a**, **g**) sham-operated group, (**b**, **h**) 4-VO-operated group, (**c**, **i**) 4-VO+PF group, (**d**, **j**) 4-VO+PF+AM630 group, (**e**, **k**) 4-VO+AM630 group or (**f**, **l**) 4-VO+HU308 group. Boxed regions in **a–f** are shown in **j–l**, respectively. Scale bar: 50 μm. **E** Neuronal cell density in CA1 region was measured by hematoxylin–eosin staining and cell counting. **F** Representative photomicrographs with a transmission electron microscope showing ultrastructural changes in hippocampus CA1 regions of rats in each group. Scale bar: 1 μm. Each bar represents mean ± SD of three independent experiments. $n = 6$ or 10 rats per group. $^{\#}P < 0.05$ versus sham group, $^{*}P < 0.05$ versus 4-VO model group, $^{\S}P < 0.05$ versus 4-VO+PF group

selective antagonist AM630 strikingly attenuated PF-induced decrease in escape latencies. Meanwhile, 4-VO rats treated with AM630 alone exhibited escape latencies even more prolonged than those seen in untreated 4-VO rats. Altogether, these results indicate that PF improves spatial learning and memory abilities in the 4-VO rat model of VD via the activation of CB_2R.

When subjected to the spatial recognition test on the 28th day after surgery, 4-VO rats crossed the platform significantly fewer times and spent a significantly smaller percentage of their total path length swimming in the fourth target quadrant than did rats in the sham operation group (Fig. 1B, C), demonstrating that 4-VO rats had significantly impaired spatial memory. However, following treatment with PF or HU308, the number of times 4-VO rats crossed the platform and the percentage of their total path length spent swimming in the platform quadrant increased significantly, and this effect of PF was blocked when combined with AM630 treatment. When 4-VO rats received only AM630, they showed an even further reduction in the number of times of crossing the platform and spent an even smaller percentage of their total swimming path in the fourth target quadrant than did the untreated 4-VO rats. Taken together, these findings indicate that PF exerts a protective effect on spatial memory abilities in this rat model of VD and that this effect occurs via the activation of CB_2R.

Effects of PF on histopathology and ultrastructure of the hippocampal CA1 area after ischemia

The hippocampal CA1 region is closely associated with high-level cognitive functions, including learning and memory and is an area of the brain that is sensitive to ischemia [27]. Histopathological study with HE staining showed a large number of neurons with high density in the hippocampal CA1 region in the brain subjected to sham-operation. These neurons had abundant cytoplasm and large round nuclei with regular shapes (Fig. 1D [a, g]). In contrast, HE staining in 4-VO rats showed a significantly reduced number of pyramidal neurons in the hippocampal CA1 region (Fig. 1E), and most neurons had smaller cell bodies, a disordered arrangement, strongly stained eosinophilic cytoplasms, and irregular triangle-shaped and polygon-shaped nuclei (Fig. 1D [b, h]). Administration of PF (Fig. 1D [c, i] or HU308 (Fig. 1D [f, l]) preserved the normal structure of neurons in the hippocampal CA1 region and prevented the loss of nerve fibers. This protective effect of PF was blocked when 4-VO rats received AM630 in addition to PF (Fig. 1D [d, j]). Further, treatment with AM630 alone further decreased the number of neurons and nerve fibers compared with that in the untreated 4-VO group, and most neurons in these AM630-treated rats were smaller and

exhibited strongly stained cytoplasm and irregular and darkly stained nuclei (Fig. 1D [e, k]). The histopathological changes in entorhinal cortex was well in agreement with those in the hippocampal CA1 region of rats (Additional file 3: Figure S2).

Transmission electron microscope imaging showed, in the sham group, the ultrastructure of hippocampal CA1 neurons was intact and clear; the nuclei were round and had a uniform distribution of chromatin and obvious nucleoli; the cytoplasm contained abundant organelles with clear structures; and the mitochondria could be clearly identified (Fig. 1F [a]). In contrast, CA1 in 4-VO rats had distended neuronal cell bodies, enlarged surrounding spaces, a reduced number of organelles surrounding the nucleus and otherwise generally disintegrated organelles. Specifically, the mitochondria appeared as swollen structures with both large vacuoles, and their cristae were disrupted and even disappeared (Fig. 1F [b]). Conversely, in 4-VO rats that received treatment with PF or HU308, the hippocampal CA1 neurons had a relatively intact and clear structure in which the chromatin was distributed evenly, the organelles in the cytoplasm were abundant, the mitochondrial membrane was largely intact, the mitochondria cristae were clear, and the endoplasmic reticulum was neatly arranged (Fig. 1F [c, f]). In these neurons, a small amount of chromatin condensation was occasionally observed, and only a few mitochondria were slightly swollen. However, when 4-VO rats were treated with both PF and AM630, the beneficial effects of PF were lost; the hippocampal CA1 neuronal ultrastructures lost integrity; and the area became disordered again, similar to that seen in untreated 4-VO rats (Fig. 1F [d]). Further, in 4-VO rats that received AM630 alone, the degrees of neuronal swelling, morphological damage, and structural disorder were exacerbated compared with those in the untreated 4-VO group (Fig. 1F [e]). Altogether, these results indicate that PF exerts a neuroprotective effect by alleviating neuropathological changes in the hippocampal CA1 region in a rat model of VD through the activation of CB_2R.

Effect of PF on CB_2R expression and M1/M2 polarization markers in microglia/macrophages in the ischemic hippocampus

In ischemic brain tissue, activated microglia/macrophages are the primary participants in the neuro-inflammatory response [28]. After cerebral ischemia, persistent inflammation in the brain can further aggravate neuronal injury. However, at the late phase of cerebral ischemia, microglia/macrophages undergo a phenotypic transition, adopting either an M1 or an M2 phenotype, which exert different physiological functions

[29]. To examine whether PF can induce microglia/ macrophages to transition from the proinflammatory M1 phenotype into the anti-inflammatory M2 phenotype by promoting CB_2R expression, thereby reducing the inflammatory damage to peripheral neurons in a rat model of VD, we first measured the mRNA and protein expression levels of CB_2R in the ischemic hippocampus, based on both RT-qPCR (Fig. 2a) and Western blotting (Fig. 2b, c) studies. The results showed compared with the sham operation group, hippocampal CB_2R mRNA and protein expression levels were slightly elevated in rats of the 4-VO group. These methods also revealed that 4-VO rats that received PF showed even further increase in the expression of CB_2R mRNA and protein, similar to that seen with HU308 treatment. Compared with the PF treatment alone, 4-VO rats that also received AM630 showed significantly reduced CB_2R mRNA and protein levels, indicating that the CB_2R antagonist AM630 significantly inhibits PF-mediated up-regulation of CB_2R expression. Finally, 4-VO rats treated with AM630 alone showed significantly reduced CB_2R mRNA and protein expression compared with untreated 4-VO rats. In addition, we also found that the density of Iba1^{+} cells per field in the ischemic hippocampi was significantly reduced in PF or HU308 treatment group compared with that in the 4-VO model group (Additional file 4: Figure S3). These results suggest that PF treatment suppresses the activation of microglia/macrophages in vivo.

Next, immunofluorescence double labeling was performed with M1 marker CD68 and M2 marker CD206 to evaluate the phenotypic polarization of microglia/macrophages in the ischemic hippocampus [28]. The results of this staining were consistent with the trend found for the expression of the CB_2R. Specifically, compared with the sham operation group, the numbers of CD68-positive and CD206-positive microglia/macrophages in the hippocampal CA1 region of the 4-VO group both increased significantly (Fig. 2d). These two types of marker proteins co-localized on microglia/macrophages, suggesting that at later stages of ischemia some microglia/macrophages in the hippocampal CA1 region were undergoing the protective M1–M2 polarity transition response. However, treatment with either PF or HU308 further induced the M2 transition of hippocampal CA1 microglia/macrophages, visible as a reduced expression of the M1 marker (CD68) and a further increased expression of the M2 marker (CD206). When PF treatment was combined with AM630 in 4-VO rats, the PF-induced M2 transition of microglia/macrophages was blocked, and in 4-VO rats treated with AM630 alone, most microglia/macrophages in the hippocampal CA1 area were of the proinflammatory M1 phenotype, while the anti-inflammatory M2 marker (CD206) was hardly detectable. Altogether, these

results suggest that PF induces microglia/macrophage polarization to an anti-inflammatory M2 phenotype in the hippocampus by up-regulating CB_2R expression in a rat model of VD.

Effect of PF on expression products of microglia/macrophages in the hippocampus after ischemia

After the ischemic injury, microglia/macrophages exhibit dynamic polarization over time, switching from the phenotype of alternatively activated M2 macrophages to an M1 profile [30]. M1-like microglia/macrophages mainly express proinflammatory proteins such as iNOS, IL-1β, TNF-α and IL-6, while M2-like microglia/macrophages mainly express anti-inflammatory proteins such as IL-10, arginase-1, TGF-β1 and Ym1. Compared with the sham operation group, the mRNA (Fig. 3a) and protein (Fig. 3b) levels of M1 expression products, including IL-1β, TNF-α and IL-6, were significantly increased in the hippocampal homogenate of the 4-VO group. Further, levels of the iNOS protein (Fig. 3c, d), a rate-limiting enzyme, and its inflammatory product, NO (Fig. 3e), were significantly increased in the hippocampal homogenate. Additionally, a significant induction of the M2-associated cytokines (IL-10 and TGF-β1) and M2-associated cell surface markers (arginase-1 and Ym1) was also found (Fig. 3f). Specifically, our data show that PF or HU308 markedly decreased the levels of IL-1β, TNF-α, IL-6, iNOS and NO, emphasizing the anti-inflammatory role of PF or HU308 in ischemic injury by inhibiting M1-microglia/macrophage polarization. On the other hand, the mRNA levels of IL-10, arginase-1, TGF-β1 and Ym1 were further increased by treatment with either PF or HU308. Treatment with PF and AM630 together blocked the effects of PF on microglia/macrophage M1/M2 polarization. Further, treatment with AM630 alone further increase proinflammatory mediator expression and NO production in the hippocampi of 4-VO rats compared with that seen in untreated 4-VO rats, but showed little effect on mRNA expression of anti-inflammatory products. Taken together, the above results suggest that PF attenuates the M1 phenotype and promotes M2 microglia/macrophage polarization by inducing CB_2R expression.

Effect of PF on the mTOR/NF-κB signaling pathway in the ischemic hippocampus

During the neuroinflammatory response, phosphorylated and activated mTOR induces phosphorylation and degradation of IκBα, leading to nuclear translocation of NF-κB and activation of the NF-κB signaling pathway [31]. Through this process, mTOR mediated the transcription of its regulated M1-associated genes and accelerates the process of neuroinflammation. Western blot analysis of hippocampal tissue showed that, compared with

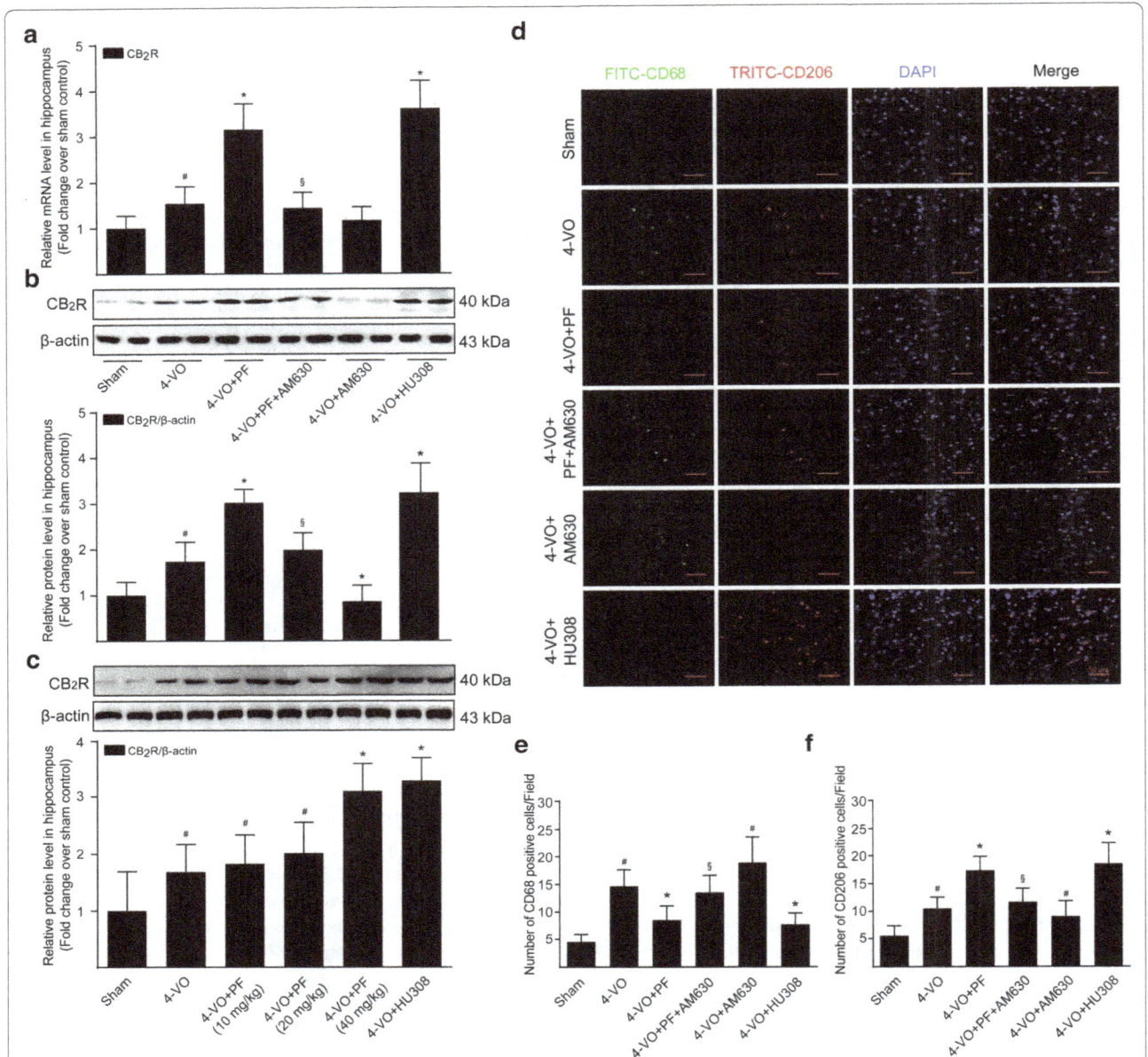

Fig. 2 Effects of paeoniflorin on the expression of CB_2R and M1/M2 polarization markers in microglia/macrophage in hippocampi of rats after cerebral ischemia. After 28 days consecutive drug treatment, **a** real-time quantitative PCR analysis of the mRNA level of CB_2R in the hippocampus tissues of rats from different groups: sham (sham operated), 4-VO (four-vessel occlusion operated), 4-VO+PF (four-vessel occlusion operated plus paeoniflorin 40 mg/kg/day), 4-VO+PF+AM630 (four-vessel occlusion operated plus paeoniflorin 40 mg/kg/day and AM630 3 mg/kg/day), 4-VO+AM630 (four-vessel occlusion operated plus AM630 3 mg/kg/day) or 4-VO+HU308 (four-vessel occlusion operated plus HU308 3 mg/kg/day). **b** Proteins were extracted from hippocampi of rats and subjected to Western blotting analysis using primary antibody specific for CB_2R. Blots were stripped and re-probed with antibody against β-actin to correct for differences in protein loading. Fold-change in the relative level of CB_2R protein is shown after normalizing with β-actin. **c** CB_2R protein level in hippocampi of rats was analyzed by Western blotting from different groups: sham (sham operated), 4-VO (four-vessel occlusion operated), 4-VO+PF (four-vessel occlusion operated plus paeoniflorin 10, 20, 40 mg/kg/day) or 4-VO+HU308 (four-vessel occlusion operated plus HU308 3 mg/kg/day). **d** Hippocampus tissue sections were co-stained for CD68 (M1 marker; green) or CD206 (M2 marker; red) and DAPI (blue). The images were observed and captured by a confocal laser scanning microscope. Scale bar: 50 μm. **e, f** Quantitative analysis of the number of CD68-positive and CD206-positive cells per visual field in the hippocampal CA1 region of rats. Each bar represents mean ± SD of three independent experiments. $n = 6$ rats per group. #$P < 0.05$ versus sham group, *$P < 0.05$ versus 4-VO model group, §$P < 0.05$ versus 4-VO+PF group

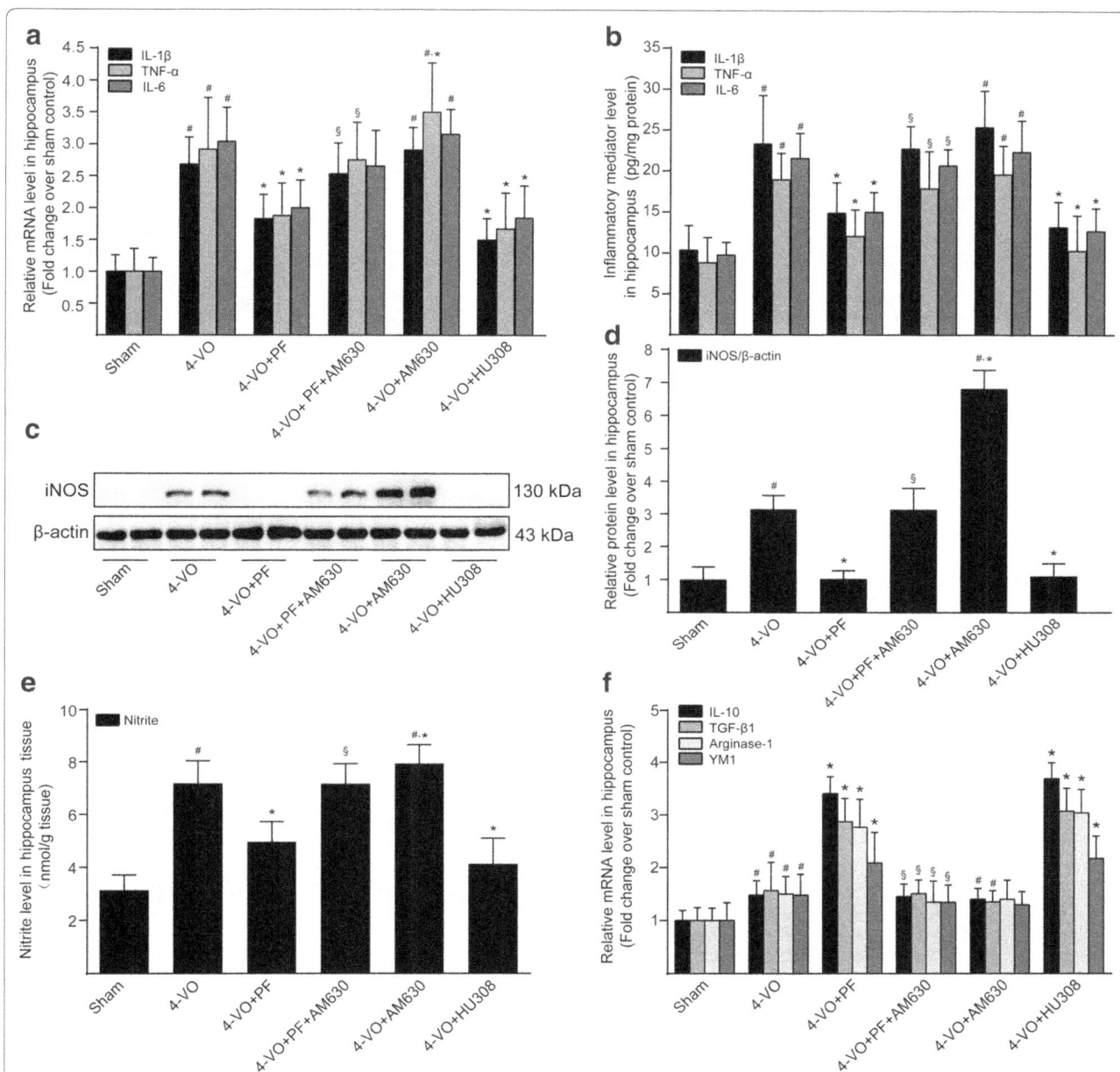

Fig. 3 Effects of paeoniflorin on expression products of microglia/macrophage in hippocampi of rats after cerebral ischemia. One week after four-vessel occlusion (4-VO) surgery, rats were intraperitoneally administered saline (4-VO), paeoniflorin (4-VO+PF; 40 mg/kg/day), paeoniflorin+AM630 (4-VO+PF+AM630; 40 + 3 mg/kg/day), AM630 (4-VO+AM630; 3 mg/kg/day) or HU308 (4-VO+HU308; 3 mg/kg/day) for consecutive 28 days. **a** After treatment, real-time quantitative PCR analysis and **b** ELISA were used to detect the mRNA and protein levels of the proinflammatory cytokines IL-1β, TNF-α and IL-6, respectively. **c** Western blotting analysis was performed to further detect iNOS protein expression level. β-Actin served as an internal control. **d** The protein level of iNOS was expressed as arbitrary densitometric unit and normalized by the value of β-actin and finally expressed relative to the protein level in the sham-operated group (defined as 1-fold). **e** The content of nitrite in the hippocampus tissues of rats were determined by the Griess reaction. **f** Real-time quantitative PCR analysis was used to detect the mRNA levels of the anti-inflammatory cytokines IL-10 and TGF-β1; and the M2-associated markers arginase-1 and Ym1. Each bar represents mean ± SD of three independent experiments. $n = 6$ rats per group. [#]$P < 0.05$ versus sham group, [*]$P < 0.05$ versus 4-VO model group, [§]$P < 0.05$ versus 4-VO+PF group

the sham operation group, 4-VO rats had significantly increased phosphorylation of mTOR (Fig. 4a, b) and IκBα (Fig. 4a, c) in cytoplasmic extracts and NF-κB p65

(Fig. 4a, d) in nuclear extracts, and they had significantly reduced expression of IκBα (Fig. 4a, c) in cytoplasmic extracts. Compared with untreated 4-VO rats, treatment

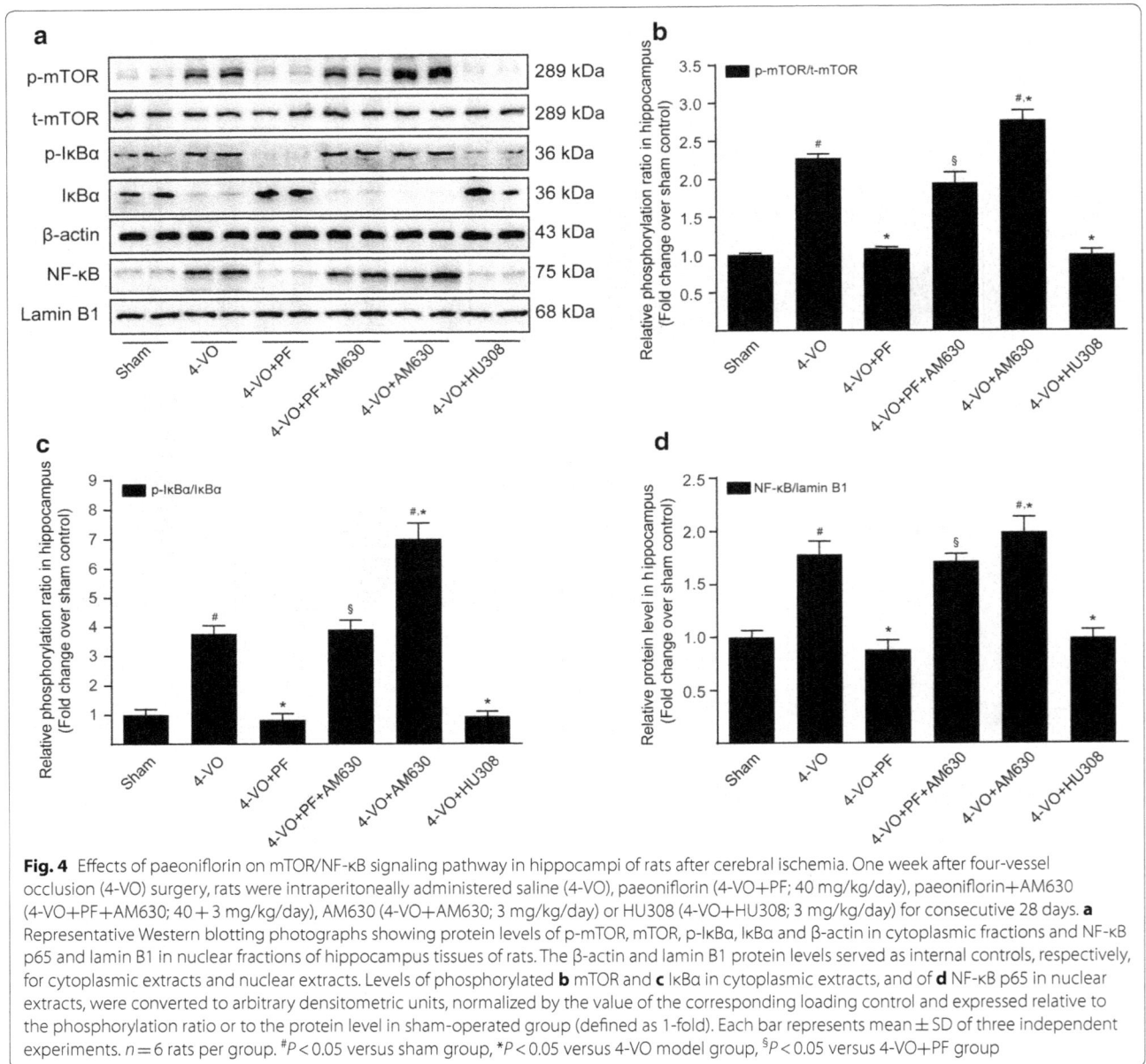

Fig. 4 Effects of paeoniflorin on mTOR/NF-κB signaling pathway in hippocampi of rats after cerebral ischemia. One week after four-vessel occlusion (4-VO) surgery, rats were intraperitoneally administered saline (4-VO), paeoniflorin (4-VO+PF; 40 mg/kg/day), paeoniflorin+AM630 (4-VO+PF+AM630; 40 + 3 mg/kg/day), AM630 (4-VO+AM630; 3 mg/kg/day) or HU308 (4-VO+HU308; 3 mg/kg/day) for consecutive 28 days. **a** Representative Western blotting photographs showing protein levels of p-mTOR, mTOR, p-IκBα, IκBα and β-actin in cytoplasmic fractions and NF-κB p65 and lamin B1 in nuclear fractions of hippocampus tissues of rats. The β-actin and lamin B1 protein levels served as internal controls, respectively, for cytoplasmic extracts and nuclear extracts. Levels of phosphorylated **b** mTOR and **c** IκBα in cytoplasmic extracts, and of **d** NF-κB p65 in nuclear extracts, were converted to arbitrary densitometric units, normalized by the value of the corresponding loading control and expressed relative to the phosphorylation ratio or to the protein level in sham-operated group (defined as 1-fold). Each bar represents mean ± SD of three independent experiments. $n = 6$ rats per group. [#]$P < 0.05$ versus sham group, [*]$P < 0.05$ versus 4-VO model group, [§]$P < 0.05$ versus 4-VO+PF group

with either PF or HU308 significantly reduced hippocampal levels of p-mTOR and p-IκBα protein in cytoplasmic extracts and of NF-κB p65 protein in nuclear extracts, and at the same time increased levels of IκBα in the cytoplasm. Treatment with both AM630 and PF together in 4-VO rats blocked effects seen with PF treatment alone, while treatment with AM630 alone in 4-VO rats further increased the expression levels of p-mTOR and p-IκBα protein in cytoplasmic extracts of the hippocampus, accelerated degradation of IκBα, and increased levels of NF-κB p65 protein in nuclear extracts. Altogether, these results indicate that PF blocks the mTOR-regulated

NF-κB signaling pathway by activating expression of the CB$_2$R in microglia/macrophages, and thereby inhibits the nuclear translocation of NF-κB and, ultimately, the transcription of M1-related inflammatory products.

Effect of PF on the PI3K/Akt signaling pathway in the ischemic hippocampus

Accumulative evidence suggests activation of the PI3K/Akt signaling pathway is involved in microglia/macrophage M2 polarization [32]. To evaluate whether PF alters M2-associated gene expression by increasing phosphorylation and activation of PI3K/Akt, hippocampus tissue lysates were prepared and subjected to Western blotting analysis using antibodies specific for PI3K and Akt, and their phosphorylated forms. The results showed that the phosphorylated levels of PI3K and Akt in the hippocampi of 4-VO rats were significantly higher than those in the sham-operated control (Fig. 5a, b). After treatment with either PF or HU308, the phosphorylation of PI3K and Akt in the hippocampus was further increased, whereas this effect of PF could be attenuated by combined treatment with AM630. Notably, 4-VO rats treated with AM630 alone did not show significantly

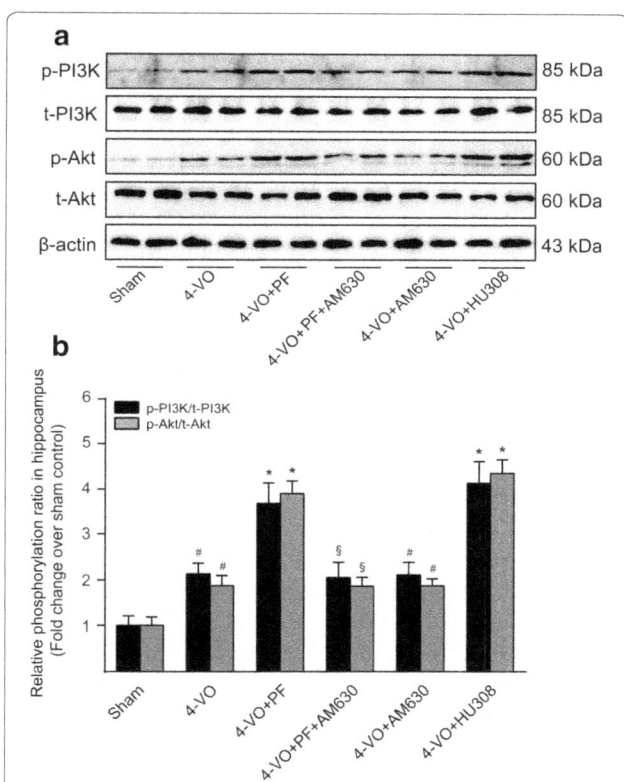

different levels of phosphorylated PI3K and Akt in the hippocampus than that seen in the untreated 4-VO group. In all cases, total PI3K and Akt protein levels did not change greatly. These results indicate that that PF activates the PI3K/Akt signaling pathway and induces transition to the anti-inflammatory M2 phenotype by up-regulating CB_2R expression in microglia/macrophages.

Discussion

Microglia/macrophage-mediated neuroinflammation is a common component of neurodegenerative disorders, including Alzheimer's disease, Parkinson's disease, multiple sclerosis and VD. Chronic activation of microglia/macrophages often occurs during early stages of these CNS inflammatory diseases. Recent studies have found that sustained activation of microglia/macrophages is not simply the result of neuropathological changes, but rather is an active contributor to these changes, as activated microglia/macrophages (M1 phenotype) can synthesize and secrete large amounts of reactive oxygen and nitrogen species, proinflammatory cytokines (e.g., IL-1, IL-6, TNF-α and NO) and proteases, can damage neuronal cells, and can participate in the progression of chronic neurodegenerative diseases [33]. In addition, when the CNS is affected by certain pathological changes, such as ischemia and inflammation, an alternatively activated M2 program is initiated. Alternative activated microglia/macrophages (M2 type) can exert functions of phagocytosis, remove damaged cell debris, and secrete neurotrophic factors and anti-inflammatory mediators (e.g., IL-10, TGF-β and brain-derived neurotrophic factor), thus playing dual roles of anti-inflammation and neuroprotection [34]. Therefore, from a therapeutic perspective, simply inhibiting all microglia/macrophage activity is not the best therapeutic option in VD. Selectively blocking the proinflammatory effects of microglia/macrophages and simultaneously inducing their transition to the phenotype of neuroprotection and regeneration may have more profound therapeutic effects.

CB_2R plays a key role in the regulation of inflammation and autoimmune diseases [35, 36]. Previous studies in primary rat cell cultures have reported that activation of CB_2R can obviously inhibit the LPS-induced transition of microglia to the M1 phenotype and thereby prevent M1-mediated inflammatory responses [37]. Further, in an animal model of VD, the selective activation of CB_2R improves memory deficit and infarct size in chronic brain hypoperfusion [38]. In support of these reports, our findings demonstrated that in the VD model rats which received either PF or a specific pharmacological CB_2R agonist HU308, hippocampal CB_2R mRNA and protein expression levels in 4-VO rats at the recovery stage of ischemia were further increased compared with

Fig. 5 Effects of paeoniflorin on PI3K/Akt signaling pathway in hippocampi of rats after cerebral ischemia. One week after four-vessel occlusion (4-VO) surgery, rats were intraperitoneally administered saline (4-VO), paeoniflorin (4-VO+PF; 40 mg/kg/day), paeoniflorin+AM630 (4-VO+PF+AM630; 40 + 3 mg/kg/day), AM630 (4-VO+AM630; 3 mg/kg/day) or HU308 (4-VO+HU308; 3 mg/kg/day) for consecutive 28 days. **a** After treatment, whole tissue lysates of hippocampus were prepared and subjected to Western blotting analysis using antibodies specific for phosphorylated forms or all forms of PI3K and Akt. β-Actin was used as a loading control. **b** The protein levels of phosphorylated PI3K and Akt were converted to arbitrary densitometricunits, normalized by the value of the corresponding total protein level and expressed relative to the phosphorylation ratio in sham-operated rats (defined as 1-fold). Each bar represents mean ± SD of three independent experiments. $n = 6$ rats per group. #$P < 0.05$ versus sham group, *$P < 0.05$ versus 4-VO model group, §$P < 0.05$ versus 4-VO+PF group

that in the untreated 4-VO group. More importantly, PF or HU308 could also suppress the M1 proinflammatory microglia/macrophage phenotype while enhance the M2 repair phenotype, characterized by lower production of IL-1, IL-6, TNF-α and iNOS, higher expression of TGF-β1 and IL-10 and had slighter damage to hippocampal neurons and nerve fibers, thereby exhibiting anti-inflammatory and neuroprotective effects in the hippocampus of rats. The M1–M2 transition of microglia/macrophages regulated by PF could be blocked by a selective CB$_2$R antagonist AM630. Taken together, the above results suggest that PF could antagonize toxic M1 responses and enhance protective M2 responses in microglia/macrophages following cerebral ischemia by activating CB$_2$R and simultaneously by up-regulating CB$_2$R expression, thereby protecting neighboring neurons indirectly.

The CB$_2$R is a G protein-coupled receptor widely distributed in the brain. Multiple downstream signaling molecules mediated by the CB$_2$R are involved in the modulation of microglia/macrophage polarity transition [39]. Among these, NF-κB is considered to be one of the most critical regulators in the activation of the microglia/macrophage M1 phenotype by controlling the transcription of M1-associated genes [40]. In the inactivated state, NF-κB is retained in the cytoplasm by binding to an inhibitory protein (IκB), but when microglia/macrophage cells are stimulated by inflammation, IκB is phosphorylated and polyubiquitinated, followed by degradation by the 26S proteasome, resulting in the dissociation of IκB from NF-κB. Subsequently, the released NF-κB translocates into the nucleus, where it binds to its cognate DNA sequence and regulates the transcription of various inflammatory mediators involved in M1 polarization, such as IL-1, IL-6, TNF-α and iNOS. At the same time, in response to the inflammatory response, the mTOR signaling pathway is also activated by phosphorylation, which can accelerate the development of inflammation through activating the NF-κB signaling pathway, resulting in ischemic necrosis of neurons. Consistent with a previous study by Li et al. who showed that administration of *trans*-caryophyllene, a CB$_2$R selective agonist, efficiently attenuates hypoxia-induced neuroinflammatory response through the NF-κB pathway in microglia [41]. Our study demonstrated that in 4-VO rats, treatment with PF or HU308 prominently inhibited the phosphorylation of mTOR and IκBα, reduced IκBα degradation, and further blocked the nuclear translocation of the NF-κB p65 subunit, thereby significantly inhibiting the expression of markers for M1 microglia/macrophages. However, this inhibitory effect of PF on mTOR/NF-κB signaling could be abolished by the simultaneous administration of AM630. Our findings suggest that PF inhibits mTOR/NF-κB signaling pathway in the hippocampus of

4-VO rats by up-regulating the CB$_2$R expression, thereby reducing the impact of the M1 microglia/macrophage phenotype and attenuating neuroinflammation. It is hard to conclude that the effect is derived from microglia rather than other cells, such as astrocytes and endothelial cells, even blood cells. Meanwhile, we conducted in vitro experiments to elucidate the effect of PF is derived from microglial cells rather than other cells. Our data from expeiments in vitro demonstrate that activation of CB$_2$R by PF facilitates the microglia phenotype switch from proinflammatory ("M1-like") to anti-inflammatory and immunomodulatory ("M2-like") via suppressing the mTOR/NF-κB signaling pathway (Additional file 5: Figure S4).

The PI3K/Akt signaling pathway is widely present in various cell types. This pathway is involved in the regulation of cell growth, proliferation and differentiation through a series of responses and is a classic anti-apoptotic and pro-survival signal transduction pathway. In recent years, studies have shown that the CB$_2$R agonist exhibits a neuroprotective effect in the CNS by activating the PI3K/Akt signaling pathway [42], which reduces cognitive impairment, increases cerebral blood flow, and inhibits neuronal apoptosis in an animal model of VD [43]. Akt is a common upstream regulator of both mTOR and NF-κB pathways. Akt activation directly phosphorylates mTOR and activates both IκB kinase and its downstream target, NF-κB. However, recent studies have found that everolimus, a small molecule mTOR inhibitor, can increase the phosphorylation of Akt and directed local microglia towards an anti-inflammatory state by shifting to an increased M2 profiles. It has been postulated that this effect may be related to the ability of everolimus to block the negative feedback effect of mTOR on Akt [10]. Moreover, PF was found to activate the PI3K/Akt signaling pathway, up-regulate Akt phosphorylation, and exert neuroprotective effects [44]. In the present study, the hippocampal phosphorylation of PI3K and Akt in 4-VO rats increased significantly with PF treatment. Meanwhile, mRNA levels of M2 microglia expression products (IL-10, arginase-1, Ym1 and TGF-β1) were also significantly increased. After treatment with both PF and the CB$_2$R selective antagonist, AM630, the activation effect of PF on the PI3K/Akt pathway was significantly inhibited. Therefore, we hypothesize that PF increases the phosphorylation levels of PI3K/Akt by up-regulating CB$_2$R expression, thereby inducing the transition of microglia/macrophages to the M2 phenotype, stimulating the secretion of neurotrophic factors and promoting brain repair and regeneration.

This present study has some limitations. First, neuroinflammation is reflected in VD model as astrogliosis and microglia activation [45]. Although CB$_2$R activation by PF on the proinflammatory microglial cells might play a vital role to ameliorate neuronal death after cerebral ischemia, we did not exclude the possibility that PF could inhibit astrogliosis after ischemic brain damage by activating CB_2R. Second, in the brain CB_2R is expressed in activated astrocytes, microglial cells, neurons and endothelial cells [46], we only focused on the anti-neuroinflammatory mechanisms of CB_2R activation by PF in activated microglia/macrophages. However, other mechanisms of CB_2R stimulation in different brain cells might exist and play a role in providing beneficial effects after PF administration, which we did not explore in this study.

Conclusion

The main findings of this study are as follows: PF exerts anti-neuroinflammation functions in a rat model of VD by specifically inducing CB_2R function in microglia/macrophages of the hippocampus and consequently reducing the activity of the mTOR/NF-κB signaling pathway, thereby inhibiting the M1 microglia/macrophage release of proinflammatory factors. Further, the present findings suggest that PF activates the PI3K/Akt signaling pathway in a CB_2R-dependent manner to promote the transition of microglia/macrophages from the M1 to M2 phenotype and stimulate M2 microglia/macrophages to secrete anti-inflammatory molecules and neuroprotective factors, thus reducing neuronal damage and further exerting neuroprotective functions. Our findings suggest that PF could be a potential therapeutic agent for the treatment of neuroinflammation-related CNS diseases, particularly VD.

Additional files

Additional file 1. The Minimum Standards of Reporting Checklist.

Additional file 2: Figure S1. Effects of paeoniflorin on histopathology and protein levels of proinflammatory cytokines in the hippocampal CA1 area of rats after cerebral ischemia. One week after four-vessel occlusion (4-VO) surgery, rats were intraperitoneally administered saline (4-VO), paeoniflorin (4-VO+PF; 10, 20, 40 mg/kg/d) or HU308 (4-VO+HU308; 3 mg/kg/d) for consecutive 28 days. (A) Rats were sacrificed after 28 days consecutive drug treatment. Representative photomicrographs of hematoxylin-eosin-stained hippocampal regions of rats are shown in different groups: (a, g) sham-operated group, (b, h) 4-VO-operated group, (c, i) 4-VO+10 mg/kg/d PF group, (d, j) 4-VO+PF+20 mg/kg/d group, (e, k) 4-VO+40 mg/kg/d group or (f, l) 4-VO+3 mg/kg/d HU308 group. Boxed regions in a–f are shown in j–l, respectively. Scale bar: 50 μm. (B) Neuronal cell density in CA1 region was measured. (C) The protein levels of proinflammatory cytokines including IL-1β, TNF-α and IL-6 in the hippocampal homogenate were measured by enzyme linked immunosorbent assay.

Additional file 3: Figure S2. Effects of paeoniflorin on histopathology of the entorhinal cortex area of rats after cerebral ischemia. Representative photomicrographs of hematoxylin-eosin-stained entorhinal cortex region of either sham-operated rats (a, g) or rats that had been subjected to four-vessel occlusion followed by the treatment with saline (4-VO; b, h), paeoniflorin (4-VO+PF; 40 mg/kg/d; c, i), paeoniflorin+AM630 (4-VO+PF+AM630; 40 + 3 mg/kg/d; d, j), AM630 (4-VO+AM630; 3 mg/

kg/d; e, k) or HU308 (4-VO+HU308; 3 mg/kg/d; f, l) for consecutive 28 days. Boxed regions in a–f are shown in j–l, respectively. Scale bar: 50 μm.

Additional file 4: Figure S3. Effects of paeoniflorin on the activation of microglial cells in hippocampi of rats after cerebral ischemia. One week after four-vessel occlusion (4-VO) surgery, rats were intraperitoneally administered saline (4-VO), paeoniflorin (4-VO+PF; 40 mg/kg/d), paeoniflorin+AM630 (4-VO+PF+AM630; 40 + 3 mg/kg/d), AM630 (4-VO+AM630; 3 mg/kg/d) or HU308 (4-VO+HU308; 3 mg/kg/d) for consecutive 28 days. After treatment, hippocampus tissue sections were co-stained for Iba1 (an activated microglia marker; green) or DAPI (blue). The images were observed and captured by a confocal laser scanning microscope. Scale bar: 50 μm.

Additional file 5: Figure S4. Effects of PF on M1/M2 polarization and mTOR/NF-κB signaling pathway in BV-2 microglia exposed to oxygen glucose deprivation (OGD). BV-2 cells were pre-incubated with DMSO (vehicle), PF (50 μM), AM630 (2 μM) or HU308 (10 μM) for 4 h followed by OGD for 6 or 24 h. (A) The cell lysates were immunoblotted with iNOS or β-actin antibody. β-Actin served as a loading control. These results are representative for three independent experiments. (B) The differences of the protein expression between the groups were analyzed with Image J. (C) The levels of nitrite in cell culture supernatants were determined by the Griess reaction. (D) Representative Western blotting photographs showing protein levels of p-mTOR, mTOR, p-IκBα, IκBα, NF-κB and β-actin in cytoplasmic fractions and NF-κB and lamin B1 in nuclear fractions of BV-2 microglia. The β-actin and lamin B1 protein levels were used as internal controls, respectively, for cytoplasmic extracts (CE) and nuclear extracts (NE). (E, F) The protein levels of phosphorylated and total mTOR and IκBα in cytoplasmic extracts and NF-κB in cytoplasmic and nuclear extracts, were converted to arbitrary densitometric units, normalized by the value of the corresponding loading controls and expressed relative to the phosphorylation ratio or to the protein levels in vechile control (defined as 1-fold). (G, H) The levels of IL-1β, IL-6, TNF-α, IL-10 and TGF-β1 in cell culture supernatants were determined by enzyme-linked immunosorbent assay. Each bar represents mean ± SD of three independent experiments. #$P < 0.05$ versus vehicle control group, *$P < 0.05$ versus OGD group, §$P < 0.05$ versus OGD+PF group.

Abbreviations
4-VO: four-vessel occlusion; BCA: bicinchoninic acid; CB_1R: cannabinoid receptor 1; CB_2R: cannabinoid receptor 2; CNS: central nervous system; Ct: threshold cycle; HE: hematoxylin and eosin; iNOS: inducible nitric oxide synthase; LPS: lipopolysaccharide; mTOR: mammalian target of rapamycin; NO: nitric oxide; NF-κB: nuclear factor-κb; PBS: phosphate buffered saline; PI3K: phosphatidylinositol-3-kinase; PF: paeoniflorin; TNF-α: tumor necrosis factor-α; VD: vascular dementia.

Authors' contributions
ZD conceived and designed the experiments. XQL and AL performed the experiments and drafted the manuscript. XY and XX collected the data. RH and TWW reviewed literature and interpreted the results. XYD conducted immunofluorescence test. DJY revised the manuscript and provided essential comments. All authors read and approved the final manuscript.

Author details
[1] Chongqing Key Laboratory of Biochemistry and Molecular Pharmacology, School of Pharmacy, Chongqing Medical University, Chongqing 400016, China. [2] College of Pharmacy and Bioengineering, Chongqing University of Technology, Chongqing 400054, China. [3] Institute of Chinese Pharmacology and Toxicology, Chongqing Academy of Chinese Materia Medica, Chongqing 400065, China. [4] Drug Review Section, China Chongqing Technical Center for Drug Evaluation and Certification, Chongqing 400014, China. [5] Institute of Life Sciences, Chongqing Medical University, Chongqing 400016, China.

Acknowledgements
Not applicable.

Competing interests
The authors declare that they have no competing interests.

All of authors consent to publication of this study in Journal of Chinese Medicine.

Funding
This work was supported by National Science and Technology Major Project (2015ZX09501004-003-007), Chongqing Integrated Demonstration Project (cstc2013jcsf10011) and Chongqing General Research and Development Project (cstc2017jxjl-jbky0013).

References

1. Sorrentino G, Migliaccio R, Bonavita V. Treatment of vascular dementia: the route of prevention. Eur J Neurol. 2008;60:217–23.
2. Black SE. Vascular cognitive impairment: epidemiology, subtypes, diagnosis and management. J R Coll Surg Edinb. 2011;41:49–56.
3. Plassman BL, Langa KM, Fisher GG, Heeringa SG, Weir DR, Ofstedal MB, et al. Prevalence of dementia in the United States: the aging, demographics, and memory study. Neuroepidemiology. 2007;29:125–32.
4. Gao YZ, Zhang JJ, Liu H, Wu GY, Xiong L, Shu M. Regional cerebral blood flow and cerebrovascular reactivity in Alzheimer's disease and vascular dementia assessed by arterial spinlabeling magnetic resonance imaging. Curr Neurovasc Res. 2013;10:49–53.
5. Jayant S, Sharma B. Selective modulator of cannabinoid receptor type 2 reduces memory impairment and infarct size during cerebral hypoperfusion and vascular dementia. Curr Neurovasc Res. 2013;10:49–53.
6. Puffenbarger RA, Boothe AC, Cabral GA. Cannabinoids inhibit LPS-inducible cytokine mRNA expression in rat microglial cells. Glia. 2000;29:58–69.
7. Ehrhart J, Obregon D, Mori T, Hou H, Sun N, Bai Y, Klein T, Fernandez F, Tan J, Shytle RD. Stimulation of cannabinoid receptor 2 (CB 2) suppresses microglial activation. J Neuroinflamm. 2005;2:29.
8. Correa F, Hernangómez M, Mestre L, Loría F, Spagnolo A, Docagne F, et al. Anandamide enhances IL-10 production in activated microglia by targeting CB2 receptors: roles of ERK1/2, JNK, and NF-κB. Glia. 2010;58:135–47.
9. Lu DY, Liou HC, Tang CH, Fu WM. Hypoxia-induced iNOS expression in microglia is regulated by the PI3-kinase/Akt/mTOR signaling pathway and activation of hypoxia inducible factor-1α. Biochem Pharmacol. 2006;72:992–1000.
10. Chen L, Zhang Y, Li D, Zhang N, Liu R, Han B, et al. Everolimus (RAD001) ameliorates vascular cognitive impairment by regulating microglial function via the mTORC1 signaling pathway. J Neuroimmunol. 2016;299:164–71.
11. Tarassishin L, Suh HS, Lee SC. Interferon regulatory factor 3 plays an anti-inflammatory role in microglia by activating the PI3K/Akt pathway. J Neuroinflamm. 2011;8:187.
12. Shi X, Cai X, Di W, Li J, Xu X, Zhang A, et al. MFG-E8 selectively inhibited Aβ-induced microglial M1 polarization via NF-κB and PI3K-Akt pathways. Mol Neurobiol. 2017;54:7777–88.
13. Liu Y, Dong Z, Xiao XQ, Tang H, Wang LL, Cheng YJ. Establishment of a high throughput screening model of cannabinoid receptor 2 agonist. Chin J Cell Mol Immunol. 2012;28:194–6.
14. Liu Y, Dong Z, Xiao XQ, Tang H, Wang LL, Cheng YJ. Construction and eukaryon expression of pIRES2-EGFP-CB2 plasmid. Laser J. 2012;1:69–71.
15. Tabata K, Matsumoto K, Watanabe H. Paeoniflorin, a major constituent of peony root, reverses muscarinic M1-receptor antagonist-induced suppression of long-term potentiation in the rat hippocampal slice. Jpn J Pharmacol. 2001;83:25–30.
16. Ohta H, Matsumoto K, Watanabe H, Shimizu M. Involvement of α1 but not α2-adrenergic systems in the antagonizing effect of paeoniflorin on scopolamine-induced deficit in radial maze performance in rats. Jpn J Pharmacol. 1993;62:199–202.
17. Yu HY, Mu DG, Chen J, Yin W. Suppressive effects of intrathecal paeoniflorin on bee venom-induced pain-related behaviors and spinal neuronal activation. Pharmacology. 2011;88:159–66.
18. Liu DZ, Xie KQ, Ji XQ, Ye Y, Jiang CL, Zhu XZ. Neuroprotective effect of paeoniflorin on cerebral ischemic rat by activating adenosine A1 receptor in a manner different from its classical agonists. Br J Clin Pharmacol. 2005;146:604–11.
19. Zhang LG, Wang LJ, Shen QQ, Wang HF, Zhang Y, Shi CG, Zhang SC, Zhang MY. Paeoniflorin improves regional cerebral blood flow and suppresses inflammatory factors in the hippocampus of rats with vascular dementia. Chin J Integr Med. 2017;23:696–702.
20. Zhang Y, Wang LL, Wu Y, Wang N, Wang SM, Zhang B, Shi CG, Zhang SC. Paeoniflorin attenuates hippocampal damage in a rat model of vascular dementia. Exp Ther Med. 2016;12:3729–34.
21. Cai JH, Rao ML, Tang M, Xiang L, Feng S, Xiao CY, Liu YJ. Protective effect of paeoniflorin on the hippocampus in rats with cerebral ischemia-reperfusion through activating cannabinoid receptor 2. Chin J Cell Mol Immunol. 2015;31:443–7.
22. Pulsinelli WA, Brierley JB. A new model of bilateral hemispheric ischemia in the unanesthetized rat. Stroke. 1979;10:267–72.
23. Pulsinelli WA, Levy DE, Duffy TE. Regional cerebral blood flow and glucose metabolism following transient forebrain ischemia. Ann Neurol. 1982;11:499–509.
24. Zhao XL, Li DP, Fang XB, Yang GR. Ultrastructural study on the hippocampal neurons of vascular dementia in rats. Prog Anat Sci. 2000;2:161–3.
25. Zhao XL, Fang XB, Li DP. Establishing vascular dementia model in rats. J Chin Med Univ. 2002;31:166–7.
26. Vorhees CV, Williams MT. Morris water maze: procedures for assessing spatial and related forms of learning and memory. Nat Protoc. 2006;1:848–58.
27. Hartman RE, Lee JM, Zipfel GJ, Wozniak DF. Characterizing learning deficits and hippocampal neuron loss following transient global cerebral ischemia in rats. Brain Res. 2005;1043:48–56.
28. Perego C, Fumagalli S, De Simoni MG. Temporal pattern of expression and colocalization of microglia/macrophage phenotype markers following brain ischemic injury in mice. J Neuroinflamm. 2011;8:174.
29. Orihuela R, McPherson CA, Harry GJ. Microglial M1/M2 polarization and metabolic states. Br J Pharmacol. 2016;173:649–65.
30. Tang Y, Le W. Differential roles of M1 and M2 microglia in neurodegenerative diseases. Mol Neurobiol. 2016;53:1181–94.
31. Zhong LM, Zong Y, Sun L, Guo JZ, Zhang W, He Y, et al. Resveratrol inhibits inflammatory responses via the mammalian target of rapamycin signaling pathway in cultured LPS-stimulated microglial cells. PLoS ONE. 2012;7:e32195.
32. Wang G, Shi Y, Jiang X, Leak RK, Hu X, Wu Y, Pu H, Li WW, Tang B, Wang Y, Gao Y. HDAC inhibition prevents white matter injury by modulating microglia/macrophage polarization through the GSK3β/PTEN/Akt axis. Proc Natl Acad Sci USA. 2015;112:2853–8.
33. Boche D, Perry VH, Nicoll JA. Activation patterns of microglia and their identification in the human brain. Neuropathol Appl Neurobiol. 2013;39:3–18.
34. Cherry JD, Olschowka JA, O'Banion MK. Neuroinflammation and M2 microglia: the good, the bad, and the inflamed. J Neuroinflamm. 2014;11:98.
35. Pazos MR, Nunez E, Benito C, Tolon RM, Romero J. Role of the endocannabinoid system in Alzheimer's disease: new perspectives. Life Sci. 2004;75:1907–15.
36. Cabral GA, Raborn ES, Griffin L, Dennis J, Marciano-Cabral F. CB2 receptors in the brain: role in central immune function. Br J Pharmacol. 2008;153:240–51.
37. Tao Y, Li L, Jiang B, Feng Z, Yang L, Tang J, et al. Cannabinoid receptor-2 stimulation suppresses neuroinflammation by regulating microglial M1/M2 polarization through the cAMP/PKA pathway in an experimental GMH rat model. Brain Behav Immun. 2016;58:118–29.
38. Jayant S, Sharma B. Selective modulator of cannabinoid receptor type 2 reduces memory impairment and infarct size during cerebral hypoperfusion and vascular dementia. Curr Neurovasc Res. 2016;13:289–302.

39. Ashton JC, Glass M. The cannabinoid CB2 receptor as a target for inflammation-dependent neurodegeneration. Curr Neuropharmacol. 2007;5:73–80.

40. Dello Russo C, Lisi L, Tentori L, Navarra P, Graziani G, Combs CK. Exploiting microglial functions for the treatment of glioblastoma. Curr Cancer Drug Targets. 2017;17:267–81.

41. Guo K, Mou X, Huang J, Xiong N, Li H. Trans-caryophyllene suppresses hypoxia-induced neuroinflammatory responses by inhibiting NF-κB activation in microglia. J Mol Neurosci. 2014;54:41–8.

42. Viscomi MT, Oddi S, Latini L, Pasquariello N, Florenzano F, Bernardi G, Molinari M, Maccarrone M. Selective CB2 receptor agonism protects central neurons from remote axotomy-induced apoptosis through the PI3K/Akt pathway. J Neurosci. 2009;29:4564–70.

43. Lou J, Teng Z, Zhang L, Yang J, Ma L, Wang F, et al. β-Caryophyllene/hydroxypropyl-β-cyclodextrin inclusion complex improves cognitive deficits in rats with vascular dementia through the cannabinoid receptor type 2-mediated pathway. Front Pharmacol. 2017;8:2.

44. Liu L, Wang SY, Wang JG. Role of PI3K/Akt pathway in effect of paeoniflorin against Aβ25-35-induced PC12 cell injury. China J Chin Mater Med. 2014;39:4045–9.

45. Cai ZY, Yan Y, Chen R. Minocycline reduces astrocytic reactivation and neuroinflammation in the hippocampus of a vascular cognitive impairment rat model. Neurosci Bull. 2010;26:28–36.

46. Onaivi ES, Ishiguro H, Gu S, Liu QR. CNS effects of CB2 cannabinoid receptors: beyond neuro-immuno-cannabinoid activity. J Psychopharmacol. 2012;26:92–103.

11

Relationship between Chinese medicine dietary patterns and the incidence of breast cancer in Chinese women in Hong Kong

Xiao Zheng[1,2], Jianping Chen[1,5*], Ting Xie[2], Zhiyu Xia[3], Wings Tjing Yung Loo[1], Lixing Lao[1], JieShu You[1], Jie Yang[5], Kamchuen Tsui[4], Feizhi Mo[1] and Fei Gao[1]

Abstract

Background: This retrospective cross-sectional study aimed to investigate the relationship between Chinese medicine (CM) dietary patterns (*hot*, *neutral*, and *cold*) and the incidence of breast cancer among Chinese women in Hong Kong.

Methods: Breast cancer cases (n = 202) and healthy controls (n = 202) were matched according to demographics. Chinese women residing in Hong Kong for the past 7 years were recruited by media advertisements (e.g., via newspapers, radio, and posters). The control participants were recruited by convenience sampling from health workshops held in clinics and communities of 15 districts of Hong Kong. After completing test–retest reliability, all participants were asked to complete diet pattern questionnaires about their food preferences and dietary patterns. The Student's unpaired *t* test, Chi square test, and logistic regression were conducted using SPSS software.

Results: Three major CM dietary patterns were identified: *hot*, *neutral*, and *cold*. The participants with breast cancer exhibited a stronger preference for *hot* food than the control group (Chi square test, $P < 0.001$). A higher frequency of breast cancer was associated with a higher frequency of dining out for breakfast (4–5 times per week, Chi square test, $P = 0.015$; 6–7 times per week, Chi square test, $P < 0.001$) and lunch (4–5 times per week, Chi square test, $P < 0.001$; 6–7 times per week, Chi square test, $P = 0.006$). The participants with no history of breast cancer consumed CM supplements and Guangdong soups (1–2 times per week, Chi square test, $P = 0.05$; >3 times per week, Chi square test, $P < 0.001$) more frequently than those with breast cancer.

Conclusions: Non-breast cancer participants adopted a *neutral* (healthy and balanced) dietary pattern, and consumed CM supplements and Guangdong soups more frequently.

Background

Breast cancer is the most common and one of the most fatal cancers in women worldwide. The number of breast cancer cases among women in Hong Kong increased from 2273 in 2004 to more than 2870 in 2009, and average incidence rate per 100,000 women between 2004 and 2009 was 386.7 [1]. In 2008, the lifetime risk of breast cancer was 1 in 20 women [2]. Breast cancer incidence was generally lower in Asia than in Europe in 2000 [3]; a key reason for this was the difference in dietary patterns between the East and the West [4]. The identification of reasonable dietary prevention methods and the development of corresponding inhibitors may be beneficial for breast cancer prevention [5]. However, little research has been conducted in this area.

The dietary patterns of women in Hong Kong have been changing with western lifestyle in recent years [6, 7]. The

*Correspondence: jpjpchen@yahoo.com; abchen@hku.hk
†Xiao Zheng and Jianping Chen are co-first authors
[1] School of Chinese Medicine, The University of Hong Kong, Hong Kong, China

intake of foods with certain properties (e.g., *hot* or *cold* features) may increase the risk of related diseases, such as cancers [8]. Although diet has been proposed as a possible cause of breast cancer [9–11], the incidence of breast cancer has not previously been related to Chinese medicine (CM)-defined dietary patterns.

The properties of CM material medica (*cold, cool, hot,* and *warm*) can be used to classify diets as *hot, neutral,* or *cold*; these types of food have different functions in the body. Under this classification, beef, shrimp, chicken, and even ice cream are *hot* foods (Additional file 1).

This study aimed to investigate the relationship between CM dietary patterns and the incidence of breast cancer among women in Hong Kong.

Methods
Study design and participants
A retrospective cross-sectional survey was conducted. Data were collected using the Food Frequency Questionnaires (FFQ) (Additional file 2) [12]. The selection of study participants was based on geographic and sociodemographic variables described previously [6, 8, 9]. The Minimum Standards of Reporting Checklist (Additional file 3) contain details of the experimental design, and statistics, and resources used in this study.

This study included female participants with breast cancer (cases), who were compared with healthy women (controls). The cases were recruited by advertisements in the local media, such as in newspapers, in booklets issued by the University of Hong Kong, on posters, and on the radio. Convenience sampling was used to recruit the control group from health workshops in clinics and communities in 15 Hong Kong districts. All participants had to fulfill the following conditions: (1) female, (2) Chinese women residing in Hong Kong, (3) 28–60 years of age, (4) living in Hong Kong for the past 7 years, (5) able to understand the questionnaire items in Chinese, and (6) provision of an informed consent. Controls were required to fulfill the following conditions: (1) no breast cancer or other gynecologic diseases; (2) no metabolic, nutritional, or other severe diseases; and (3) no serious disease after doctor consultation in the past 3 months. Case inclusion criteria were: (1) new primary breast cancer patients, and (2) a diagnosis of primary breast cancer through biopsy and/or discharge report. Participants were excluded from the study if they had (1) other prior cancer diagnosis, (2) treatments with psychotropic drugs, (3) any medical conditions that limited their physical activity, and (4) not completed the questionnaire.

Sample size
We conducted a pilot study with 37 participants whose total diet comprised mainly *hot* foods and an expected

odds ratio (OR) of 2.32 according to the formula of OR was found. For the pilot study, we invited 37 people from the oncology outpatient clinic and the general outpatient clinic in the School of Chinese Medicine, University of Hong Kong, to complete the questionnaire: 20 were breast cancer cases and 17 were not. After the pilot study, we analyzed the responses and calculated the consumption of 12 kinds of *hot* foods including beef, mutton, shrimp, soft drinks, and milk. Of the breast cancer cases, 45.8% consumed *hot* foods regularly, whereas only 26.7% of the controls did so. We chose 10% as the estimated prevalence of *hot* food consumption for control group and calculated the estimated prevalence of *hot* food consumption for breast cancer group as 0.2 the expected OR of 2.32 to estimate the sample size of our research. The estimated sample size was calculated as about 207 participants in each group. Taking into account the nullified questionnaires, 202 participants were eventually included out of the total 207 participants recruited in each group.

Questionnaire
A self-administered FFQ was used to collect the dietary intake information. This questionnaire was adapted from the Fred Hutchinson Cancer Research Center Food Questionnaire, which is based on Western dietary patterns [13, 14]. Two CM experts and a group of laypeople approved the revised questionnaire as suitable to assess the average dietary patterns of Chinese women in Hong Kong. The FFQ consisted of 74 food items (Additional file 4). A commonly used portion size was specified for each food based on the conventional food intake and dietary patterns of Hong Kong women.

The questionnaire consists of two sections. The first section assessed sociodemographic information, including age, working status, education level, weight, height, and marital status. The second section contained the CM FFQ items, which measured consumption of very common foods. The FFQ consists of 74 items scored on a 5-point scale, ranging from 1 (not consumed at all) to 5 (consumed very often). It comprises nine subscales of food consumption frequency for CM-defined foods, and a general preference score for three kinds of food (*cold, neutral,* and *hot* foods, classified according to CM). A total score for each subscale was obtained by summing the relevant item scores. Higher scores indicated higher consumption frequencies [15]. We modified the semantic expression of several items to adapt those items to the dietary patterns and habits of the women in Hong Kong. Our pilot study of 37 participants demonstrated that the version could be read and understood by local Chinese women.

The questionnaire design was single-blind to participants to ensure the validity of participants' stated consumption of their preferred and most frequently eaten foods. Different kinds of food were included and randomized to ensure the aim of the survey was not revealed to the cases or controls. Completed questionnaires were collected individually to ensure the responses were not misinterpreted owing to communication gaps between the researchers and the participants.

Study procedures

Test–retest reliability was examined using pre-survey responses. Two weeks after completing the first questionnaire, we asked the same participants to complete the same questionnaire to confirm the instrument's validity and test–retest reliability. Analysis of homogeneity in this pilot study result was used to test the consistency of the 37 completed questionnaires (20 cases and 17 controls). The results produced a P value of 0.915, which indicated that the questionnaire responses were statistically the same for the two tests. Each participant was asked to appraise each item for its relevance in evaluating the content, and to suggest any items that should be added to improve the questionnaire's validity. All items had a content validity index of clarity greater than 80%.

Every potential participant was interviewed by a trained research doctor at the clinic center of the School of Chinese Medicine, University of Hong Kong. Participants completed a self-administered questionnaire and had a face-to-face consultation for the same research doctor to check the questionnaire.

Three important steps were taken throughout the process to ensure the quality of investigation. First, to ensure consistency of the survey across sites and over time, the same interviewer used the same procedures and standards to investigate all women. Second, each questionnaire was checked by the same researcher carefully and those questionnaires with missing data on foods or dietary patterns were excluded. Third, to prevent input error, we used a double data entry method by different researchers to enter all data into SPSS.

Measurement

According to CM theory, different foods possess different *cold*, *neutral*, and *hot* properties and have different nutritional constituents, each with their own *cold*, *neutral*, and *hot* properties. These food properties are based on the functions the foods perform after consumption. All vegetables, meat, fruits, and grains are classified according to one of these three properties, as summarized in Additional file 1. Participants' final overall food preference score of *hot*, *neutral*, or *cold* was determined by the average score for all the foods listed. For example, if the overall FFQ score for *neutral* food was the highest, then the overall preference score for food was considered *neutral*. The *hot* and *cold* preference scores were calculated in the same manner.

Additionally, participants were asked to indicate the frequency of (1) eating out for breakfast, lunch, and dinner (0–1 time/week; 2–3 times/week; 4–5 times/week, and 6–7 times/week); (2) CM intake, CM supplement intake, and Chinese soup consumption (seldom, sometimes, often); and (3) Chinese-style food (i.e., Guangdong *dim sum*/tea drinking) and Western-style food consumption (i.e., fast food) (<once/week; 1–2 times/week; >3 times/week). Demographic information such as age, marital status, current height and weight (to obtain body mass index), and education level was also collected.

Data analysis

The statistics program SPSS version 16.0 (SPSS Inc., Chicago, IL, USA) was used for data analysis. Descriptive statistics were calculated; continuous variables were presented as mean ± standard deviation, and categorical variables were presented as frequencies. The mean difference between continuous variables was tested using Student's t test for independent samples. The association between categorical variables was tested using the Chi square test. A binary logistic regression model was used to evaluate the association of different food preferences with the likelihood of having breast cancer. Results were presented as ORs and corresponding 95% confidence intervals, with age as a variable in the logistic regression. All P values were based on two-tailed tests, with $P < 0.05$ considered statistically significant.

Regarding the validity and reliability assessment of the questionnaire, we examined test–retest reliability by inviting participants in the pilot study to complete the questionnaire a second time. We compared both test results using ANOVA, which produced a value of 0.915, showing high test–retest reliability. All the pilot study participants were interviewed about the interpretability of the questionnaire, and the interpretability was reported to be good.

Results

Sociodemographic characteristics of participants

The case and control groups were similar in terms of body mass index, occupation, education, marital status, age at first menstrual cycle, and family history of cancer (Table 1).

When age was treated as a continuous variable, there was a significant difference between the case and control groups ($P < 0.001$): participants in the control group were 2.4 years younger. However, when age was categorized according to five different age groups, there was no significant difference between the case and control groups ($P = 0.061$). Because there was a marginally significant difference in age between the two groups, we considered age a confounder in multivariate analysis of variance (MANOVA).

Table 1 Socio-demographic characteristics of participants (*N* = 404,%)

Socio-demographic characteristics	Controls (*n* = 202)	Cases (*n* = 202)	*P* values
Age			0.061
Mean ± SD	45.35 ± 6.765	47.75 ± 6.17	
≤34	14 (6.9)	7 (3.5)	
35–41	39 (19.3)	25 (12.4)	
42–48	76 (37.6)	72 (36.6)	
49–55	62 (30.7)	78 (39.0)	
≥56	11 (5.4)	18 (9.0)	
BMI			0.132
Underweight (<18.5)	17 (8.5)	19 (9.5)	
Normal weight (18.5–24.9)	143 (71.1)	156 (78.4)	
Overweight (25–29.9)	33 (16.4)	21 (10.6)	
Obesity (≥30)	8 (4)	3 (1.5)	
Occupational type			0.589
Full-time	119 (59.5)	113 (55.9)	
Part-time	14 (7.0)	22 (10.9)	
Housewife	66 (33.0)	66 (32.7)	
Others	1 (0.5)	1 (0.5)	
Educational level			0.063
Primary	21 (10.4)	24 (11.9)	
Secondary	92 (45.5)	115 (56.9)	
Tertiary or above	87 (43.1)	62 (30.7)	
Others	2 (1.0)	1 (0.5)	
Marital status			0.389
Single	33 (16.3)	25 (12.4)	
Married or cohabited	155 (76.7)	158 (78.2)	
Divorced	14 (6.9)	19 (9.4)	
Family tumor history			0.318
Yes	87 (43.1)	97 (48.0)	
No	115 (56.9)	105 (52.0)	

BMI body mass index. The following factors are related to breast cancer incidence and were measured by the questionnaire: age, race, BMI, educational level, marital status, religion, family tumor history, and occupation. The two groups were comparable on these factors, although no significant between-group differences were found

Characteristics of food preferences based on CM theory

Tables 2 and 3 showed that there was a significant between-group difference in the frequency distribution of the preferences for the three food types ($P < 0.001$). We analyzed the between-group differences in food preferences of *hot*, *neutral*, and *cold* using logistic regression with age as a variable. The consumption of *hot* foods such as roast meat, shrimp, shellfish, soft drinks, popcorn/fries, and candies was significantly different between groups. Participants with a strong preference for roast meat, shrimp, shellfish, and popcorn/fries had 6-, 9.2-, 13.3-, and 7.6-times higher risk, respectively, of having breast cancer compared with participants with an average preference for these foods. Women who preferred soft drinks had a 4.9-times higher risk of having breast cancer compared with women who had an average

Table 2 Frequency distribution of preference for foods with hot, neutral and cold characteristics (N = 404, %)

Groups	Food nature			*P* value
	Hot (warm)	Neutral	Cold (cool)	
Controls	14 (6.9)	121 (59.9)	67 (33.2)	<0.001*
Cases	53 (26.4)	103 (50.8)	46 (22.8)	

The *P* value was <0.05, indicating a statistically significant between-group difference. The results showed a possible association between consumption of *hot* foods and a higher risk of breast cancer

* *P* value was calculated by Chi square test

preference. Higher preferences for nuts and freshwater fish (*neutral)* and tofu and squid (*cold)* showed a lower OR for breast cancer (Table 4).

Table 3 Specific frequency distribution of preference for foods with *hot, neutral* and *cold* characteristics (*N* = 404, %)

Food nature	Food	Breast cancer	Very preferred	Preferred	Average	Not preferred	Not very preferred	Statistical significance
Hot	Spicy food	No	14 (6.9)	50 (24.8)	82 (40.6)	43 (21.3)	13 (6.4)	0.655
		Yes	19 (9.4)	55 (27.2)	68 (33.7)	46 (22.8)	14 (6.9)	
	Roast meat	No	5 (2.5)	59 (29.2)	113 (55.9)	22 (10.9)	3 (1.5)	0.237
		Yes	12 (5.9)	68 (33.7)	104 (51.5)	17 (8.4)	1 (0.5)	
	Beef	No	16 (8.0)	58 (28.9)	83 (41.3)	29 (14.4)	15 (7.5)	0.534
		Yes	24 (12.1)	48 (23.6)	87 (43.2)	31 (15.1)	12 (6.0)	
	Mutton	No	8 (4.0)	32 (16.0)	83 (41.0)	50 (24.5)	29 (14.5)	0.777
		Yes	11 (5.6)	33 (16.3)	72 (35.7)	51 (25.0)	35 (17.3)	
	Chicken	No	36 (17.8)	102 (50.5)	55 (27.2)	8 (4.0)	1 (0.5)	0.138
		Yes	56 (27.8)	82 (40.4)	54 (26.8)	8 (4.0)	2 (1.0)	
	Salmon/tuna	No	30 (14.9)	87 (43.3)	57 (28.4)	19 (9.5)	7 (3.5)	0.687
		Yes	37 (18.2)	76 (37.4)	65 (32.3)	18 (9.1)	6 (3.0)	
	Shrimp	No	13 (6.5)	53 (26.4)	84 (41.3)	38 (18.9)	14 (7.0)	*<0.001**
		Yes	44 (21.9)	60 (29.9)	73 (6.3)	19 (9.5)	5 (2.5)	
	Shellfish	No	9 (4.5)	37 (18.3)	97 (48.0)	48 (23.8)	11 (5.4)	*<0.001**
		Yes	31 (15.2)	56 (27.8)	73 (36.4)	39 (19.2)	3 (1.5)	
	Dark Chinese tea	No	30 (14.9)	76 (37.6)	73 (36.1)	15 (7.4)	8 (4.0)	0.071
		Yes	31 (15.2)	73 (36.0)	67 (33.0)	30 (14.7)	2 (1.0)	
	Coffee/tea with milk	No	38 (18.8)	52 (25.7)	52 (25.7)	44 (21.8)	16 (7.9)	0.678
		Yes	43 (21.5)	54 (26.5)	56 (27.5)	32 (16.0)	17 (8.5)	
	Soft drinks	No	3 (1.5)	10 (5.0)	65 (32.2)	92 (45.5)	31 (15.3)	*0.001**
		Yes	10 (5.0)	30 (14.9)	72 (35.8)	65 (32.3)	24 (11.9)	
	Milk	No	10 (5.0)	49 (24.4)	91 (44.8)	35 (17.4)	17 (8.5)	*0.014**
		Yes	25 (12.2)	37 (18.3)	90 (44.7)	43 (21.3)	7 (3.6)	
	Alcohol	No	0 (0.0)	4 (2.0)	21 (10.4)	58 (28.7)	117 (57.9)	0.257
		Yes	3 (1.5)	2 (1.0)	17 (8.5)	66 (32.5)	114 (56.5)	
	Beer	No	2 (1.0)	23 (11.4)	64 (31.7)	48 (23.8)	64 (31.7)	0.075
		Yes	6 (3.0)	15 (7.5)	47 (23.1)	65 (32.2)	69 (34.2)	
	Popcorn/fries	No	3 (1.5)	34 (16.8)	79 (39.1)	57 (28.2)	29 (14.4)	*0.035**
		Yes	15 (7.6)	32 (15.7)	86 (42.4)	46 (22.7)	23 (11.6)	
	Chocolate	No	25 (12.4)	61 (30.3)	82 (40.8)	26 (12.9)	7 (3.5)	0.842
		Yes	25 (12.4)	64 (31.8)	72 (35.8)	31 (15.4)	9 (4.5)	
	Candies	No	3 (1.5)	21 (10.4)	93 (46.0)	67 (33.2)	18 (8.9)	0.250
		Yes	7 (3.5)	33 (16.4)	80 (39.8)	65 (32.3)	16 (8.0)	
	Deep boiled soup	No	59 (29.2)	98 (48.5)	38 (18.8)	5 (2.5)	2 (1.0)	0.759
		Yes	56 (27.9)	104 (51.7)	38 (18.9)	2 (1.0)	1 (0.5)	
	Western soup	No	13 (6.5)	73 (36.3)	81 (40.3)	22 (10.9)	12 (6.0)	0.059
		Yes	18 (9.0)	51 (25.4)	86 (42.8)	37 (18.4)	9 (4.5)	
Neutral	Fruits and vegetables	No	44 (21.6)	131 (64.8)	25 (12.6)	2 (1.0)	0 (0.0)	0.452
		Yes	41 (20.2)	121 (60.1)	37 (18.1)	3 (1.6)	0 (0.0)	
	Pork	No	15 (7.5)	95 (46.8)	83 (41.3)	5 (2.5)	4 (2.0)	0.690
		Yes	18 (9.0)	94 (46.5)	86 (42.5)	2 (1.0)	2 (1.0)	
	Pork with fat	No	4 (2.0)	17 (8.4)	70 (34.7)	66 (32.7)	45 (22.3)	0.121
		Yes	4 (2.0)	32 (16.0)	72 (35.5)	63 (31.0)	31 (15.5)	
	Geese/duck	No	5 (2.5)	45 (22.3)	101 (50.0)	36 (17.8)	15 (7.4)	0.209
		Yes	13 (6.5)	55 (27.0)	92 (45.5)	31 (15.5)	11 (5.5)	
	Fresh water fish	No	19 (9.4)	79 (39.1)	80 (39.6)	16 (7.9)	7 (3.5)	0.140
		Yes	10 (5.0)	63 (31.3)	100 (49.3)	20 (10.0)	9 (4.5)	

Table 3 continued

Food nature	Food	Breast cancer	Very preferred	Preferred	Average	Not preferred	Not very preferred	Statistical significance
	Nuts	No	39 (19.5)	84 (41.5)	64 (31.5)	10 (5.0)	5 (2.5)	*0.020**
		Yes	26 (12.6)	65 (32.2)	88 (43.7)	18 (9.0)	5 (2.5)	
	Boiling soup	No	37 (18.3)	98 (48.5)	57 (28.2)	6 (3.0)	4 (2.0)	0.233
		Yes	31 (15.5)	90 (44.5)	61 (30.0)	16 (8.0)	4 (2.0)	
Cold	Fruits and vegetables	No	38 (19.0)	117 (58.0)	45 (22.5)	1 (0.5)	0 (0.0)	0.323
		Yes	30 (14.9)	11 (56.9)	53 (26.1)	4 (2.1)	0 (0.0)	
	Sea fish	No	35 (17.3)	97 (48.0)	58 (28.7)	10 (5.0)	2 (1.0)	0.963
		Yes	31 (15.5)	102 (50.5)	57 (28.0)	9 (4.5)	3 (1.5)	
	Squid	No	27 (13.6)	59 (29.1)	85 (42.2)	25 (12.6)	5 (2.5)	0.219
		Yes	19 (9.5)	45 (22.1)	96 (47.7)	36 (17.6)	6 (3.0)	
	Products made from bean	No	53 (26.4)	103 (50.7)	39 (19.4)	5 (2.5)	2 (1.0)	*0.019**
		Yes	39 (19.1)	87 (43.2)	67 (33.2)	8 (4.0)	1 (0.5)	
	Light Chinese tea	No	28 (13.9)	82 (40.6)	64 (31.7)	23 (11.4)	5 (2.5)	0.148
		Yes	33 (16.1)	64 (31.7)	78 (38.7)	26 (13.1)	1 (0.5)	
	Herbal tea	No	4 (2.0)	40 (19.8)	111 (55.0)	39 (19.3)	8 (4.0)	0.582
		Yes	5 (2.5)	36 (17.7)	101 (50.0)	47 (23.2)	13 (6.6)	

The P value was <0.05, indicating a statistically significant between-group difference. The results showed a possible association between consumption of *hot* foods and a higher risk of breast cancer

* P values were calculated by Chi square tests

Association between CM dietary patterns or habits and risk of breast cancer

A higher frequency of eating out for breakfast (4–5 times per week, $P = 0.015$; 6–7 times per week, $P < 0.001$) and lunch (4–5 times per week, $P < 0.001$; 6–7 times per week, $P = 0.006$) was positively associated with the risk of breast cancer. In general, participants who dined out for breakfast and lunch (at least four times per week) had at least twice the risk of having breast cancer compared with participants who dined out 0–1 time per week (Table 5). A higher frequency of Guangdong *dim sum*/tea drinking was positively associated with a higher risk of breast cancer. Participants who ate *dim sum* more than three times per week were 2.8 times higher in frequency to be at risk of breast cancer than those who ate it less than once a week (1–2 times per week, $P = 0.05$; >3 times per week, $P < 0.001$) (Table 6).

Consumption of CM supplements, Chinese soup, and risk of breast cancer

The results indicated significant positive associations of the consumption of CM supplements and Chinese soup with a lower risk of breast cancer (Table 7).

Discussion

CM theory offers a way of classifying food based on its properties. When the balance of *Yin* and *Yang* in the body is upset, many diseases can develop, including breast cancer [14, 16]. Although different from modern nutritional classification theories, CM-based food classification could help people to improve their dietary patterns by eating more *neutral* or *cold* pattern foods and reducing consumption of high-risk *hot* foods to prevent breast cancer. Different food characteristics can alter the balance of *Yin* and *Yang* in the body. Numerous experimental studies have demonstrated that some food based on CM classifications may reduce the risk of cancer [8, 16–20]. However, no epidemiological research has reported a relationship between CM-defined dietary patterns and breast cancer morbidity.

In this study, participants with breast cancer shared a preference for a *hot*-patterned diet containing fried foods and meat rather than vegetables. This may have contributed to their breast cancer. The participants with breast cancer also had a relatively higher frequency of dining out, eating fast food, and consuming soft drinks, coffee, milk, and other foods classified as *hot* according to CM theory. In CM, *hot* food is defined as food that is high in energy and low in fiber, such as beef and prawns, or food that is fried or roasted [8, 21]. This is consistent with the etiology and pathogenesis of breast cancer in Western medicine [22]. It was demonstrated that carcinogenic substances found in foods according to Western medicine mostly belong to foods classified as *hot* according to CM, such as barbecued foods, red meat, fatty meat, and prawns [23–27].

Table 4 Odds ratio and its corresponding 95% confidence intervals of having breast cancer by eating different food

	Controls N = 202	Cases N = 202	OR	95% CI	P value
Shrimp					
Average	84	73	1.00	Reference	
Much preferred	13	44	3.90	1.95–7.79	<0.001*
Preferred	53	60	1.30	0.80–2.12	0.285
Not preferred	38	19	0.58	0.31–1.08	0.086
Not preferred much	14	5	0.41	0.14–1.20	0.094
Shellfish					
Average	97	73	1.00	Reference	
Much preferred	9	31	4.58	2.05–10.21	<0.001*
Preferred	37	56	2.01	1.20–3.36	0.007*
Not preferred	48	39	1.08	0.64–1.82	0.773
Not preferred much	11	3	0.36	0.10–1.35	0.116
Soft drinks					
Average	65	72	1.00	Reference	
Much preferred	3	10	3.01	0.79–11.41	0.092
Preferred	10	30	2.71	1.23–5.97	0.011*
Not preferred	92	65	0.64	0.40–1.01	0.056
Not preferred much	31	24	0.70	0.37–1.31	0.264
Milk					
Average	91	90	1.00	Reference	
Much preferred	10	25	2.53	1.15–5.57	0.018*
Preferred	49	37	0.76	0.46–1.28	0.306
Not preferred	35	43	1.24	0.73–2.12	0.425
Not preferred much	17	7	0.42	0.17–1.05	0.058
Popcorn/fries					
Average	79	86	1.00	Reference	
Much preferred	3	15	4.59	1.28–16.46	0.011*
Preferred	34	32	0.87	0.49–1.53	0.618
Not preferred	57	46	0.74	0.45–1.22	0.235
Not preferred much	29	23	0.73	0.39–1.36	0.321
Nuts					
Average	64	88	1.00	Reference	
Much preferred	39	26	0.49	0.27–0.88	0.016*
Preferred	84	65	0.56	0.36–0.89	0.013*
Not preferred	10	18	1.31	0.57–3.02	0.528
Not preferred much	5	5	0.73	0.20–2.62	0.745
Products made from bean					
Average	39	67	1.00	Reference	
Much preferred	53	39	0.43	0.24–0.76	0.003*
Preferred	103	87	0.49	0.30–0.80	0.004*
Not preferred	5	8	0.93	0.29–3.05	1.000
Not preferred much	2	1	0.29	0.026–3.32	0.555

A statistically significant OR (odds ratio) >1 indicates a risk factor; an OR <1 indicates a prevention factor

* indicates a statistically significant between-group diference

Depending on the seasons and individual constitution, people in Hong Kong will choose different foods, herbs, or soups to adjust the functions of the organs and balance the *Yin* and *Yang* of the body [28, 29]. Our findings suggested that frequent consumption of Chinese herbs or Chinese soup is inversely associated with the risk of breast cancer. CM dietary herbs (supplements) or Chinese herbal medicine may play a crucial role in

Table 5 Adjusted odds ratio and its corresponding 95% confidence intervals of having breast cancer by dining out patterns (fast food)

	Controls $n = 202$	Cases $n = 202$	Adjusted OR	95% CI	P value
Breakfast					
0–1 times per week	113	81	1.00	Reference	
2–3 times per week	39	34	1.22	0.71–2.09	0.479
4–5 times per week	19	30	2.20	1.16–4.18	0.015*
6–7 times per week	31	56	2.52	1.49–4.25	<0.001*
Lunch					
0–1 times per week	68	40	1.00	Reference	
2–3 times per week	56	59	1.70	0.99–2.91	0.053
4–5 times per week	31	44	3.24	1.80–5.80	<0.001*
6–7 times per week	47	59	2.13	1.24–3.69	0.006*

Adjusted for age and body mass index (BMI)

* The P value was <0.05, indicating a statistically significant between-group difference

Table 6 Adjusted odds ratio and its corresponding 95% confidence intervals of having breast cancer by frequency of Guangdong drinking tea

	Controls $n = 202$	Cases $n = 202$	Adjusted OR	95% CI	P value
Guangdong tea (Yum Cha)					
Less than once per week	142	109	1.00	Reference	
1–2 times per week	46	56	1.59	1.00–2.52	0.05*
>3 times per week	12	35	3.80	1.88–7.66	<0.001*

The P value was <0.05, indicating a statistically significant between-group difference

* Adjusted for age and body mass index (BMI)

Table 7 Adjusted odds ratio and its corresponding 95% confidence intervals of having breast cancer by the dietary patterns of Chinese medicine and related supplement and soup intake

	Controls $n = 202$	Cases $n = 202$	Adjusted OR	95% CI	P value
Chinese medicine					
Seldom	98	112	1.00	Reference	
Sometimes	61	51	0.73	0.46–1.16	0.183
Often	43	36	0.73	0.44–1.23	0.240
Food supplement					
Seldom	119	140	1.00	Reference	
Sometimes	35	32	0.78	0.45–1.33	0.358
Often	47	26	0.47	0.28–0.81	0.005*
Chinese soup					
Seldom	91	115	1.00	Reference	
Sometimes	83	69	0.66	0.43–1.00	0.051
Often	28	16	0.45	0.23–0.89	0.019*

The P value was <0.05, indicating a statistically significant between-group difference

* Adjusted for age and body mass index (BMI)

preventing the incidence, recurrence, and metastasis of breast cancer. Many experimental studies have demonstrated that some foods representative of the CM classifications could reduce the risk of cancer [30–32], and that there is a relationship between the use of CM herbs or related Chinese herbal medicine and the reduced incidence of breast cancer [33].

The design and conduct of this study had some limitations. This study did not examine other factors related to breast cancer, such as whether or not participants exercised regularly or whether they used oral contraceptives. In addition, because the control group was recruited from health workshops, and included both healthy and unhealthy women, there may be a health worker effect resulting in selection bias. Because of limited resources, we recruited only 37 people to our pilot study. This sample size was not large enough to conduct a factor analysis to assess the internal consistency of the questionnaire. Because this questionnaire was the first to analyze dietary patterns in terms of *hot*, *neutral*, and *cold* characteristics as defined by CM, there was no other standard questionnaire and results for comparison. The evidence strength in terms of epidemiology is also insufficient.

Conclusions

Non-breast cancer participants adopted a healthy and balanced (*neutral*) dietary pattern, along with consumption of CM supplements and Guangdong soups.

Abbreviations

CM: Chinese medicine; FFQ: Food Frequency Questionnaires; CSCMHKU: Clinic Center of School of Chinese Medicine, The University of Hong Kong; BMI: body mass index.

Authors' contributions

JPC conceived and designed the study. XZ, JSY, JY, FZM and KCT recruited the participants. WTYL revised the questionnaire. XZ and TX collected the data. ZYX, LXL and JSY performed the data analysis. FG performed the literature search. JPC and XZ wrote the manuscript. TX, ZYX, JSY, JY, KCT and FG revised the manuscript. All authors read and approved the final manuscript.

Author details

[1] School of Chinese Medicine, The University of Hong Kong, Hong Kong, China. [2] Department of Dermatology, Guangzhou University of Chinese Medicine, Guangzhou 510020, China. [3] School of Public Health, Peking University, Beijing, China. [4] The Hong Kong Associate of Chinese Medicine, Hong Kong, China. [5] Chengdu University of Traditional Chinese Medicine, Chengdu 510020, China.

Acknowledgements

Thanks a lot of Prof. Y Tong for the application IRB, Ms. Xue Huitian and Ms. Wong Mei Kuen for the provision of statistics. We are grateful to all the study participants for their contributions and support. Incident breast cancer cases for this study were collected by the School of Chinese Medicine, the University of Hong Kong.

Competing interests

The authors declare that they have no competing interests.

References

1.   Hospital Authority: Hong Kong Cancer Registry web site. http://www3.ha.org.hk/cancereg/statistics.html.

2.   Wang L, Wang J, Wang M, et al. Using Internet search engines to obtain medical information: a comparative study. J Med Internet Res. 2012;14:e74.

3.   Sasco AJ. Breast cancer and the environment. Horm Res. 2003;60(Suppl 3):50.

4.   Li C, Zhao X, Toline EC, Siegal GP, Evans LM, Ibrahim-Hashim A, Desmond RA, Hardy RW. Prevention of carcinogenesis and inhibition of breast cancer tumor burden by dietary stearate. Carcinogenesis. 2011;4:1–8.

5.   Evans LM, Toline EC, Desmond R, Siegal GP, Hashim AI, Hardy RW. Dietary stearate reduces human breast cancer metastasis burden in athymic nude mice. Clin Exp Metastasis. 2009;26:415–24.

6.   Leung J. The dieting phenomenon in Hong Kong: the changing attitudes towards dieting among young women in Hong Kong. In: Civic exchange. 6; 2002.

7.   Crozier SR, Robinson SM, Godfrey KM, Cooper C, Inskip HM. Women's dietary patterns change little from before to during pregnancy. J Nutr. 2009;139:1956–63.

8.   Lee MM, Shen JM. Dietary patterns using traditional Chinese medicine principles in epidemiological studies. Asia Pac J Clin Nutr. 2008;17(Suppl 1):79–81.

9.   Pierce JP. Diet and breast cancer prognosis: making sense of the women's healthy eating and living and women's intervention nutrition study trials. Curr Opin Obstet Gyn. 2009;21(1):86–91.

10. Martinez-Chacin RC, Keniry M, Dearth RK. Analysis of high fat diet induced genes during mammary gland development: identifying role players in poor prognosis of breast cancer. BMC Res Notes. 2014;18(7):543.

11. De Lorgeril M, Salen P. Do statins increase and Mediterranean diet decrease the risk of breast cancer? BMC Med. 2014;5(12):94.

12. Hu FB, Rimm E, Smith-Warner SA. Reproducibility and validity of dietary patterns assessed with a food-frequency questionnaire. Am J Clin Nutr. 1999;69(2):243–9.

13. Kroenke Candyce H, Fung Teresa T, Hu Frank B, Holmes Michelle D. Dietary patterns and survival after breast cancer diagnosis. J Clin Oncol. 2005;23(36):9295–303.

14. Zhang CX, Ho SC, Fu JH, Cheng SZ, Chen YM, Lin FY. Dietary patterns and breast cancer risk among Chinese women. Cancer Causes Control. 2011;22(1):115–24.

15. Lv N, Brown JL. Chinese American family food systems: impact of Western influences. J Nutr Educ Behav. 2010;42(2):106–14.

16. Miller PE, Morey MC, Hartman TJ, Snyder DC, Sloane R, Cohen HJ, Demark-Wahnefried W. Dietary patterns differ between urban and rural older, long-term survivors of breast, prostate, and colorectal cancer and are associated with body mass index. J Acad Nutr Diet. 2012;112(6):824–31.

17. Pierce JP, Faerber S, Wright FA, Newman V, Flatt SW, Kealey S, Rock CL, Hryniuk W, Greenberg ER. Feasibility of a randomized trial of a high-vegetable diet to prevent breast cancer recurrence. Nutr Cancer. 1997;28(3):282–8.

18. Moran LJ, Hutchison SK, Norman RJ, Teede HJ. Lifestyle changes in women with polycystic ovary syndrome. Cochrane Database Syst Rev. 2011;16(2):CD007506.

19. Brunner EJ, Rees K, Ward K, Burke M, Thorogood M. Dietary advice for reducing cardiovascular risk. Cochrane Database Syst Rev. 2007;17(4):CD002128.

20. Schatzkin A. Dietary change as a strategy for preventing cancer. Cancer Metastasis Rev. 1997;16(3–4):377–92.

21. Huang LP, Zhu MF, Yu RY, Du JQ, Liu HN. Study on discrimination mode of cold and hot properties of traditional Chinese medicines based on biological effects. China J Chin Mater Med. 2014;39(17):3353–8.

22. Reuss-Borst M, Kötter J, Hartmann U, Füger-Helmerking G, Weiß J. Nutrition patterns in German breast cancer patients. Dtsch Med Wochenschr. 2011;136(12):575–81.

23. Zhang CX, Ho SC, Fu JH, Cheng SZ, Chen YM, Lin FY. Dietary patterns and breast cancer risk among Chinese women. Cancer Cause Control. 2011;22(1):115–24.

24. Cui X, Dai Q, Tseng M, Shu XO, Gao YT, Zheng W. Dietary patterns and breast cancer risk in the shanghai breast cancer study. Cancer Epidemiol Biomark. 2007;16:1443–8.

25. Zhang CX, Ho SC, Chen YM, Lin FY, Fu JH, Cheng SZ. Meat and egg consumption and risk of breast cancer among Chinese women. Cancer Cause Control. 2009;20:1845–53.

26. Andrici J, Eslick GD. Hot food and beverage consumption and the risk of esophageal cancer: a meta-analysis. Am J Prev Med. 2015;49(6):952–60.

27. Turner LB. A meta-analysis of fat intake, reproduction, and breast cancer risk: an evolutionary perspective. Am J Hum Biol. 2011;23(5):601–8.

28. Ou B, Huang D, Hampsch-Woodill M, Flanagan JA. When east meets west: the relationship between yin-yang and antioxidation–oxidation. Faseb J. 2003;17(2):127–9.

29. Wang J, Tang YL. On the concept of health in traditional Chinese medicine and its characteristics and advantages. Chin J Med Hist. 2011;40(1):13–4.

30. Fornier MN. Approved agents for metastatic breast cancer. Semin Oncol. 2011;38(Suppl 2):S3–10.

31. Cuzick J, DeCensi A, Arun B, Brown PH, Castiglione M, Dunn B, Forbes JF, Glaus A, Howell A, von Minckwitz G, Vogel V, Zwierzina H. Preventive therapy for breast cancer: a consensus statement. Lancet Oncol. 2011;12(5):496–503.

32. Molokhia EA, Perkins A. Preventing cancer. Prim Care. 2008;35(4):609–23.

33. Dayal HH, Kalia A. Preventing breast cancer in postmenopausal women by achievable diet modification: a missed opportunity in public health policy. Breast. 2010;19(5):309–11.

12

Application of metabolomics in toxicity evaluation of traditional Chinese medicines

Li Duan[1†], Long Guo[2,4†], Lei Wang[2], Qiang Yin[5], Chen-Meng Zhang[1], Yu-Guang Zheng[2] and E.-Hu Liu[3*]

Abstract

Traditional Chinese medicines (TCM) have a long history of use because of its potential complementary therapy and fewer adverse effects. However, the toxicity and safety issues of TCM have drawn considerable attention in the past two decades. Metabolomics is an "omics" approach that aims to comprehensively analyze all metabolites in biological samples. In agreement with the holistic concept of TCM, metabolomics has shown great potential in efficacy and toxicity evaluation of TCM. Recently, a large amount of metabolomic researches have been devoted to exploring the mechanism of toxicity induced by TCM, such as hepatotoxicity, nephrotoxicity, and cardiotoxicity. In this paper, the application of metabolomics in toxicity evaluation of bioactive compounds, TCM extracts and TCM prescriptions are reviewed, and the potential problems and further perspectives for application of metabolomics in toxicological studies are also discussed.

Keywords: Traditional Chinese medicines, Toxicity, Metabolomics, Toxicity mechanisms

Background

Traditional Chinese medicines (TCM) have been used for the treatment of a variety of diseases for thousands of years in China since they are relatively inexpensive, widely available and have reliable therapeutic efficacy [1–3]. Accompanying with hot discussions on development of multidrug therapy for multi-gene diseases, TCM are receiving increasing attention worldwide because it is well accepted that TCM exert their curative effects via multiple components on multiple targets in clinic [4–6].

Many people believe that TCM are safe because they derive from natural origin. However, this belief has been greatly challenged in recent years. In fact, the toxicity and safety issues of TCM has aroused increasing concern to international community, such as identification of plant materials, preparation method, and the potential to interact with other herbal medicines and conventional drugs [7–10]. Moreover, the traditional safety assessment methods may not accurately assess safety knowledge of

TCM due to the complexity of its constituents and action mechanisms.

Systems biology is a biology-based interdisciplinary field of study that focuses on complex interactions within biological systems, using a holistic approach to biological research [11]. Indeed, the holistic properties of systems biology are in agreement with TCM theory in nature [12, 13]. The omics approaches, such as genomics, transcriptomics, proteomics and metabolomics, have greatly facilitated the systematic study of complex systems, especially TCM and herbal medicines [14–16].

Metabolomics, first put forward by professor Nicholson in 1999 [17], is defined as systematically qualitative and quantitative analysis of metabolites in a given organism or biological sample. It allows the quantitative measurement of large numbers of low-molecular-weight (< 1 kDa) endogenous metabolites, including lipids, amino acids, peptides, nucleic acids, organic acids, vitamins, and carbohydrates, which play important roles in biological systems and represent attractive candidates to understand phenotypes [18–20]. Metabolomics is suitable for observing abnormal changes of endogenous metabolites before the appearance of physiological or pathological damages. As a systemic approach, metabolomics adopts a "top-down" strategy to reflect the function of organisms from

*Correspondence: liuehu2011@163.com
†Li Duan and Long Guo contributed equally to this work
[3] State Key Laboratory of Natural Medicines, China Pharmaceutical University, Nanjing 210009, China

terminal symptoms of metabolic network and understand metabolic changes of a complete system caused by interventions in a holistic context [21].

Recently, metabolomics has been widely applied to the modern researches of TCM including theory of TCM, syndrome, efficacy and toxicity since the metabolome represents the physiological or pathological status of organisms [22–25]. It was deemed that metabolomic analysis is an efficacious and noninvasive method to evaluate toxicity of TCM and explore toxicity mechanisms through correlations of physiological changes and metabolic changes [26, 27]. In this review, we summarized the metabolomics analytical techniques widely used in the study of TCM, and focusing on the application of metabolomics in the toxicological evaluation of TCM.

Metabolomic technology and data analysis

Modern metabolomic technologies allow for qualitative and quantitative measurement of a vast number of metabolites in complex biological systems. The main analytical techniques in metabolomics, which have widespread applications in the assessments of efficacy and toxicology of TCM, are proton nuclear magnetic resonance spectroscopy (^{1}H NMR) and mass spectrometry (MS) [28].

^{1}H NMR is a non-destructive technique, which provides high-throughput and automated analysis of crude extracts, and quantitatively detects different metabolites in different groups, as well as offers structural information [29]. The advantages of ^{1}H NMR in metabolomic analysis include simple and nondestructive sample preparation, fast analysis rate, and non-selective judgment. However, ^{1}H NMR fails to obtain valid data when the concentrations of metabolites in complex sample are quite low [30]. Therefore, in most cases, MS is preferred in metabolomic analysis because of its advantages of unparalleled sensitivity, high resolution and structural specificity [31]. In practical applications, MS requires combining with different separation techniques such as gas chromatography (GC–MS), liquid chromatography (LC–MS), capillary electrophoresis (CE–MS) and ultra-performance liquid chromatography (UPLC–MS) for a pre-separation. GC–MS is particularly suitable for the detection of thermally stable volatile metabolites. Hence, the application range of GC–MS is limited as most non-volatile metabolites cannot be analyzed directly [32]. Compared to GC–MS, the utilization of LC–MS is more frequent in metabolomic analysis, LC can isolate different kinds of metabolites in a complex system and MS can provide structural information to help to identify metabolites. LC–MS can provide more details of submerged portions than ^{1}H NMR, and can detected molecules with different proper polarity [33]. The ability of LC–MS

to analyze various kinds of metabolites depends on the ionization source and the chromatographic method that is used to separate a complex mixture of analytes. Nowadays, two-dimensional LC method has been successfully applied in metabolomic analysis of TCM and due to its enhanced selectivity, peak capacity and high resolution compared with one-dimensional LC [34]. Normally, the selection of metabolomic technology depends on the research purpose and the properties of samples. In fact, due to the large number and the wide concentration range of metabolites, and the complexity of TCM, integrated metabolomic approaches have been frequently used to provide sensitive, accurate and reliable results [35].

Sample preparation, including its source, storage and extraction, has significant effects on the results of metabolomic analysis. Plasma, serum, urine and tissue are usually biological samples in metabolomic analysis [36]. To decrease the changes of potential metabolites in metabolomic samples, biological samples usually can be restored in -80 °C. For ^{1}H NMR analysis, the change of pH and ionic strength caused by the change of the chemical shift is the primary problem, and the addition of pH buffer during the sample extraction can solve the problem [37]. Compared with ^{1}H NMR, the samples extraction for MS-based metabolomics are more complicated. For LC–MS analysis, biological samples are complex and contain various endogenous and exogenous acidic, basic, and neutral compounds with high polarity. The samples usually require to be centrifuged and diluted with deionized water before metabolomic analysis [38]. For GC–MS analysis, most potential biomarkers in biological samples are high polar and nonvolatile, thus the samples must be derivatized before analysis [39].

Data analysis are crucial since the data matrix generated in metabolomic study is generally large and complex. Data preprocessing is the first step of metabolomic data analysis. The main objective of data preprocessing is to transform the data in such way that the samples in the dataset are more comparable in order to ease and improve the data analysis [40]. ^{1}H NMR data preprocessing usually includes baseline correction, alignment, binning, normalization and scaling [41]. For MS data preprocessing, many softwares such as MetAlign, MZmine and XCMS have been developed to process raw data [42]. Multivariate statistical methods are professional approaches for analyzing and maximizing information retrieval from complex metabolomic data. The multivariate statistical methods can be classified into two groups, namely unsupervised methods and supervised methods. Unsupervised methods mainly include principal component analysis (PCA), hierarchical cluster analysis (HCA), K-means and statistical total correlation spectroscopy.

PCA can summarize the information in an experimental data set using a small number of orthogonal latent variables obtained by searching the direction of maximum variance in the data set. However, PCA does not always extract hidden information that explains system behavior. Supervised methods, such as partial least squares discriminant analysis (PLS-DA), orthogonal partial least squares discriminant analysis (OPLS-DA), quadratic discriminant analysis and linear discriminant analysis can reveal the most important factors of variability characterizing the metabolomic datasets [43]. The commonly used softwares for metabolomic multivariate statistical analysis are Shimadzu Class-VP software and SIMCA-P software. The identification of metabolites and the pathway analysis of metabolites are also essential components of metabolomic data analysis. The updating commercial software is crucial for identifying potential metabolites, while accurate mass, isotopic pattern, fragments information, and available biochemical databases are also necessary. Presently, a number of metabolites databases such as Human Metabolome Database (HMDB), Kyoto Encyclopedia of Genes and Genomes (KEGG), Biochemical Genetic and Genomic (BiGG), ChemSpider and PubChem Compound, are emerging and have been applied in the identification of metabolites and biomarkers. For metabolic pathway analysis, KEGG, Ingenuity Pathway Analysis, Cytoscape and Reactome Pathway Database are commonly used databases and softwares. The flowchart of typical metabolomic experiment including sample preparation, metabolomic technology, data analysis and pathway analysis is shown in Fig. 1.

Metabolomics in toxicity evaluation of TCM

Metabolomic analysis is an effectively and noninvasive method for evaluating toxicology of TCM and exploring toxicity mechanisms through correlations of physiological changes and metabolic changes. The metabolomic researches on hepatotoxicity, nephrotoxicity, cardiotoxicity and other toxicity induced by bioactive compounds, TCM extracts and TCM prescriptions were summarized in Tables 1, 2, 3 and 4, respectively.

Metabolomics in hepatotoxicity evaluation of TCM

Metabolomics is a useful tool to evaluate toxicity and identify toxicological biomarkers of bioactive compounds from TCM. Triptolide, a bioactive diterpenoid compound isolated from *Tripterygium wilfordii*, exhibits diverse biological activities such as anti-inflammatory, immune-modulatory and anti-proliferative activities [44]. However, the further clinical research and application of triptolide is confined by its severe toxicity on the liver, kidney and reproductive systems [45]. Zhao et al. developed a LC–MS based metabolomic method to investigate the hepatotoxicity of triptolide in mice. Mice were administered triptolide by gavage to establish the acute liver injury model. Metabolomic results showed that a total of thirty metabolites were significantly changed by triptolide treatment and the abundance of twenty-nine metabolites was correlated with toxicity. Pathway analysis indicated that the mechanism of triptolide induced hepatotoxicity was related to alterations in multiple metabolic pathways, including glutathione metabolism, tricarboxylic acid cycle, purine metabolism, glycerophospholipid

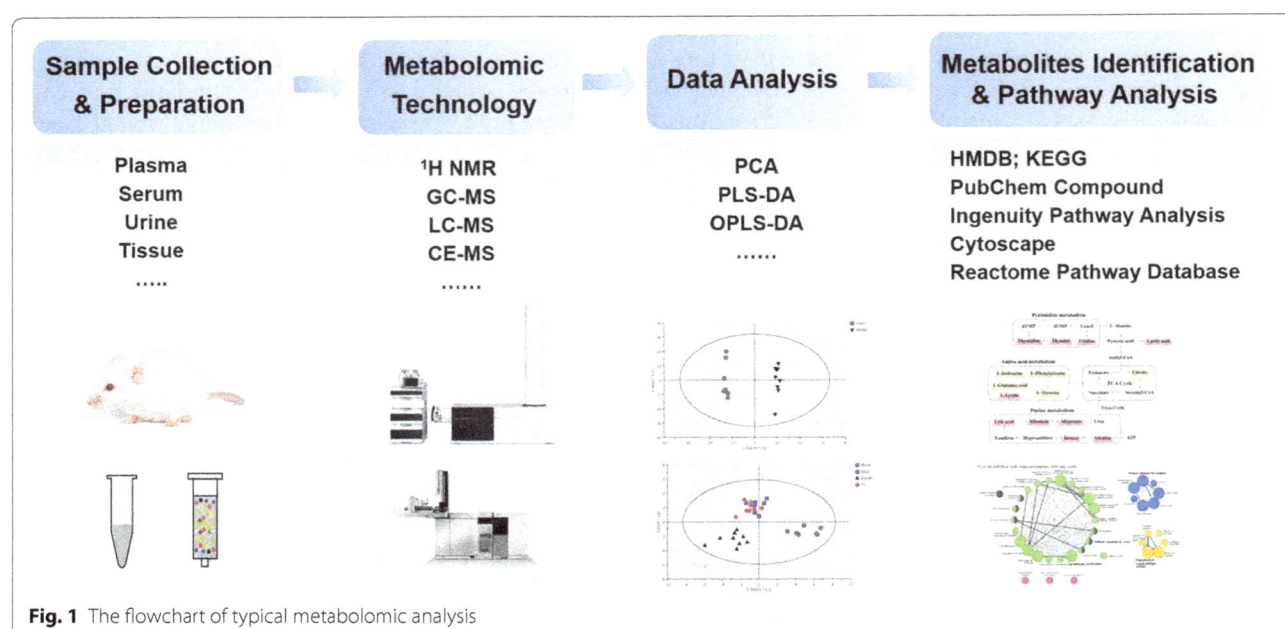

Fig. 1 The flowchart of typical metabolomic analysis

Table 1 The applications of metabolomics in hepatotoxicity evaluation of TCM

TCM	Toxicity	Animals	Samples	Metabolomic technology	Data analysis	Metabolic pathways	References
Triptolide	Hepatotoxicity	Mice	Serum, liver	LC–MS	PCA, PLS-DA	Glutathione metabolism, tricarboxylic acid cycle, purine metabolism, glycerophospholipid metabolism, taurine and hypotaurine metabolism, pantothenate and coenzyme A biosynthesis, pyrimidine metabolism, amino acid metabolism	[45, 46]
Dioscorea bulbifera Rhizome	Hepatotoxicity	Rats	Plasma, urine, feces	GC–MS	OPLS-DA	Amino acid metabolism, bile acid metabolism, purine metabolism, pyrimidine metabolism, lipid metabolism, energy metabolism	[49]
		Rats	Urine	^{1}H NMR	PLS-DA	Amino acid metabolism, fatty acid metabolism, energy metabolism	[50]
Xanthii Fructus	Hepatotoxicity	Rats	Urine	LC–MS	PCA, PLS-DA, OPLS-DA	Mitochondrial inability, fatty acid metabolism, amino acids metabolism	[52, 53]
Polygoni multiflori radix	Chronic hepatotoxicity	Rats	Serum	GC–MS	PCA, PLS-DA	Amino acid metabolism, fatty acid metabolism, oxidative injury	[55]
Realgar	Hepatotoxicity	Rats	Urine	LC–MS, ^{1}H NMR	PCA, OPLS-DA	Citric acid cycle, tryptophan metabolism, porphyrin metabolism	[57]
	Sub-chronic hepatotoxicity	Mice	Plasma, urine	^{1}H NMR	PCA	Energy metabolism, amino acids metabolism, gut bacteria metabolism	[58]

metabolism, taurine and hypotaurine metabolism, pantothenate and coenzyme A biosynthesis, pyrimidine metabolism and amino acid metabolism [46]. Recently, another LC–MS based metabolomic approach was developed to discover hepatotoxic and nephrotoxic potential biomarkers of triptolide. The metabolic profiles of liver, kidney and plasma were characterized by HPLC Q/TOF MS. The metabolite profiles of the liver, kidney and

plasma of toxic and therapeutically dosed mice showed significant differences. Two toxic markers, mono-hydroxylated metabolite of triptolide, tri-hydroxylated and dehydrogenated metabolite of triptolide, were detected both in mice plasma and human liver microsomes following incubation with triptolide. The two metabolites could be potential diagnosis markers for hepatotoxicity and nephrotoxicity induced by triptolide [45]. The

Table 2 The applications of metabolomics in nephrotoxicity evaluation of TCM

TCM	Toxicity	Animals	Samples	Metabolomic technology	Data analysis	Metabolic pathways	References
Aristolochic acid	Nephrotoxicity	Rats	Urine	GC–MS	PCA, PLS-DA	Energy metabolism, gut microbiota, purine metabolism	[60]
		Rats	Urine	LC–MS	OPLS-DA	Tricarboxylic acid cycle, gut microflora metabolism, amino acid metabolism, purine metabolism, bile acid biosynthesis	[61]
Strychni Semen	Nephrotoxicity	Rats	Serum, urine	^{1}H NMR	OPLS-DA	Glycolysis, lipid and amino acid metabolism	[64]
Arisaematis Rhizoma	Nephrotoxicity	Rats	Serum, urine	^{1}H NMR	PLS-DA	Glycolysis–gluconeogenesis, tricarboxylic acid cycle, fatty acid metabolism, gut microflora metabolism	[66]
Pharbitidis Semen	Nephrotoxicity	Rats	Serum, kidney	LC–MS	PCA	Phospholipids metabolism, amino acid metabolism, sphingolipids biosynthesis and metabolism	[68]
		Rats	Urine	LC–MS	PCA	Amino acid metabolism, citric acid cycle, bile acid metabolism	[69]
Alismatis Rhizoma	Chronic nephrotoxicity	Rats	Urine	LC–MS	PCA	Amino acid metabolism, Purine metabolism, bile acid metabolism, sphingolipids metabolism	[71]

metabolomic analysis could provide an integral understanding of the mechanism of the hepatotoxicity, and it may be useful for further prediction and diagnosis of liver injury during clinical use of triptolide.

Compared with the limited applications in toxicity evaluation of bioactive compounds, metabolomics was widely applied to toxicity evaluation of the TCM extracts. Dioscorea bulbifera Rhizome, the dried root of *Dioscorea bulbifera* L., has been known to have many bioactivities such as anti-tumor, anti-bacterial, anti-feedant, antifungal and anti-salmonella [47]. However, experimental studies and clinical reports indicated that Dioscorea bulbifera Rhizome could cause toxicity, particularly in the liver [48]. A multisample integrated metabolomic strategy was employed to precisely describe the status and mechanism of hepatotoxicity induced by Dioscorea bulbifera Rhizome. Comparison of metabolomic profiles of rat plasma, urine, and feces by GC–MS, a total of fifty-five metabolites distributed in 33 metabolic pathways were identified. Correlation network analysis revealed that the hub metabolites of hepatotoxicity were mainly associated with amino acid metabolism, bile acid metabolism, purine metabolism, pyrimidine metabolism, lipid metabolism and energy metabolism [49]. In another study, liver toxicity induced by Dioscorea bulbifera Rhizome was investigated by ^{1}H NMR. The metabolomic results revealed that the levels of taurine, creatine,

betaine, dimethylglycine, acetate, glycine were elevated, whereas, the levels of succinate, 2-oxoglutarate, citrate, hippurate and urea were reduced. With molecular function analysis of these changed metabolites, the hepatotoxicity of Dioscorea bulbifera Rhizome was involved in hepatic mitochondrial injury [50].

Xanthii Fructus is the mature fruit with involucres of *Xanthium sibirium* Patr. and widely used for the treatment of sinusitis, headache, rheumatism, and skin itching [51]. Xue et al. performed an integrated metabolomic study using ^{1}H NMR combined with multivariate statistical analysis to elucidate the hepatotoxicity of Xanthii Fructus. When rats were treated with Xanthii Fructus at 30.0 g/kg, the hepatotoxicity was reflected in the changes observed in serum biochemical profiles and by the histopathological examination of the liver. The results demonstrated that atractyloside, carboxyatractyloside and 40-desulphate-atractyloside were the major hepatotoxicity constituents in Xanthii Fructus. Moreover, the hepatotoxicity of Xanthii Fructus mainly associated with mitochondrial inability, fatty acid metabolism, and some amino acids metabolism [52]. The urinary metabolic perturbations associated with toxicity induced by Xanthii Fructus were also studied using UPLC–MS. The results showed that the metabolic characters in Xanthii Fructus treated rats were perturbed in a dose dependent manner and ten metabolites including

Table 3 The applications of metabolomics in cardiotoxicity evaluation of TCM

TCM	Toxicity	Animals	Samples	Metabolomic technology	Data analysis	Metabolic pathways	References
Periplocin	Cardiotoxicity	Neonatal rats	Cardiomyocytes	LC–MS	PCA, PLS-DA, Support Vector Machine	Amino acid metabolism, energy metabolism, sphingolipid metabolism	[73]
Aconitum alkaloids	Cardiotoxicity	Rats	Plasma	^{1}H NMR, GC–MS	PCA	Energy metabolism, fatty acid metabolism, amino acid metabolism, purine metabolism	[74]
Aconiti kusnezoffii Radix	Cardiotoxicity	Rats	Urine	LC–MS	PCA, PLS-DA, OPLS-DA	Pentose and glucuronate interconversions, tryptophan metabolism, amino sugar and nucleotide sugar metabolism, taurine and hypotaurine metabolism, ascorbate and aldarate metabolism, fructose and mannose metabolism, starch and sucrose metabolism	[77]
Aconiti Radix	Cardiotoxicity	Rats	Urine	LC–MS	PCA, PLS-DA, OPLS-DA	pentose and glucuronate interconversions, amino acid metabolism, starch and sucrose metabolism, amino sugar and nucleotide sugar metabolism, purine metabolism, tryptophan metabolism, taurine and hypotaurine metabolism, fructose and mannose metabolism, fatty acid metabolism	[78, 79]
Aconiti Lateralis Radix Praeparata	Cardiotoxicity	Rats	Plasma	LC–MS	PCA, PLS-DA, OPLS-DA	Sphingolipid metabolism, aminoacyl-tRNA biosynthesis, tryptophan metabolism	[80]
		Mices	Heart	LC–MS	PCA, PLS-DA	Phospholipid metabolism, Sphingolipid metabolism, saturated fatty acid oxidation, unsaturated fatty acid peroxidation	[81]
Pinelliae Rhizoma	Cardiotoxicity	Rats	Serum	LC–MS	PCA, PLS-DA	Phospholipid metabolism, amino acid metabolism, carnitine metabolism	[83]

Table 4 The applications of metabolomics in other toxicity evaluation of TCM

TCM	Toxicity	Animals	Samples	Metabolomic technology	Data analysis	Metabolic pathways	References
Triptolide	Reproduction toxicity	Mice	Serum, testis	GC–MS	PLS-DA	Lipid metabolism, energy metabolism	[85]
Cinnabar	Neurotoxicity	Rats	Brain	^{1}H NMR	PCA	Glutamate metabolism, membrane disruption, energy metabolism, oxidative injury	[87]
Kunsui Radix	Inflammation, irritation to the skin, tumor-promotion	Rats	Urine	^{1}H NMR	PCA	Tricarboxylic acid cycle, anaerobic glycolysis, amino acids metabolism	[89]
Coptidis Rhizome	Diarrhea	Rats	Serum, urine	^{1}H NMR, GC–MS	PCA, OPLS-DA	Gut microflora metabolism, energy metabolism, amino acids metabolism	[90]
Niuhuang Jiedu Tablet	Hepatotoxicity, nephrotoxicity	Rats	Urine	^{1}H NMR	PCA, PLS-DA	Energy metabolism, choline metabolism, amino acid metabolism, gut flora disorder	[92]
Zhusha Anshen Wan	Hepatotoxicity, nephrotoxicity	Rats	Serum, urine	^{1}H NMR	PLS-DA	Energy metabolism, lipid metabolism, choline metabolism	[93]
Shuanghuanglian injection	Hemolytic anemia	Dogs	Serum	^{1}H NMR	PCA	Cell membranes metabolism, lipid metabolism, energy metabolism, amino acid metabolism, gut microflora metabolism	[95]

6-hydroxy-5-methoxyindole glucuronide/5-hydroxy-6-methoxyindole glucuronide, 4,6-dihydroxyquinoline, 3-methyldioxyindole, phenylalanine, indoxyl sulfate, hippuric acid, uridine, l-phenylalanyl-l-hydroxyproline, sebacic acid, and arachidonic acid were preliminarily identified as potential toxicity biomarkers [53].

Polygoni Multiflori Radix, the dried root of *Polygonum multiflorum* Thunb, is commonly used to prevent or treat non-alcoholic fatty liver disease, hyperlipidemia or related hepatic diseases in clinic. Currently, several clinical cases associated with hepatotoxicity of Polygoni Multiflori Radix including toxic hepatitis and acute hepatitis have been reported [54]. Xia et al. used an untargeted metabolomic strategy to investigate the chronic hepatotoxicity induced by Polygoni Multiflori Radix in rats. Ten potential endogenous metabolites including glycine, 13-eicosenoic acid, lactic acid, octadecanoic acid, proline, 2-furoic acid, cholesterol, alanine, docosahexaenoic acid, and lysine were identified. The ten potential biomarkers were involved in three metabolic pathways, amino acid metabolism, fatty acid metabolism and oxidative injury. The results indicated that Polygoni Multiflori Radix-induced liver damage

is dosage dependent and disruption in amino acid and energy metabolism might lead to subsequent oxidative damage in the liver of rats [55].

Realgar, an ore crystal containing more than 90% tetra-arsenic tetrasulfide, has been used for the treatment of carbuncles, boils, insect-and snake-bites, intestinal parasitosis, convulsive epilepsy and psoriasis [56]. As an arsenical, realgar is known as a poison and paradoxically as a therapeutic agent. Using a combined LC–MS and ^{1}H NMR based metabolomic approach, Huang et al. investigated the hepatotoxicity induced by realgar in rats. Thirty-six potential biomarkers were discovered, and these metabolites were distributed in citric acid cycle, tryptophan metabolism, and porphyrin metabolism. Glycine and serine were proposed as key metabolites related to realgar-induced disturbance [57]. In another study, a ^{1}H NMR-based metabolomic approach was employed to investigate the subchronic hepatotoxicity of realgar on mice. The change trends of metabolites in urine and plasma from mice subchronic exposed to realgar are similar to those acute exposed to realgar, which indicate the acute and sub-chronic toxic mechanisms of realgar are same. The disturbed metabolic pathways include energy metabolism, amino acids metabolism and gut bacteria metabolism [58].

Metabolomics in nephrotoxicity evaluation of TCM

Aristolochic acid is a mixture of structural-related nitrophenanthrene carboxylic acid derivatives existed in *Aristolochia, Bragantia and Asarum* genus, such as Aristolochiae Fructus, Stephaniae tetrandrae Radix and Asari Ridix et Rhizoma [59]. Aristolochic acid is a toxicant that can cause a common and rapidly progressive interstitial nephropathy called aristolochic acid nephropathy. The pathophysiology and underlying mechanisms of the aristolochic acid nephropathy have been studied using metabolomic approach by different analysis methods. Hu et al. employed a GC–MS based metabolomic technique to analyze urinary metabolites in aristolochic acid treated rats. Eight metabolites were selected as potential metabolic biomarkers including methylsuccinic acid, nicotinamide, 3-hydroxyphenylacetic acid, citric acid, creatinine, uric acid, glycolic acid, and gluconic acid. The identified metabolites suggested that the pathways of energy metabolism, gut microbiota, and purine metabolism were associated with aristolochic acid induced nephrotoxicity [60]. In another LC–MS based urinary metabolomic study, the results suggested that the nephrotoxicity of aristolochic acid could be characterized via systemic disturbance of metabolic network including tricarboxylic acid cycle, gut microflora metabolism, amino acid metabolism, purine metabolism and bile acid biosynthesis, which were partly consistent with the results of GC–MS based metabolomic study [61].

Strychni Semen, the dried ripe seeds of *Strychnos nux-vomica* Linn., was commonly used to relieve rheumatism, induce analgesia, remove stasis, clear heat, and alleviate swelling in China [62]. However, the clinical applications of Strychni Semen is limited by its severe toxicity, especially nephrotoxicity. Fan et al. established a ^{1}H NMR based metabolomic method to evaluate the toxicity induced by Strychni Semen. The results indicated that Strychni Semen induced disruptions in glycolysis, lipid and amino acid metabolism, and the toxic effects were aggravated in liver and kidney tissues as dosing time was prolonged [63]. A cell metabolomic strategy was also developed to investigate the nephrotoxicity of Strychni Semen. A total of 10 biomarkers and 24 related metabolic pathways were screened. The possible mechanisms of Strychni Semen nephrotoxicity might be cellular component disruption, oxidative damage, metabolic waste accumulation and the disturbance of energy and ion transport systems [64]. Metabolomics could be an efficient means to elucidate the mechanism of Strychni Semen-induced nephrotoxicity and might contribute to investigation of possible nephrotoxic mechanisms of other TCM.

Arisaematis Rhizoma, the dried rhizomes of *Arisaema erubescens* Schott, *Arisaema heterophyllum* BI. and *Arisaema amurense* Maxim., has been widely used due to its various effects including analgesic, sedative, stomachic, anticoagulant, antiemetic, anti-inflammatory and antitumor activities [65]. A ^{1}H NMR based metabolomic approach complemented with serum chemistry and histopathology has been applied to investigate the nephrotoxicity of Arisaematis Rhizoma. The results indicated that thirteen metabolites in urine and six metabolites in serum were significantly altered, suggesting disturbances in energy metabolism, perturbation of the gut microflora environment, membrane damage, folate deficiency and injury of kidneys produced by Arisaematis Rhizoma [66].

Pharbitidis Semen, the dried mature seeds of *Pharbitis nil* (L.) Choisy or *Pharbitis purpurea* (L.) Voigt, is widely used for treatment of edema, simple obesity and lung fever in China and some east Asian countries. Several animal and clinical studies have reported the nephrotoxicity of Pharbitidis Semen [67]. Recently, a LC–MS based metabolomic approach was employed to delineate the comprehensive mechanism of nephrotoxicity induced by Pharbitidis Semen. The results indicated that certain metabolic pathways, such as lysophosphatidylcholines formation and sphingolipids cycle were accelerated [68]. Ma et al. performed another LC–MS based urinary metabolomics to investigate the nephrotoxicity induced by Pharbitidis Semen. The results indicated that ethanol extract of Pharbitidis Semen should be responsible for the nephrotoxicity and eight metabolites were identified. According to the identified metabolites, the underlying regulations of Pharbitidis Semen perturbed metabolic pathways were amino acid metabolism, citric acid cycle and bile acid metabolism [69].

Alismatis Rhizoma, the dried rhizome of *Alisma orientale* (Sam.) Juz., has been widely used as diuretic, antinephrolithic, hypolipidemic, antiatherosclerotic, antidiabetic and anti-inflammatory in China [70]. However, overdose or long-term usage of Alismatis Rhizoma can cause nephrotoxicity. Yu et al. employed a LC–MS based metabolomic approach to investigate the nephrotoxicity of Alismatis Rhizoma in rats. The results indicated that significant changes in thirteen metabolite biomarkers were detected in the urine after treatment of Alismatis Rhizoma. The metabolomic method could discriminate the extract treated rats from the control rats on days 60, 120, and 180 after treatment. While serious organic renal damage was not observed on histopathology until day 180. The results indicated that LC–MS based metabolomic analysis is an useful tool for predicting the chronic nephrotoxicity induced by Alismatis Rhizoma [71].

Metabolomics in cardiotoxicity evaluation of TCM

Periplocin, a digitalis-like cardiac glycoside from Periplocae Cortex, has been used widely in clinic for its cardiotonic, anti-inflammatory and anti-tumor effects [72]. To evaluate the cardiotoxicity of periplocin, Li et al. reported an UPLC Q/TOF MS method to reveal the metabolic profiles on neonatal rat cardiomyocytes exposed to periplocin. Eleven biomarkers associated with cardiotoxicity including carnitine, acetylcarnitine, lysoPC, proline, glutamic acid, pyroglutamic acid, leucine, pantothenic acid, tryptophan, indoleacrylic acid and citric acid were identified. The metabolic pathway analysis indicated that these metabolites were associated with amino acid metabolism, energy metabolism and sphingolipid metabolism, which contributes to the cardiotoxicity mechanism of periplocin [73].

Herbal medicines derived from *Aconitum* species, including Aconiti kusnezoffii Radix, Aconiti Radix and Aconiti Lateralis Preparata Radix have a long history of clinical use. These herbs have been shown to exhibit biological effects on various diseases, including rheumatic fever, painful joints, bronchial asthma, gastroenteritis, collapse, syncope, diarrhea, edema and tumors. Modern research revealed that *Aconitum* herbs have potent toxicity, and *Aconitum* alkaloids are not only the active ingredients but also toxic components [74]. Aconitine, mesaconitine, and hypaconitine are the main *Aconitum* alkaloids derived from Aconiti lateralis Radix praeparata, the lateral root of *Aconitum carmichaelii* Debx. These alkaloids have analgesic, antipyretic, and local anesthetic activities and have beneficial effects against rheumatosis and rheumatoid arthritis. But the strong toxicity and the narrow margin between therapeutic and toxic doses limited clinical application of the *Aconitum* alkaloids. Sun et al. investigated the metabolic changes in rats caused by the aconitine, mesaconitine, and hypaconitine using ^{1}H NMR and GC–MS. Compared with control group, the results revealed larger deviations in the aconitine and mesaconitine groups and smaller deviations in hypaconitine group, illustrating the different toxicity mechanisms of these alkaloids. Metabolomic analysis indicated that most of the metabolic biomarkers were related to tricarboxylic acid cycle [75].

Aconiti kusnezoffii Radix, the root of *Aconitum kusnezoffii* Reichb., was reported to induce toxicity to heart and central nervous system [76]. Recently, Yan et al. proposed a UPLC Q/TOF MS based metabolomic approach to characterize the phenotypically biochemical perturbations and potential mechanisms of Aconiti kusnezoffii Radix-induced toxicity. The urinary metabolomics revealed serious toxicity to heart and liver. Thirteen metabolites were identified and validated as phenotypic toxicity biomarkers of Aconiti kusnezoffii Radix. These

biomarkers were responsible for pentose and glucuronate interconversions, tryptophan metabolism, amino sugar and nucleotide sugar metabolism, taurine and hypotaurine metabolism, ascorbate and aldarate metabolism, fructose and mannose metabolism, and starch and sucrose metabolism [77].

The potential cardiotoxicity of Aconiti Radix (the mother roots of *Aconitum carmichaelii* Debx) was frequently reported because of its narrow therapeutic window. A metabolomic method was performed to characterize the potential mechanisms of Aconiti Radix-induced cardiotoxicity by UPLC Q/TOF MS. Seventeen biomarkers were identified in urinary samples, which were associated with pentose and glucuronate interconversions, alanine, aspartate, and glutamate metabolism [78]. Meanwhile, the levels of the identified toxicity biomarkers were modulated to the normal ranges by Glyeyrrhizae Radix, Paeoniae Alba Radix and Zingiberis Rhizoma. The results indicated that these three compatible herbal medicines could be the effective detoxifying substances against the toxicity of Aconiti Radix [79].

Aconiti Lateralis Radix Praeparata, the lateral or daughter root of *Aconitum carmichaelii* Debx, has a potential cardiotoxicity with a relatively narrow margin of safety. Wang et al. reported a LC–MS metabolomic approach to investigate and compare the metabolic changing of Aconiti Lateralis Radix Praeparata, Aconiti Radix and the processed products. The data demonstrated that both Aconiti Lateralis Radix Praeparata and Aconiti Radix could lead to serious cardiotoxicity in a time- and dose-dependent manner. Sphingolipid metabolism, aminoacyl-tRNA biosynthesis and tryptophan metabolism mainly contributed to the toxicity of Aconiti Lateralis Radix Praeparata and Aconiti Radix [80]. Cai et al. further employed a lipidomics strategy to explore the cardiotoxic mechanisms of Aconiti Lateralis Radix Praeparata and find out potential tissue-specific biomarkers by HPLC Q/TOF MS. Fourteen lipid metabolites, which are primarily involved in phospholipid metabolism, sphingolipid metabolism, saturated fatty acid oxidation and unsaturated fatty acid peroxidation, were identified and considered as the potential biomarkers of the cardiotoxicity induced by Aconiti Lateralis Radix Praeparata [81].

Pinelliae Rhizoma, the dried tuber of *Pinellia ternata* (Thunb.) Breit., is commonly used for treatment of cough, vomiting, infection and inflammation [82]. Zhang et al. proposed a UPLC Q/TOF MS metabolomic approach to elucidate the toxicity of Pinelliae Rhizoma extract in rats. The results indicated that oral administration of Pinelliae Rhizoma did not induce obvious liver and kidney toxicity, but caused certain cardiotoxicity. The identified seven endogenous metabolites indicated the perturbations of phospholipid metabolism, amino acid metabolism and carnitine metabolism in Pinelliae Rhizoma treated rats [83]. According to the TCM theory, processing can reduce the toxicity of Pinelliae Rhizoma. Using the metabolomic approach, Su et al. investigated the mechanisms of raw Pinelliae Rhizoma induced toxicity and toxicity-reducing effect of processing. Consistent with the above report, the metabolomic results also indicated that raw Pinelliae Rhizoma could cause cardiotoxicity. Inhibition of mTOR signaling and activation of the TGF-β pathway contributed to raw Pinelliae Rhizoma-induced cardiotoxicity, and free radical scavenging might be responsible for the toxicity-reducing effect of processing [84].

Metabolomics in other toxicity evaluation of TCM

In addition to the above-mentioned hepatotoxicity, nephrotoxicity and cardiotoxicity, reproduction toxicity of triptolide is also the main obstacle for its clinical applications. Ma et al. developed a GC–MS based metabolomic approach to evaluate the mechanism of triptolide-induced reproductive toxicity in male mice and identify potential biomarkers for the early detection of spermatogenesis dysfunction. The results indicated that the testicular toxicity of triptolide may be caused by abnormal lipid and energy metabolism in testis via down-regulation of peroxisome proliferator-activated receptor mediated [85].

Cinnabar, a traditional mineral medicine containing more than 96% mercuric sulfide, has been used as a sedative and soporific for more than 2000 years. It was reported that cinnabar can impact central nervous system and cause neurotoxicity through blood–brain barrier [86]. Wei et al. investigated the neurotoxicity of cinnabar in rats by ^{1}H NMR based metabolomics combined with multivariate pattern recognition. The metabolite variations induced by cinnabar were characterized by increased levels of glutamate, glutamine, myo-inositol, and choline, as well as decreased levels of γ-amino-n-butyrate, taurine, N-acetylaspartate and N-acetylaspartylglutamate in tissue extracts of the cerebellum and cerebrum. The results indicated that cinnabar induced glutamate excitotoxicity, neuronal cell loss, osmotic state changes, membrane fluidity disruption, and oxidative injury in the brain [87].

Kunsui Radix, the dried root of *Euphorbia kansui* T. N. Liou ex T. P. Wang, was widely used for treatment of edema, ascites, and asthma [88]. The clinical application of Kunsui Radix is greatly restricted since it can induce toxic symptoms such as stomachache, diarrhea, dehydration and respiratory failure. The metabolites responsible for the toxicity of Kunsui Radix were evaluated by ^{1}H NMR based metabolomics. The toxicity of Kunsui Radix

accumulated with dosing time, and persisted even when treatment was stopped. The metabolomic results revealed that the levels of alanine, lactate, taurine, betaine, hippurate, phenylalanine and glucose were increased, while the levels of succinate, citrate, glycine, creatine and creatinine were decreased. The corresponding biochemical pathways alterations included inhibited tricarboxylic acid cycle, increased anaerobic glycolysis, and perturbed amino acids metabolism [89].

Coptidis Rhizome has been used as a heat-clearing and detoxifying agent in China for 2000 years. Coptidis Rhizome is relatively safe in normal dosage, but an extensive dosage can cause side effects such as diarrhea. A combination of ^{1}H NMR and GC–MS based metabolomic approach was applied to discover the endogenous metabolites which related to the diarrheal induced by Coptidis Rhizome. In the study, twelve marker metabolites from ^{1}H NMR and eight from GC–MS were identified, among those metabolites, hippurate, acetate, alanine, glycine and glutamate were likely to break the balance of gut microbiota, whereas, lactate and 2-ketoisovalerate were associated with energy metabolism [90].

TCM is generally used in the form of prescriptions (the combination of several different herbal medicines). The bioactive constituents and fundamental mechanisms of most TCM prescriptions remain unclear due to the complex components of remedies. Metabolomics could provide a holistic view and deeper insight into the efficacy and toxicity of TCM prescriptions. It might also be a promising approach to investigate the detoxification of Chinese medicines and reasonable combination of TCM prescriptions. Niuhuang Jiedu Tablet, composed of Realgar, Bovis Calculus Artificialis, Borneolum Synthcticum, Gypsum Fibrosum, Rhei Radix et Rhizoma, Scutellariae Radix, Platycodonis Radix and Glycyrrhizae Radix et Rhizoma, is an effective TCM prescription used for treatment of acute tonsillitis, pharyngitis, periodontitis and mouth ulcer [91]. In the prescription, significant level of realgar is a potentially toxic element. Xu et al. proposed a ^{1}H NMR based metabolomic approach to investigate the toxicity of realgar after being counterbalanced by other herbal medicines in Niuhuang Jiedu Tablet. The results showed that it was more secure and much less toxic for counterbalanced realgar in Niuhuang Jiedu Tablet. The effective material bases of toxicity alleviation to realgar were Rhei Radix et Rhizoma, Scutellariae Radix, Platycodonis Radix and Glycyrrhizae Radix et Rhizoma, which regulated energy metabolism, choline metabolism, amino acid metabolism and gut flora disorder affected by realgar exposure [92].

Zhusha Anshen Wan, composed of cinnabar, Coptidis Rhizoma, Angelicae Sinensis Radix, Rehmanniae Radix, Glycyrrhizae Radix et Rhizoma, is a widely used

TCM prescription for sedative therapy. Cinnabar is the chief component of Zhusha Anshen Wan and possesses certain toxicity. A metabolomic analysis suggested that Zhusha Anshen Wan may be more secure and much less toxic than cinnabar alone, and the four combined herbal medicines of Zhusha Anshen Wan had the effects of protecting from the toxicity induced by cinnabar alone [93].

Shuanghuanglian injection, composed of Lonicerae japonicae Flos, Scutellariae Radix and Forsythiae Fructus suspensa, is a commonly used TCM preparation with known antimicrobial properties [94]. It was reported that the adverse drug reactions of Shuanghuanglian injection occurred in approximately 2.22–2.56% after clinical exposure and the main adverse drug reactions were hypersensitive response, hemolytic anemia, haematuria and jaundice. The toxicological effects of Shuanghuanglian injection after intravenous administration in Beagle dogs were investigated by a ^{1}H NMR-based metabolomic approach. The results revealed increases in serum choline, phosphocholine, ketone body and lactate, but decreases in trimethylamine N-oxide, taurine, leucine, valine, glycine and glutamine, and these findings may underlie the toxicity mechanisms of Shuanghuanglian injection [95].

Conclusions and perspectives

In recent years, metabolomics analysis has increased markedly in efficacy, quality control, action of mechanism, and active components discovery of TCM. Meanwhile, the toxicity of TCM have attracted a wide range of concerns and aroused many toxicity studies on TCM. Nevertheless, there is no standard and objective basis for TCM toxicity evaluation and no standard for safety assessment up to now, which seriously hinders the toxicological researches of TCM. As a systemic approach, metabolomics focuses on the analysis of global metabolites and their functions in the biological system. It allows quantitative measurement of large numbers of low-molecular endogenous metabolites involved in metabolic pathways, and thus reflects fundamental metabolism status of body. The systematic study of metabolomics is in agreement with TCM theory and may be the best approach to fit the holistic concept of TCM. Therefore, metabolomic analysis is a suitable tool to systematically evaluate toxicity, find potential biomarkers and explore the toxicological mechanisms of TCM.

Despite its potential and advantages, there are still great challenges for the metabolomic applications on toxicology of TCM. Firstly, high sensitivity of metabolites to various genetic and environmental factors might lead to difficult interpretation of data analysis. Secondly, there are still substantial shortcomings for the existing metabolomic techniques to analyze the full spectrum of

metabolites. Thirdly, it is difficult to establish relationships between metabolomic results with genomics, proteomics and clinical data. Although there are still many challenges for the development of metabolomics in toxicity evaluation and it is a long way to get it into clinical application, we believe that the comprehensive metabolomic approach is a potentially powerful tool to evaluate toxicology and explore toxicological mechanisms of TCM. It is expectable that with the development of various analytical techniques, metabolomics will play an increasingly critical role in TCM toxicology research and be beneficial to the modernization of TCM.

Abbreviations

TCM: traditional Chinese medicines; ^{1}H NMR: proton nuclear magnetic resonance spectroscopy; MS: mass spectrometry; GC: gas chromatography; GC–MS: gas chromatography–mass spectrometry; LC: liquid chromatography; LC–MS: liquid chromatography–mass spectrometry; CE: capillary electrophoresis; CE–MS: capillary electrophoresis–mass spectrometry; UPLC: ultra-performance liquid chromatography; UPLC–MS: ultra-performance liquid chromatography–mass spectrometry; PCA: principal component analysis; HCA: hierarchical cluster analysis; PLS-DA: partial least squares discriminant analysis; OPLS-DA: orthogonal partial least squares discriminant analysis; HMDB: human metabolome database; KEGG: Kyoto Encyclopedia of Genes and Genomes; BiGG: biochemical genetic and genomic; HPLC Q/TOF MS: high performance liquid chromatography coupled with quadrupole time-of-flight mass spectrometry; UPLC Q/TOF MS: ultra-performance liquid chromatography coupled with quadrupole time-of-flight mass spectrometry.

Authors' contributions

LD, LG and LW drafted the manuscript. CMZ, QY and YGZ collected and analyzed relevant literatures. EHL conceived and designed the review. All authors read and approved the final manuscript.

Author details

College of Chemistry and Material Science, Hebei Normal University, Shijiazhuang 050024, China. ^{2} School of Pharmacy, Hebei University of Chinese Medicine, Shijiazhuang 050200, China. ^{3} State Key Laboratory of Natural Medicines, China Pharmaceutical University, Nanjing 210009, China. ^{4} Hebei Key Laboratory of Chinese Medicine Research on Cardio-cerebrovascular Disease, Hebei University of Chinese Medicine, Shijiazhuang 050200, China. ^{5} Department of Management, Xinjiang Uygur Pharmaceutical Co., Ltd., Wulumuqi 830001, China.

Acknowledgements

The authors greatly appreciate financial support from the National Key Research and Development Program of China (2017YFC1701105 and 2017YFC1701103), National Natural Science Foundation of China (81673569, 81803685, 81803697), National Modern Agricultural Industrial Park of China (NO. njf [2017] 110), a Project Funded by the Priority Academic Program Development of Jiangsu Higher Education Institutions, Natural Science Foundation of Hebei Province (H2018205185, H2018423032) and Research Foundation of Hebei Provincial Administration of Traditional Chinese Medicine (2018108).

Competing interests

The authors declare that they have no competing interests.

Consent for publication

All of authors consent to publication of this work in Chinese Medicine.

Funding

National Key Research and Development Program of China (2017YFC1701105 and 2017YFC1701103), National Natural Science Foundation of China (81673569, 81803685, 81803697), National Modern Agricultural Industrial Park of China (NO. njf [2017] 110), a Project Funded by the Priority Academic Program Development of Jiangsu Higher Education Institutions, Natural Science Foundation of Hebei Province (H2018205185, H2018423032), Research Foundation of Hebei Provincial Administration of Traditional Chinese Medicine (2018108).

References

1. Cheung F. TCM: made in China. Nature. 2011;480:S82–3.
2. Chan K, Zhang H, Lin ZX. An overview on adverse drug reactions to traditional Chinese medicines. Br J Clin Pharmacol. 2015;80:834–43.
3. Lin AX, Chan G, Hu Y, Ouyang D, Ung COL, Shi L, et al. Internationalization of traditional chinese medicine: current international market, internationalization challenges and prospective suggestions. Chin Med. 2018;13:9.
4. Wang L, Zhou GB, Liu P, Song JH, Liang Y, Yan XJ, et al. Dissection of mechanisms of Chinese medicinal formula Realgar-Indigo naturalis as an effective treatment for promyelocytic leukemia. Proc Natl Acad Sci USA. 2008;105:4826–31.
5. Li P, Qi LW, Liu EH, Zhou JL, Wen XD. Analysis of chinese herbal medicines with holistic approaches and integrated evaluation models. Trends Analyt Chem. 2008;27:66–77.
6. Liu P, Yang H, Long F, Hao HP, Xu X, Liu Y, et al. Bioactive equivalence of combinatorial components identified in screening of an herbal medicine. Pharm Res. 2014;31:1788–800.
7. Liu SH, Chuang WC, Lam W, Jiang Z, Cheng YC. Safety surveillance of traditional Chinese medicine: current and future. Drug Saf. 2015;38:117–28.
8. Jeong TY, Park BK, Cho JH, Kim YI, Ahn YC, Son CG. A prospective study on the safety of herbal medicines, used alone or with conventional medicines. J Ethnopharmacol. 2012;143:884–8.
9. Zheng RS, Wang WL, Tan J, Xu H, Zhan RT, Chen WW. An investigation of fungal contamination on the surface of medicinal herbs in China. Chin Med. 2017;12:2.
10. Ouedraogo M, Baudoux T, Stévigny C, Nortier J, Colet JM, Efferth T, et al. Review of current and "omics" methods for assessing the toxicity (genotoxicity, teratogenicity and nephrotoxicity) of herbal medicines and mushrooms. J Ethnopharmacol. 2012;140:492–512.
11. Kitano H. Systems biology: a brief overview. Science. 2002;295:1662–4.
12. Zhang A, Sun H, Wang P, Han Y, Wang X. Future perspectives of personalized medicine in traditional Chinese medicine: a systems biology approach. Complement Ther Med. 2012;20:93–9.
13. Wang X, Zhang A, Sun H, Wang P. Systems biology technologies enable personalized traditional Chinese medicine: a systematic review. Am J Chin Med. 2012;40:1109–22.
14. Uzuner H, Bauer R, Fan TP, Guo DA, Dias A, El-Nezami H, et al. Traditional Chinese medicine research in the post-genomic era: good practice, priorities, challenges and opportunities. J Ethnopharmacol. 2012;140:458–68.
15. Dong L, Xu J, Zhang L, Yang J, Liao B, Li X, et al. High-throughput sequencing technology reveals that continuous cropping of American ginseng results in changes in the microbial community in arable soil. Chin Med. 2017;12:18.
16. Suo T, Wang H, Li Z. Application of proteomics in research on traditional Chinese medicine. Expert Rev Proteomics. 2016;13:873–81.
17. Nicholson JK, Lindon JC, Holmes E. Metabonomics: understanding the metabolic responses of living systems to pathophysiological stimuli via multivariate statistical analysis of biological NMR spectroscopic data. Xenobiotica. 1999;29:1181–9.
18. Wood PL. Mass spectrometry strategies for clinical metabolomics and lipidomics in psychiatry, neurology, and neuro-oncology. Neuropsychopharmacology. 2014;39:24–33.
19. Gu H, Du J, Carnevale Neto F, Carroll PA, Turner SJ, Chiorean EG, et al. Metabolomics method to comprehensively analyze amino acids in different domains. Analyst. 2015;140(8):2726–34.
20. Liu LY, Zhang HJ, Luo LY, Pu JB, Liang WQ, Zhu CQ, et al. Blood and urinary metabolomic evidence validating traditional chinese medicine diagnostic classification of major depressive disorder. Chin Med. 2018;13:53.
21. Holmes E, Loo RL, Stamler J, Bictash M, Yap IK, Chan Q, et al. Human metabolic phenotype diversity and its association with diet and blood pressure. Nature. 2008;453:396–400.
22. Zhang AH, Sun H, Qiu S, Wang XJ. Recent highlights of metabolomics in chinese medicine syndrome research. Evid Based Complement Alternat Med. 2013;2013:402159.
23. Dai M, Wang F, Zou Z, Xiao G, Chen H, Yang H. Metabolic regulations of a decoction of Hedyotis diffusa in acute liver injury of mouse models. Chin Med. 2017;12:35.
24. Wang M, Chen L, Liu D, Chen H, Tang DD, Zhao YY. Metabolomics highlights pharmacological bioactivity and biochemical mechanism of traditional Chinese medicine. Chem Biol Interact. 2017;273:133–41.
25. Tang JF, Li WX, Zhang F, Li YH, Cao YJ, Zhao Y, et al. Discrimination of Radix Polygoni Multiflori from different geographical areas by UPLC-QTOF/MS combined with chemometrics. Chin Med. 2017;12:34.
26. Shi J, Cao B, Wang XW, Aa JY, Duan JA, Zhu XX, et al. Metabolomics and its application to the evaluation of the efficacy and toxicity of traditional Chinese herb medicines. J Chromatogr B Analyt Technol Biomed Life Sci. 2016;1026:204–16.
27. Lao YM, Jiang JG, Yan L. Application of metabonomic analytical techniques in the modernization and toxicology research of traditional Chinese medicine. Br J Pharmacol. 2009;157:1128–41.
28. Zhang A, Sun H, Wang P, Han Y, Wang X. Modern analytical techniques in metabolomics analysis. Analyst. 2012;137:293–300.
29. Nagana Gowda GA, Raftery D. Recent advances in NMR-based metabolomics. Anal Chem. 2017;89:490–510.
30. Markley JL, Brüschweiler R, Edison AS, Eghbalnia HR, Powers R, Raftery D, et al. The future of NMR-based metabolomics. Curr Opin Biotechnol. 2017;43:34–40.
31. Ernst M, Silva DB, Silva RR, Vêncio RZ, Lopes NP. Mass spectrometry in plant metabolomics strategies: from analytical platforms to data acquisition and processing. Nat Prod Rep. 2014;31:784–806.
32. Naz S, Moreira dos Santos DC, García A, Barbas C. Analytical protocols based on LC–MS, GC–MS and CE–MS for nontargeted metabolomics of biological tissues. Bioanalysis. 2014;6:1657–77.
33. Chaleckis R, Meister I, Zhang P, Wheelock CE. Challenges, progress and promises of metabolite annotation for LC–MS-based metabolomics. Curr Opin Biotechnol. 2018;55:44–50.
34. Li Z, Chen K, Guo MZ, Tang DQ. Two-dimensional liquid chromatography and its application in traditional Chinese medicine analysis and metabonomic investigation. J Sep Sci. 2016;39:21–37.
35. Yan Y, Du C, Li Z, Zhang M, Li J, Jia J, et al. Comparing the antidiabetic effects and chemical profiles of raw and fermented chinese Ge-Gen-Qin-Lian decoction by integrating untargeted metabolomics and targeted analysis. Chin Med. 2018;13:54.
36. Vuckovic D. Current trends and challenges in sample preparation for global metabolomics using liquid chromatography-mass spectrometry. Anal Bioanal Chem. 2012;403:1523–48.
37. Gil RB, Lehmann R, Schmitt-Kopplin P, Heinzmann SS. 1H NMR-based metabolite profiling workflow to reduce inter-sample chemical shift variations in urine samples for improved biomarker discovery. Anal Bioanal Chem. 2016;408:4683–91.
38. Sitnikov DG, Monnin CS, Vuckovic D. Systematic assessment of seven solvent and solid-phase extraction methods for metabolomics analysis of human plasma by LC–MS. Sci Rep. 2016;6:38885.
39. Tong K, Li ZL, Sun X, Yan S, Jiang MJ, Deng MS, et al. Metabolomics approach reveals annual metabolic variation in roots of *Cyathula officinalis* Kuan based on gas chromatography–mass spectrum. Chin Med. 2017;12:12.
40. Martínez-Arranz I, Mayo R, Pérez-Cormenzana M, Mincholé I, Salazar L, et al. Enhancing metabolomics research through data mining. J Proteomics. 2015;127:275–88.
41. Smolinska A, Blanchet L, Buydens LM, Wijmenga SS. NMR and pattern recognition methods in metabolomics: from data acquisition to biomarker discovery: a review. Anal Chim Acta. 2012;750:82–97.
42. Eliasson M, Rännar S, Madsen R, Donten MA, Marsden-Edwards E, Moritz T, et al. Strategy for optimizing LC–MS data processing in metabolomics: a design of experiments approach. Anal Chem. 2012;84:6869–76.

43. Gromski PS, Muhamadali H, Ellis DI, Xu Y, Correa E, Turner ML, et al. A tutorial review: metabolomics and partial least squares-discriminant analysis–a marriage of convenience or a shotgun wedding. Anal Chim Acta. 2015;879:10–23.

44. Li XJ, Jiang ZZ, Zhang LY. Triptolide: progress on research in pharmacodynamics and toxicology. J Ethnopharmacol. 2014;155:67–79.

45. Wang Z, Qu L, Li M, Zhang J. Identification of hepatotoxic and nephrotoxic potential markers of triptolide in mice with delayed-type hypersensitivity. J Pharm Biomed Anal. 2018;160:404–14.

46. Zhao J, Xie C, Mu X, Krausz KW, Patel DP, Shi X, et al. Metabolic alterations in triptolide-induced acute hepatotoxicity. Biomed Chromatogr. 2018;32:e4299.

47. Mbiantcha M, Kamanyi A, Teponno RB, Tapondjou AL, Watcho P, Nguelefack TB. Analgesic and Anti-Inflammatory Properties of Extracts from the Bulbils of *Dioscorea bulbifera* L. var sativa (Dioscoreaceae) in Mice and Rats. Evid Based Complement Alternat Med. 2011;2011:912935.

48. Zhao DS, Wu ZT, Li ZQ, Wang LL, Jiang LL, Shi W, et al. Liver-specific metabolomics characterizes the hepatotoxicity of *Dioscorea bulbifera* rhizome in rats by integration of GC–MS and ^{1}H-NMR. J Ethnopharmacol. 2018;226:111–9.

49. Zhao DS, Jiang LL, Fan YX, Wang LL, Li ZQ, Shi W, et al. Investigation of dioscorea bulbifera rhizome-induced hepatotoxicity in rats by a multisample integrated metabolomics approach. Chem Res Toxicol. 2017;30:1865–73.

50. Liu Y, Huang R, Liu L, Peng J, Xiao B, Yang J, et al. Metabonomics study of urine from Sprague-Dawley rats exposed to Huang-yao-zi using (1)H NMR spectroscopy. J Pharm Biomed Anal. 2010;52:136–41.

51. Han T, Li HL, Zhang QY, Han P, Zheng HC, Rahman K, et al. Bioactivity-guided fractionation for anti-inflammatory and analgesic properties and constituents of *Xanthium strumarium* L. Phytomedicine. 2007;14(12):825–9.

52. Xue LM, Zhang QY, Han P, Jiang YP, Yan RD, Wang Y, et al. Hepatotoxic constituents and toxicological mechanism of *Xanthium strumarium* L. fruits. J Ethnopharmacol. 2014;152:272–82.

53. Lu F, Cao M, Wu B, Li XZ, Liu HY, Chen DZ, et al. Urinary metabonomics study on toxicity biomarker discovery in rats treated with Xanthii Fructus. J Ethnopharmacol. 2013;149:311–20.

54. Liu Y, Wang Q, Yang J, Guo X, Liu W, Ma S, et al. Polygonum multiflorum Thunb.: a review on chemical analysis, processing mechanism, quality evaluation, and hepatotoxicity. Front Pharmacol. 2018;9:364.

55. Xia XH, Yuan YY, Liu M. The assessment of the chronic hepatotoxicity induced by Polygoni Multiflori Radix in rats: a pilot study by using untargeted metabolomics method. J Ethnopharmacol. 2017;203:182–90.

56. Liu J, Lu Y, Wu Q, Goyer RA, Waalkes MP. Mineral arsenicals in traditional medicines: orpiment, realgar, and arsenolite. J Pharmacol Exp Ther. 2008;326:363–8.

57. Huang Y, Tian Y, Li G, Li Y, Yin X, Peng C, et al. Discovery of safety biomarkers for realgar in rat urine using UFLC-IT-TOF/MS and 1H NMR based metabolomics. Anal Bioanal Chem. 2013;405:4811–22.

58. Huo T, Fang Y, Zhao L, Xiong Z, Zhang Y, Wang Y, et al. ^{1}HNMR-based metabonomic study of sub-chronic hepatotoxicity induced by realgar. J Ethnopharmacol. 2016;192:1–9.

59. Michl J, Ingrouille MJ, Simmonds MS, Heinrich M. Naturally occurring aristolochic acid analogues and their toxicities. Nat Prod Rep. 2014;31:676–93.

60. Hu X, Shen J, Pu X, Zheng N, Deng Z, Zhang Z, et al. Urinary time- or dose-dependent metabolic biomarkers of aristolochic acid-induced nephrotoxicity in rats. Toxicol Sci. 2017;156(1):123–32.

61. Zhao YY, Tang DD, Chen H, Mao JR, Bai X, Cheng XH, et al. Urinary metabolomics and biomarkers of aristolochic acid nephrotoxicity by UPLC-QTOF/HDMS. Bioanalysis. 2015;7:685–700.

62. Tang HB, Cai HL, Li HD, Zhang LJ, Li XL, Tang JH, et al. HPLC-DAD method for comprehensive quality control of Semen Strychni. Pharm Biol. 2013;51(11):1378–83.

63. Fan Y, Liu S, Chen X, Feng M, Song F, Gao X. Toxicological effects of Nux Vomica in rats urine and serum by means of clinical chemistry, histopathology and ^{1}H NMR-based metabonomics approach. J Ethnopharmacol. 2018;210:242–53.

64. Gu L, Hou P, Zhang R, Liu Z, Bi K, Chen X. An analytical strategy to investigate Semen Strychni nephrotoxicity based on simultaneous HILIC-ESI-MS/MS detection of Semen Strychni alkaloids, tyrosine and tyramine in HEK 293t cell lysates. J Chromatogr B Analyt Technol Biomed Life Sci. 2016;1033–1034:157–65.

65. Huang CF, Yang RS, Liu SH, Hsieh PC, Lin-Shiau SY. Evidence for improved neuropharmacological efficacy and decreased neurotoxicity in mice with traditional processing of Rhizoma Arisaematis. Am J Chin Med. 2011;39:981–98.

66. Dong G, Wang J, Guo P, Wei D, Yang M, Kong L. Toxicity assessment of Arisaematis Rhizoma in rats by a (1)H NMR-based metabolomics approach. Mol BioSyst. 2015;11:407–17.

67. Tian LQ, Zhang ZL, Zhang BS. Research on the pharmacology, toxicity and clinical application of morning glory seed. Chin J Nat Med. 2004;3:146–7.

68. Ma C, Bi K, Su D, Ji W, Zhang M, Fan X, et al. Serum and kidney metabolic changes of rat nephrotoxicity induced by Morning Glory Seed. Food Chem Toxicol. 2010;48:2988–93.

69. Ma C, Bi K, Zhang M, Su D, Fan X, Ji W, et al. Metabonomic study of biochemical changes in the urine of Morning Glory Seed treated rat. J Pharm Biomed Anal. 2010;53:559–66.

70. Zhang LL, Xu W, Xu YL, Chen X, Huang M, Lu JJ. Therapeutic potential of Rhizoma Alismatis: a review on ethnomedicinal application, phytochemistry, pharmacology, and toxicology. Ann N Y Acad Sci. 2017;1401:90–101.

71. Yu Y, Ma C, Bi K, Yang G, Xie P, Wang J, et al. A metabonomic analysis of urine from rats treated with rhizoma alismatis using ultra-performance liquid chromatography/mass spectrometry. Rapid Commun Mass Spectrom. 2011;25:2633–40.

72. Li Y, Li J, Zhou K, He J, Cao J, An M, et al. A review on phytochemistry and pharmacology of Cortex Periplocae. Molecules. 2016;21:E1702.

73. Li A, Guo X, Xie J, Liu X, Zhang Z, Li Y, et al. Validation of biomarkers in cardiotoxicity induced by Periplocin on neonatal rat cardiomyocytes using UPLC-Q-TOF/MS combined with a support vector machine. J Pharm Biomed Anal. 2016;123:179–85.

74. Nyirimigabo E, Xu Y, Li Y, Wang Y, Agyemang K, Zhang Y. A review on phytochemistry, pharmacology and toxicology studies of Aconitum. J Pharm Pharmacol. 2015;67:1–19.

75. Sun B, Li L, Wu S, Zhang Q, Li H, Chen H, et al. Metabolomic analysis of biofluids from rats treated with Aconitum alkaloids using nuclear magnetic resonance and gas chromatography/time-of-flight mass spectrometry. Anal Biochem. 2009;395:125–33.

76. Sui Z, Li Q, Zhu L, Wang Z, Lv C, Liu R, et al. An integrative investigation of the toxicity of *Aconiti kusnezoffii* radix and the attenuation effect of its processed drug using a UHPLC-Q-TOF based rat serum and urine metabolomics strategy. J Pharm Biomed Anal. 2017;145:240–7.

77. Yan Y, Zhang A, Dong H, Yan G, Sun H, Wu X, et al. Toxicity and detoxification effects of herbal Caowu via ultra performance liquid chromatography/mass spectrometry metabolomics analyzed using pattern recognition method. Pharmacogn Mag. 2017;13:683–92.

78. Dong H, Zhang A, Sun H, Wang H, Lu X, Wang M, et al. Ingenuity pathways analysis of urine metabolomics phenotypes toxicity of Chuanwu in Wistar rats by UPLC-Q-TOF-HDMS coupled with pattern recognition methods. Mol BioSyst. 2012;8:1206–21.

79. Dong H, Yan GL, Han Y, Sun H, Zhang AH, Li XN, et al. UPLC-Q-TOF/MS-based metabolomic studies on the toxicity mechanisms of traditional Chinese medicine Chuanwu and the detoxification mechanisms of Gancao, Baishao, and Ganjiang. Chin J Nat Med. 2015;13:687–98.

80. Wang X, Wang H, Zhang A, Lu X, Sun H, Dong H, et al. Metabolomics study on the toxicity of aconite root and its processed products using ultra-performance liquid-chromatography/electrospray-ionization synapt high-definition mass spectrometry coupled with pattern recognition approach and ingenuity pathways analysis. J Proteome Res. 2012;11:1284–301.

81. Cai Y, Gao Y, Tan G, Wu S, Dong X, Lou Z, et al. Myocardial lipidomics profiling delineate the toxicity of traditional Chinese medicine Aconiti Lateralis radix praeparata. J Ethnopharmacol. 2013;147:349–56.

82. Wu J, Cheng Z, He S, Shi J, Liu S, Zhang G, et al. Pinelliae rhizoma, a toxic chinese herb, can significantly inhibit CYP3A activity in rats. Molecules. 2015;20:792–806.

83. Zhang ZH, Zhao YY, Cheng XL, Dai Z, Zhou C, Bai X, et al. General toxicity of *Pinellia ternata* (Thunb.) Berit. in rat: a metabonomic method for profiling of serum metabolic changes. J Ethnopharmacol. 2013;149:303–10.

84. Su T, Tan Y, Tsui MS, Yi H, Fu XQ, Li T, et al. Metabolomics reveals the mechanisms for the cardiotoxicity of Pinelliae Rhizoma and the toxicity-reducing effect of processing. Sci Rep. 2016;6:34692.

85. Ma B, Qi H, Li J, Xu H, Chi B, Zhu J, et al. Triptolide disrupts fatty acids and peroxisome proliferator-activated receptor (PPAR) levels in male mice testes followed by testicular injury: a GC–MS based metabolomics study. Toxicology. 2015;336:84–95.

86. Liu J, Shi JZ, Yu LM, Goyer RA, Waalkes MP. Mercury in traditional medicines: is cinnabar toxicologically similar to common mercurials? Exp Biol Med. 2008;233:810–7.

87. Li X, Pei F, Wei L, Zhang P, Wu Y, Xue R. H-1 NMR-based metabolomics and neurotoxicity study of cerebrum and cerebellum in rats treated with cinnabar, a traditional chinese medicine. OMICS. 2015;19:490–8.

88. Shen J, Kai J, Tang Y, Zhang L, Su S, Duan JA. The chemical and biological properties of Euphorbia kansui. Am J Chin Med. 2016;44:253–73.

89. Tang B, Ding J, Wu F, Chen L, Yang Y, Song F. ^{1}H NMR-based metabonomics study of the urinary biochemical changes in Kansui treated rat. J Ethnopharmacol. 2012;141:134–42.

90. Zhou Y, Liao Q, Lin M, Deng X, Zhang P, Yao M, et al. Combination of ^{1}H NMR- and GC–MS-based metabonomics to study on the toxicity of Coptidis Rhizome in rats. PLoS ONE. 2014;9:e88281.

91. Xu W, Wang H, Chen G, Li W, Xiang R, Zhang X, et al. A metabolic profiling analysis of the acute toxicological effects of the realgar (As_2S_2) combined with other herbs in Niuhuang Jiedu Tablet using ^{1}H NMR spectroscopy. J Ethnopharmacol. 2014;153:771–81.

92. Xu W, Wang H, Chen G, Li W, Xiang R, Pei Y. ^{1}H NMR-based metabonomics study on the toxicity alleviation effect of other traditional Chinese medicines in Niuhuang Jiedu tablet to realgar (As2S2). J Ethnopharmacol. 2013;148:88–98.

93. Wang H, Bai J, Chen G, Li W, Xiang R, Su G, et al. A metabolic profiling analysis of the acute hepatotoxicity and nephrotoxicity of Zhusha Anshen Wan compared with cinnabar in rats using ^{1}H NMR spectroscopy. J Ethnopharmacol. 2013;146:572–80.

94. Tang Y, Wang Z, Huo C, Guo X, Yang G, Wang M, et al. Antiviral effects of Shuanghuanglian injection powder against influenza A virus H5N1 in vitro and in vivo. Microb Pathog. 2018;121:318–24.

95. Yan G, Zhao Y, Deng P, Lv L, Wang Y, Bu Q, et al. Investigation of toxicological effects of Shuanghuanglian injection in Beagle dogs by metabonomic and traditional approaches. Exp Biol Med. 2010;235:1356–64.

13

Psoriasis therapy by Chinese medicine and modern agents

Shikang Meng[1], Zibei Lin[1], Yan Wang[2], Zhenping Wang[3], Ping Li[2,4*] and Ying Zheng[1*] 🄳

Abstract

Psoriasis is a chronic, painful, disfiguring and non-contagious skin disease that has globally affected at least 200 million patients. In general, mild to moderate psoriasis patients will be treated by chemical drugs or Chinese medicine, while targeting systemic biological drugs have been successfully developed with good efficacy but high cost burden to patients with severe psoriasis. Since the underlying mechanisms of psoriasis are not well understood, in this review, psoriasis pathogenesis and clinical therapeutic principles by modern medicine and Chinese medicine are extensively described. Based on the data from the China Food and Drug Administration, the majority of chemical drugs are utilized as the topical formulations, while Chinese medicines are mainly delivered by an oral route, suggesting that the market for topical preparations of Chinese medicine to treat psoriasis is worth to exploration. Moreover, considering the unique clinical therapeutic theory and successful clinical application of Chinese medicine in the treatment of psoriasis, we believe that development of new small molecule drugs based on Chinese medicine will be a promising strategy to reduce therapeutic costs and improve safety for psoriatic patients.

Keywords: Psoriasis, Therapy, Chinese medicine

Background

Psoriasis

Psoriasis is a chronic, painful, disfiguring and non-infectious skin disease that is believed to be an autoimmune inflammation disorder with unclear underlying mechanism [1]. Psoriasis negatively affects the quality of life of patients [2]. People of different ages and in different countries develop psoriasis. Patients with psoriasis are not often successfully surveyed because of the inconvenience of the disease, and the statistics of prevalence in different places may not be accurate. From a survey in China of 6 provinces, the overall prevalence of psoriasis was 0.47% [3]. According to current investigation, the outburst of psoriasis was not associated with gender, but mainly with the climate of the environment; that is,

dry cold weather will more likely to induce psoriasis [4, 5]. Approximately 3% of people around the world have psoriasis, which is near the most common autoimmune skin disease in adults. By simple estimation, there are at least two hundred million psoriasis patients in the world [2]. Therefore, it is not just a simple health problem in a country or a region but a serious global challenge. Of note, about half of the adult patients had been reported to be sick in their childhood and they mostly fell ill around 10 years old [6, 7].

Psoriasis could be divided into five types [2]. Psoriasis vulgaris is the most common type of psoriasis. It is initially red papules or rash, then, expands gradually or merged into a flake. The surface is covered with multilayer gray or silver white scales; Intertriginous psoriasis usually appears at the folding parts of the human body such as armpits, groin and reproductive areas, generally without any scales to be seen, the only the erythema. Guttate psoriasis usually arises in the torso among children and the onset of the disease is often related to streptococcal infection of the upper respiratory tract. Pustular psoriasis is generally seen in the palm of the hands and fingertips. The main feature of this kind is that the

*Correspondence: liping411@163.com; yzheng@umac.mo
[1] State Key Laboratory of Quality Research in Chinese Medicine, Institute of Chinese Medical Science, University of Macau, Macau, China
[4] Department of Pathophysiology, Beijing Key Laboratory of Clinic and Basic Research with Traditional Chinese Medicine on Psoriasis, Beijing Institute of Traditional Chinese Medicine, 23 Meishuguan Back Street, Dongcheng, Beijing 100010, People's Republic of China

aggregated pustules are always filled with non-infectious pus. Erythrodermic psoriasis is the most serious type of all psoriases. It could bring about the lowering of body temperature, hypoproteinemia and high output heart failure. Generally, large areas of burn-like erythema and skin peeling are seen on the patients' bodies.

Modern understanding of pathologic mechanisms of psoriasis

Twenty-five years ago, people thought that, psoriasis was caused of excessive proliferation of skin cells and the chronic inflammation was just the side effect. In 1994, Krueger, a cell biologist at the Rockefeller University, started working on the origins of psoriasis. His team administered a compound that could target the immune-related cells without affecting the normal skin function of patients. The results showed a great improvement of the skin condition, and some individual cases with mild trauma were even cured. This experiment proved that psoriasis was mainly caused by immune system cells and was not the side effect of cell proliferation. The research of Krueger involved first separating the different roles of keratinocytes and T cells [8].

The main characteristics of psoriasis are excessive proliferation of keratinocytes and being easy to relapse. It is reported that this disease might involve many tissues in the muscles, joints, alimentary tract and even eyes [9]. The cardiovascular performance and abnormal metabolism phenomenon among psoriasis patients marks the important role of fat cells and vascular reconstruction related to skin inflammation, which might be mediated by sub-populations of inflammatory monocytes [9]. Nevertheless, the external factors including bacterial infection, trauma, mental pressure and genetic factors, will all lead to the onset of psoriasis [2]. Before all other symptoms are seen, at the cellular level, the accumulation of inflammatory cells headed by a large number of activated T cells and antigen presenting cells (APCs) as well as plasmacytoid dendritic cells (DCs) appear at the beginning of the disease. This is the reason why psoriasis is considered to be an autoimmune inflammatory disease [1]. According to the research progress of immunologists and psoriasis specialists in the past 20 years, the skin is essentially an active immune organ. It also becomes the carrier of several chronic inflammatory diseases like rheumatoid arthritis and systemic lupus erythematosus [10]. In recent years, studies on the relationship between autoimmune diseases and the IL-17/IL-23 axis continuously keep growing.

IL-17 is a proinflammatory cytokine produced by activated T cells, leading to the generation of inflammation [11]. IL-23 belongs to the IL-12 family and is mainly produced by activated dendritic cells, which is a heterodimer consisting of two subunits, P40 and P19. The formation pathway of Th17 cells is also called the IL-23/IL-17 inflammatory reaction axis. The general process is as follows. The initial T cells differentiate into Th17 cells with the collective effect of TGF-β and IL-6. IL-23 could improve the proliferation of Th17 cells and mediate the immune response, including secreting IL-17A, IL-17F, and IL-22. Among them, IL-22 would take part in the proinflammatory response by inducing the production of proinflammatory cytokines and chemokines [12]. Generally, activation of the IL-23/IL-17 axis could quickly gather the neutrophils and produce oxygen free radicals as well as other inflammatory mediators. As reported, autoimmune disorders were mediated by the harmful regulation of the IL-23/IL-17 axis, and this fact will create a new orientation of autoimmune disease treatment. While precisely targeting IL-23 P40, a subunit shared with IL-12, some reports showed a theoretical safety concern that it might make patients more susceptible to bacterial and other types of infections because IL-12 would induce the Th1 cells secreting IFN-γ, which is involved in anti-pathogen immune defenses [13]. Therefore, they prefer more targeting of P19 selectively. However, some other reports held their view that precisely targeting IL-23 P19 but not IL-23 P40 could lead to the blocking of the organ specific autoimmune pathologic response whose long-term immune protection cannot be guaranteed [14]. Now, the clinical results of anti-P40 treatment have already shown a good effect against psoriasis [15]. Increasing evidence has shown that the IL-23/IL-17 axis takes part in the development of psoriasis [16].

Many IL-23+ dendritic cells exist at the skin lesions of psoriasis. The mRNAs expression levels of subunits of IL-23 are also relatively higher [17]. The mRNA levels of Th17 type cytokines and some other kinds of chemokines were improved at the same time [18]. According to the latest articles, IFN-γ also had an strong activity inducing the hyperproliferation of keratinocytes by activating monocytes, DCs, and endothelial cells in psoriasis patients [19]. Meanwhile, IL-5 was reported to inhibit AMPs and IL-4 was reported to inhibit epidermal cornification without inducing epidermal hyperplasia in the incidence of psoriasis [20].

In summary, IL-23 secreted by dendritic cells mediate the activation of Th17 lymphocytes and the production of Th17 type cytokines, which might be the initial factor of psoriasis. At the skin lesions of psoriasis, the accumulation of cytokines, such as IL-2 and TNF-alpha, will promote the development of psoriasis. Lymphocytes in skin lesions will produce many kinds of cytokines, forming a mighty cell network headed by Th1- and Th17-type cytokines, which is also important in the pathology of psoriasis.

Chemical and biological drugs

Historical development

A 100 years ago, humans treated psoriasis mainly with coal tar topically. This effective therapy had been used for many years, although it is inconvenient. In 1925, a combination treatment of coal tar and UV light exposure was put into application, called "Goeckerman therapy", which is rarely used now. From 1950 to 1970, methotrexate, corticosteroids, and psoralen with UVB treatment were put into application successively. In 1993, vitamin D3 analogs were used topically for psoriasis treatment. It had a good therapeutic effect, a high body tolerance, and the fewest side effects at that time. Acitretin was introduced in 1996 as a systemic drug and was commonly used for severe psoriasis, such as pustular and erythrodermic psoriasis. In 2003, the first systemic biologic drug in the world, Amevive, was approved by the US FDA. After 14 weeks of treatment, the Psoriasis Area Severity Index (PASI) standard ratio, which is an index combining the severity and percentage of the affected area used to express the condition of psoriasis, reached 21% [2]. Following that, many systemic biologic drugs were released, including Enbrel in 2004, Remicade in 2006, Humira in 2008 and Stelara in 2009. Among all the biologics, Stelara has even become the therapeutic standard for judging new psoriasis systemic biologic drugs, because after 28 weeks of treatment, the PASI 75 standard ratio, which is the percentage of patients achieving a reduction of at least 75% in their baseline PASI at a given time, could reach approximately 80% [21, 22].

Current treatment

Currently, there are many types of treatments for psoriasis of different degrees, as shown in Table 1. Mild to moderate psoriasis patients will usually use topical drugs, regulating gene transcription, to inhibit the proliferation of cells and boost the differentiation of keratinocytes. In terms of severe psoriasis patients, physical treatment combined with oral systemic drugs that regulate epidermal cell differentiation and proliferation such as Methotrexate, Acitretin or Cyclosporine were applied [23]. Ultraviolet radiation b (UVB) exposure at a wavelength of 311 nm has now become the major physical therapy for the treatment of psoriasis. Its remission period is short, but long-term application causes skin aging, pigmentation, skin cancer and increasing the risk of cataracts. When treating severe psoriasis vulgaris by irradiating 3–4 times a week, and the efficacy could reach 80% [24].

Biologics that work against IL-17, IL-23, or TNF-α are usually injected as systemic drugs because of their good efficacy and safety. The efficacy is outstanding and fits nearly all conditions of psoriasis. Biologics work quickly, have a long duration, have a long treatment cycle and do not produce relapse. There are still a few limitations about patient applicability. Generally, the age should be between 18 and 65 years; psoriasis should be diagnosed for more than 6 months; the psoriasis affected area should be at least 10% and the PASI score should be over 12 during the baseline period. There should be no potential or active tuberculosis before screening. However, the biggest reason hindering the promotion of biologics is their high cost. Although only administered once every 8 weeks, the cost of the therapy of each time reached ~2100 dollars. Therefore, only patients with severe psoriasis are recommended for biologics.

Over all, the final purpose of any kind of psoriasis treatment was to eliminate all the symptoms on the skin. The minimum requirement for therapy evaluation was set to be over 50% reduction of the PASI baseline [25]. If this goal could not be reached, then the therapy should be modified by the way of adjusting the dosage, turning to another treatment or using a combination therapy.

Table 1 Common medication of psoriasis

Psoriasis degree	Suitable formulation	Common drugs	Drug action	Formulation features
Mild Moderate	Topical drugs	Corticosteroids Retinoids Calcineurin inhibitors Vitamin D analogues	Regulate genes transcription Inhibit the proliferation of cells Boost the differentiation of keratinocytes, etc.	Avoidance of first pass metabolism Avoidance of extreme condition in GI Reduction of systemic toxicity Direct access to target of skin High patient compliance Limitation in molecular weight/Log P of drugs
Severe	Systemic chemical drugs (oral)	Methotrexate Acitretin Cyclosporine	Immunosuppressive effect Anti-inflammatory Inhibit PDE-4, etc.	Convenient, Safe Slow absorbing velocity Unfit to unconscious patients
	Biologics (injection)	Ustekinumab Secukinumab Etanercept Stelara	Target IL-17, IL-23, TNF-α	High targeting specificity Few adverse reactions Safe Extremely expensive

In terms of moderate to severe psoriasis, phototherapy combined with systemic oral drugs or biologics is usually recommended. Griffths et al. [26] reported that a combination of retinoid and PUVA was more effective than each given alone, and this combination had the potential for lowering the cumulative UVA dosage. They also reported that phototherapy combined with a vitamin D3 analog such as calcipotriol was more effective than either alone. Roman et al. [27] reported a successful case with a complete clearance using a combination of acitretin and apremilast on patients with severe palmoplantar psoriasis. AbuHilal et al. [28] reported several cases using apremilast combined with other therapy, including NB-UVB, methotrexate and acitretin, of which 81% achieved PASI 75 at week 12 after the combination was applied.

Common topical chemical drugs

According to the statistical induction of CFDA about domestic psoriasis chemical drugs, as shown in Table 2, among all 890 drug products recorded in the market, only 169 of them are systemic drugs, while most of them are topical formulations, including creams, ointments and solutions [29]. The most common topical chemical drugs are listed and described below.

Corticosteroids, such as Fluocinonide, are used for the treatment of itching and noninvasive skin diseases. These anti-inflammatory anti-allergy drugs could inhibit the proliferation of connective tissue, reduce the permeability of capillaries and cell membranes, reduce inflammatory exudation, and inhibit the formation and release of histamine and other inflammatory mediators.

Retinoids, such as tazarotene, regulate the abnormal differentiation of keratinocytes, alleviate proliferation and speed up the inflammation subsiding. The specific performance after treatment include down-regulation of cell differentiation markers to reduce over-differentiation, inhibition of cell proliferation markers, reduction of the expression of inflammatory markers and up-regulation of tazarotene induced genes to against the proliferation.

Calcineurin inhibitors, such as tacrolimus, belong to macrolide antibiotics. It is a kind of new powerful immunosuppressive agent that are fit for patients who cannot receive traditional therapy and those severe patients who cannot tolerate the treatment program. On a molecular level, tacrolimus is combined with the cellular protein, FKBP12. The FKBP12-tacrolimus complex will specifically combine and inhibit calcineurin, which will inhibit the calcium ion-dependent message conduction pathway in cells, preventing the transcription of the discontinuous lymphokine gene.

Vitamin D analogs, such as calcipotriol, have a strong affinity to the calcitriol receptor. They can decrease the content and distribution of IL-6 as well as the amount of T lymphocytes in the activated epidermis in psoriasis patients. The mechanisms for inhibiting the hyperplasia and inducing the differentiation of skin cells are still not clear and are possibly influenced through the JAT/STAT signaling pathway.

Psoriasis therapy based on "treatment from blood aspect"

Different from previous understanding of psoriasis, in ancient books of traditional Chinese medicine (TCM), for the psoriasis-like diseases, pathogenesis was thought to be the exogenous evils invading and battling in human blood. As recorded in the ancient book *Zhu Bing Yuan Hou Lun* "Blood dryness symptom, caused by all evils, pathogenic wind and dampness attacking and stalling between skin and fascia, together with evil cold, defeated positive Qi of the blood" [30]. Pathogenic wind dries the fluid in the blood, by which skin and muscle could not be nourished and moisturized. As the same sayings in *The essence of medicine is the secret of the heart of surgery* [31]:"Psoriasis, either skin suffered from pathogenic wind, or lost nourishment from blood dryness".

After 1949, a number of experts, such as Dr. Bing-nan Zhao, Ren-kang Zhu and Qi-fengJin, advocated "treatment of psoriasis from the blood aspect". For example, Zhao [32, 33] proposed the evil fire should be caused by internal heat from emotional stress, which blocked Qi movement, and excessive Qi gathered together to produce fire. As a result, the evil fire entered and stalled in blood circulation; or by stagnated heat derived from Qi dysfunction between the spleen and stomach, due to an improper diet, which caused disease when suffering from exogenous evil fire once again. During a long disease course, *Yin* and blood were exhausted, which led to pathogenic wind blowing or blood circulation stagnation. At last Qi and blood coagulated and blocked the meridians, which resulted in skin and muscle loss of nourishment.

The enrichment and development of psoriasis vulgaris based on "treatment from blood aspect"

"Treatment from blood aspect" is the principal diagnosis system of psoriasis vulgaris, which can be used as an overall differentiation system together with other differentiation methods such as six climatic evils, visceral syndrome, and/or poisonous pathogenic. For example, Zhu [34] first proposed that the treatment of psoriasis should be based on the principle "Treatment from blood aspect, combined with other ways", and advocated that the differentiation of psoriasis should combine with other syndrome differentiation systems, such as expelling wind and detoxification. Jin [35] stated the pathogenesis of psoriasis should be mainly divided into four aspects, including invasion of exogenous pathogenic

Table 2 Chemical drugs for topical delivery to treat psoriasis

Drug	Formulas approved by FDA	Dosage	Indications	Adverse reactions and precautions
Beclometasone Dipropionate[a]	Cream (41)[e], ointment (1), spray (8), plasters (2)	2–4 times/day, less than 45 mg/week	Contact eczema, atopic dermatitis, neurodermatitis, pruritus, psoriasis, sclerosing atrophic moss, lichen planus, discoid lupus erythematosus, seborrheic dermatitis, hypertrophic scars	Short-term application: burning, tingling, itching
Fluocinonide[a]	Cream (72), ointment (1), tincture (27), liniments (1)	2–3 times/day, less than 12.5 mg/week		Long-term application: skin telangiectasia, skin atrophy, atrophy pattern, secondary purpura, ecchymosis, skin fragility, hirsutism, folliculitis, milia, skin bleaching, systemic adverse reactions (absorbed too much)
Halcinonide[a]	Cream (27), ointment (10), solution (37)	Twice/day		
Hydrocortisone Butyrate[a]	Cream (11)	Twice/day		
Triamcinolone Acetonide[a]	Spray (5), cream (86), paste (2), ointment (22)	2–3 times/day		
Methoxsalen[b]	Solution (12)	Once/day, apply UVA 2–4 h later	Psoriasis vulgaris and acne vulgaris	Erythema, skin pigmentation, itching, redness, blisters, pain, scaling
Tazarotene[b]	Cream (2), gel (3)	Apply half an hour before sleep, then wash off.		Itching, erythema, burning sensation, skin irritation, dryness and edema
Tretinoin[b]	Cream (35)	1–3 times/day		Burning, erythema and desquamation, but gradually disappear
Tacrolimus[b]	Ointment (4)	Twice/day	Patients unfit traditional therapies due to potential risk	Rosacea, edema at the site of administration
Calcipotriol[c]	Ointment (2)	1–2 times/day, less than 100 g/week	Psoriasis vulgaris	Pruritus, burning sensation, tingling, dry skin, erythema, contact dermatitis, eczema
Biphenyl benzazole[d]	Gel (5), solution (8), spray (1), cream (39), film (1)	Once/day	Hand skin fungi, yeasts, molds, fungal skin diseases caused by pityrosporum and infections caused by Corynebacterium parvum	Pain and peripheral edema, contact dermatitis, erythema, pruritus, rash, urticaria, blisters, peeling, eczema, dry skin, skin irritation, skin impregnation, burning sensation
Clotrimazole[d]	Solution (32), cream (102), liniments (7), film (3)	2–3 times/day	Tinea corporis, tinea corporis, tinea capitis, tinea pedis, tinea versicolor, tinea capitis, and candidiasis parvitis and candidal vulvovaginitis	Itching, tingling, erythema, edema
Econazole Nitrate[d]	Solution (9), spray (4), cream (42)	Twice/day		Itching, tingling, erythema, edema
Terbinafine Hydrochloride[d]	Cream (37), liniments (2), spray (7), gel (11)	Once/day		Burning sensation, rash, pruritus

[a] Corticosteroids

[b] Small molecule inhibitors

[c] V_D analogues

[d] Broad spectrum antimicrobials

[e] Cream (41) means 41 cream formulations had been proved by CFDA

factors, entrance of heat into the blood phase, obstruction of heat-toxins on the collaterals and *Yin* deficiency and blood dryness. Therefore, the syndrome falls into four categories: blood heat, dampness heat, blood dryness and blood stasis. Zhang [36] suggested that except for blood heat, blood dryness and blood stasis, there were still dampness heat and heat-toxin syndromes. The former one usually occurred in exudation type of psoriasis, and latter one was caused by acute tonsillitis or upper respiratory tract infection. Xu [37] reported the aeropathic factors were the invasion of pathogenic wind, cold, dampness, heat and dryness, and the intrinsic factors were congenital blood heat, improper diet and emotional hurt. In the early stages, blood symptoms such as blood heat, blood dryness and blood stasis were the main clinical manifestations. However, after a long disease course, the function of Zang and Fu declined, among them, and the liver and kidney showed the most prominent damage. Ma [38] thought psoriasis was caused by blood stasis and heat-toxin. Cooling-Blood and detoxification should be used in the early onset, and after a long duration, promoting-blood circulation and detoxification was available. In short, all the methods are beneficial supplements to the "treatment from blood aspect".

In addition, understanding the pathogenesis of blood aspect got improved and was supplanted with considering different physical states. If the disease exacerbated in winter, complicated with lassitude, lack of *qi* and no desire to speak, spontaneous perspiration, drowsiness, thin and weak pulse, cold limbs, low back cold, tastelessness and lusterless complexion, it should be treated by warming *yang* based on "treatment from blood aspect" to improve the curative effect. If chronic plaque psoriasis with skin lesions, less sweat and feeling oppressed was accompanied by physical obesity, dizziness, drowsiness, heavy body fat, elevated blood lipids and other characteristics, except the existence of blood stasis symptoms, the patients had phlegm blocking and disharmony between *Ying* and *Wei*, with phlegm and blood stasis. Here, "Warming *Yang* and harmony *Ying*, cooling blood and improving blood circulation" therapy should be applied under the guidance of cold and hot medicine equivalence.

Research progress on the syndrome evolution of psoriasis vulgaris based on "treatment from blood aspect"

The "treatment from blood aspect" of psoriasis vulgaris should pay attention to the conversion and evolution of syndromes. First, Deng [39] reported that there are three basic syndromes, including blood heat, blood dryness and blood stasis, by large-scale epidemiological survey. Second, the distribution of the three syndromes was closely related to the stage of the disease. Blood heat syndromes were commonly seen in a progressive stage,

blood dryness in the extinction stage and blood stasis in a stationary stage. However, some of patients showed three instability syndromes, such as blood heat with blood dryness, blood dryness with blood stasis, as well as blood stasis with blood heat. Among them, the conversion of blood heat with blood dryness syndrome was the most common transformation type.

Li et al. [40] employed a cross-sectional survey of 500 cases of psoriasis vulgaris in the Central China region. The results showed that the main syndromes of patients are blood stasis, blood dryness, blood heat, blood heat with blood stasis, blood heat with blood dryness and blood stasis with blood dryness. In all cases, patients with six types of blood syndrome in stable and unstable stages accounted for 91%. Among them, the blood stasis syndrome accounted for 57%. In the progression stage, TCM syndromes were blood heat and blood heat with blood stasis, while in stationary stages, it was blood stasis with blood dryness, then in extinction stage it was blood dryness. Meanwhile, the longer course it took, the more blood stasis and dryness syndromes appeared.

Zhang et al. [41] employed a cross-sectional survey on 2651 cases of psoriasis vulgaris in three hospitals of Traditional Chinese medicine in the Beijing area. The data demonstrated that the blood heat syndrome is the most common in psoriasis vulgaris, followed by blood dryness and blood stasis. The distribution of syndromes is closely related to the stage of the disease. The syndromes of blood heat, blood dryness and blood stasis are commonly seen in progression, catagen and the stationary stage, respectively. The PASI score, severity index of the disease is closely related to the syndrome distribution. With aggravation of the disease, the PASI value increased, the proportion of both blood heat and blood stasis syndrome also increased, while the proportion of blood dryness syndrome decreased.

Treatment of psoriasis with traditional Chinese medicines

The syndrome differentiation and treatment of psoriasis mainly involve removing pathogenic heat from the blood and toxic material from the body, promoting blood circulation and removing blood stasis, nourishing blood and removing toxins, where the central idea of treatment is "treatment from blood aspect". Therefore, Chinese medicines for regulating blood conditions are considered to be effective, including Chinese medicines that can cool blood, nourish blood and promote blood circulation. Cooling-blood Chinese medicines are divided into those that can cool blood to be antipyretic and those that can cool blood to stop bleeding. Among all the blood-regulating Chinese medicines, those most widely used for treating psoriasis in practice are *Arnebiae Radix* (Zicao),

Paeoniae Radix Alba (Baishao), *Paeoniae Radix Rubra* (Chishao), *Spatholobi Caulis* (Jixueteng), *Moutan Cortex* (Danpi), *Curcumae Rhizoma* (E'zhu) and *Salviae Miltiorrhizae Radix and Rhizoma* (Danshen). In addition, since psoriasis has the characteristics of toxin-damage of the choroid, antipyretic-detoxicate Chinese medicines are used frequently [42].

Current clinical practice of anti-psoriatic traditional Chinese medicines

Various remedies used to treat psoriasis were recorded in Chinese medicinal classics, like *TaiPingShengHui Formulas* and *PuJi Formulas*, which can be divided into two parts as formulas for topical or for oral use, respectively. Topical remedies involve preparations manufactured into traditional dosage forms, like creams, oils, unguentum, plaster and lotion decoctions, while oral drugs involve those prepared into decoctions, tablets and pulvis, etc. The use of traditional herbal compound prescriptions for psoriasis treatment is under the guideline of "treatment from blood aspect". Therefore, herbs that are targeted to "blood" and detoxification are usually used. A clinical study on 675 cases [43] made a comparison between *Yinxieling Ointment*, a topical prescription [Mustard gas, R*adix Sangusorbae* (Diyu), *Radix Scutellariae* (Huangqin), *Cortex Phellodendri* (Huangbai)] and Dichlorodiethyl sulfide, and they found comparatively equal efficacy. For oral prescriptions, the clinical efficacy of *HuoXueSanYu Decoction* [44] [*Rhizoma Sparganii* (Sanleng), *Curcumae Rhizoma* (E'zhu), *Semen Persicae* (Taoren), *Flos Carthami* (Honghua), *Spatholobi Caulis* (Jixueteng), *Ramulus Euonymi* (Guijianyu), *Herba Hedyotis* (Baihuasheshecao), *Salviae Miltiorrhizae Radix and Rhizoma* (Danshen), and *Pericarpium Citri Reticulatae* (Chenpi)] were found to be comparable to acitretin (10 mg, b.i.d.), for the treatment of psoriasis vulgaris. *JiaWeiHuangLianJieDu Decoction* [45] [*Radix Scutellariae* (Huangqin), *Cortex Phellodendri* (Huangbai), *Rhizoma-Coptidis* (Huanglian), etc.] was reported to alleviate the symptoms in 45 of 50 psoriatic subjects.

In most cases, the formula for anti-psoriatic treatment consists of different kinds of herbs, which are used as adjuvant therapy or joint with other drug as combined treatment. Anti-psoriatic herb compound prescriptions commonly combine with Narrow Bound Ultra Violet B(NB-UVB) light to achieve higher efficacy. A study [46] analyzed the effect of *Tuiyin Decoction* combined with NB-UVB, where one group used combined therapy and two control groups applied NB-UVB or *Tuiyin Decoction*, respectively, and efficiency rates were revealed to 95.3, 67.4 and 72.1%, respectively, indicating that joint treatment has much higher efficacy. Some psoriasis cases are also treated by chemical drugs jointly with Chinese herbal

formulas, such as corticosteroids, calcineurin inhibitors and so on. A study [47] demonstrated that calcipotriol betamethasone ointment combined with *PSORI-CM01 Decoction* [*Paeoniae Radix Rubra* (Chishao), *Rhizoma Curcumae* (Erzhu), *Sarcandra* (Caoshanhu), *Radix Glycyrrhiza* (Gancao), *Fructus Mume* (Wumei), *Arnebiae Radix* (Zicao), and *Rhizoma Smilacis Glabrae* (Tufuling)] performed better efficacy and a lower relapse rate than combined with an oral placebo. *ZaoShiKuShen Decoction* [48] [*Radix Sophorae Flavescentis* (Kushen), *Coix chinensis Tod.* (Yiyiren), *Rhizoma Smilacis Glabrae* (Tufuling), *Cortex Phellodendri* (Huangbai), etc.] was jointly applied with 0.03% Tacrolimus, which showed 14% higher efficacy than that of 0.03% tacrolimus alone in a 100-patient clinical trial.

Some of the traditional prescriptions or active ingredients extracted from Chinese herbs have been developed into hospital agents with good efficacy. For instance, an *Indigo naturalis* composite ointment [consisting of *Indigo naturalis* (Qingdai), *Scutellaria baicalensis Georgi* (Huangqin) and *Cortex phellodendri* (Huangbai)] exhibited a successful treatment on pediatric psoriasis [49]. New Pulian Ointment consisting of Huangqin and Huangbai has successfully been used to treat psoriasis of blood-heat syndrome [50]. Herose capsules consisting of (*Rhizoma Zingiberis* (Ganjiang), *Radix Salviae Miltiorrhizae* (Danshen), *Radix Astragali* (Huangqi), *Ramulus Cinnamomi* (Guizhi), *Radix Paeoniae Alba* (Baishao), *Radix Codonopsis Pilosula* (Dangshen) and *Semen Coicis* (Yiyiren)) were reported to have better efficacy on plaque psoriasis [51].

In addition, drugs approved by CFDA have also been studied, which contained herbal prescriptions and active composites extracted from herbs in various dosage forms, such as tablets, pills, creams, ointments, patches and injections. In the 34 approved drugs, the majority of them were orally administered two or three times per day, while 17 of them were the same extraction prepared in different dosage forms, such as formula Fufangqingdai, which has been prepared into tablets (Approved Number: Z20150034), pills (Approved Number: Z61020964), condensed pills (Approved Number: Z20080269) and capsules (Approved Number: Z20010157). There were also two injections, one containing *Radix Sophorae Flavescentis* (Kushen) (Approved Number: Z14021231), another involving *Fructus Psoraleae* (Buguzhi) (Approved Number: Z41022361) and six topical agents. However, from 2004 to June 2012, the National Adverse Drug Reaction Monitoring Center has revealed 344 cases that appeared to have adverse reactions in that digestive system, skin and its affiliated glands, and the nervous system after being treated with systemic administered prescriptions, and 23 severe cases involved medicinal liver damage and gastrointestinal bleeding. Compared to systemic preparations, those for topical use showed less adverse events including hotness, redness, dryness or itching on the administered skin, which are usually reversible or self-healing.

Modern studies on anti-psoriatic extraction from Chinese medicines

With huge potential for treating psoriasis, novel drugs involving pure ingredients extracted from Chinese herbs also have been explored. Curcumin, which is an active constituent in *Curcuma longa* L., has been developed into various kinds of formulations due to its inhibition of several inflammatory enzymes. Studies have found that it exerted anti-psoriatic action probably via suppressing the expression of VEGF and iNOS [52]. Additionally, curcumin was reported to show anti-inflammatory and growth suppressive effects in TNF-α treated HaCaT cells through inhibition of the NF-κB and MAPK pathways [53]. Curcuminoid C3 complex capsules are an oral drug candidate, which is under a phase II clinical trial to assess its safety and efficacy [54]. Fufangezhu Oil Cream [55] and ethanolic extract of 'Ezhu' [56] were both applied in animal tests and showed better efficacy. Topical nano-emulsion of turmeric oil was employed in both in vivo and in vitro animal experiments and was found to have high potential to treat psoriasis [57]. Our previous work has applied curcumin-load PLGA nanoparticles hydrogel topically to treat psoriatic mice with good bioactivity [58].

Moreover, we have performed extensive studies to understand the underlying mechanisms of single constituents isolated from effective Chinese medicines on psoriasis treatment. For example, our recent studies revealed that indirubin, the active component of *Indigo naturalis* (Qingdai), significantly mitigated psoriatic lesions induced by imiquimod in mice. Meanwhile, it could suppress infiltration of inflammatory cells, proliferation of epidermal cells and expression of pre-inflammatory factors. In addition, in vitro studies demonstrated the inhibition effect on the expression of IL-17A and phosphorylation of STAT3 and JAK3, indicating that the expression of IL-17A from γδ T cells and immuno-inflammatory reactions can be inhibited by indirubin probably via mediating the JAK3/STAT3 signaling pathway [59]. *Paeonia lactiflora Pall.* (Shaoyao), whose active compound is paeoniflorin, can significantly alleviate imiquimod-induced psoriatic lesions and inhibit the infiltration of inflammatory cells as well as the proliferation and differentiation of epidermal cells. Furthermore, it mainly targeted the regulation of Th cell factor expression, and inhibited the excretion of relevant cytokines probably via modulating the phosphorylation of STAT3

[60]. Astilbin, the active composite extracted from *rhizoma Smilacis Glabrae* (Tufuling), showed suppressive effects on the differentiation of Th 17 cells and γδ T cells. Therefore, the content of IL-17 in lesions and peripheral blood was mediated. However, the specific underlying molecular mechanics remains unclear [61]. *Tripterygium wilfordii Hook.* (Leigongteng) is a traditional medicinal herb that has been used for several centuries in China. Multi-glycoside from this herb could effectively disturb the formation of skin lesions in imiquimod-induced mice and inhibit the proliferation of epithelial cells and infiltration of T cells in lesion sites via downmodulating Th 17 function [62]. *Arnebiae Radix* (Zicao), a blood-regulating herb, and its ingredient β, β-dimethyl acryloyl alkannin has demonstrated suppressing psoriasis-activated dendritic cells and inhibiting mRNA expression of inflammatory factors due to curbing the TLR7/8 pathway [63, 64].

Conclusions and perspectives

Psoriasis not only affects people with itching and pain but also causes serious distress in their daily lives. Because of the abnormal appearance and texture of the skin, it is likely that psoriasis patients will be less likely to take part in social activities because of depression, so apparent skin treatment is more important. According to the CFDA data, the chemical formulations of psoriasis treatments are mainly topical drugs, while the traditional Chinese medicine formulations are mainly oral systemic drugs, suggesting that the market of topical preparations of Chinese medicine for the treatment of psoriasis is still waiting for exploration. At present, the most effective drug is biologics, but their cost, relative to chemical drugs or traditional Chinese medicine, is too high to be used for long term treatment. Looking for new technologies to reduce production costs is definitely a development trend for monoclonal antibody drugs. On the other hand, compared to chemical and biological treatments, traditional Chinese medicine and their active extracts are much cheaper with fewer adverse reactions, which is more suitable for the treatment of less severe psoriasis. Therefore, the topical use of Chinese medicine or their small-molecule extractions for the treatment of psoriasis is a potentially promising new area for future exploration.

Authors' contributions
SM finished the Background section, Chemical and biological drugs section, 2 Tables and is the major contributor in writing the manuscript. YW provided Chinese medicine understanding of psoriasis and medication principles. ZL elaborated the application of different Chinese medicine on psoriasis. ZW provided a few studies, ideas and some revised opinion. YZ and PL, as corresponding authors, are responsible for guiding the writing orientation. All authors read and approved the final manuscript.

Author details
[1] State Key Laboratory of Quality Research in Chinese Medicine, Institute of Chinese Medical Science, University of Macau, Macau, China. [2] Beijing

Hospital of Traditional Chinese Medicine, Affiliated with Capital Medical University, Beijing, China. [3] Department of Dermatology, School of Medicine, University of California, San Diego, La Jolla, CA, USA. [4] Department of Pathophysiology, Beijing Key Laboratory of Clinic and Basic Research with Traditional Chinese Medicine on Psoriasis, Beijing Institute of Traditional Chinese Medicine, 23 Meishuguan Back Street, Dongcheng, Beijing 100010, People's Republic of China.

Acknowledgements
We are grateful for the financial support from the Research Committee of University of Macau (Ref. Nos. MYRG2016-00090-ICMS-QRCM & MYRG2014-00040-ICMS-QRCM).

Competing interests
The authors declare that they have no competing interests.

Consent for publication
Not applicable.

Funding
Research Committee of University of Macau (Ref. Nos. MYRG2016-00090-ICMS-QRCM & MYRG2014-00040-ICMS-QRCM).

References
1. Baumgarth N, Bevins CL. Autoimmune disease: skin deep but complex. Nature. 2007;449(7162):551–3.
2. Organization WH. Global report on psoriasis. 2016. WHO Library Cataloguing-in-Publication Data 2016.
3. Xiao-lan D, Ting-lin W, Yi-wei S, Xiao-yan W, Cheng Z, Shan T, Ying L, Guang-hui P, Jun-e A, Shu-qi X. Prevalence of psoriasis in China: an epidemiological survey in six Provinces. Chin J Derm Venerol. 2010;24(7):598–601.
4. Rachakonda TD, Schupp CW, Armstrong AW. Psoriasis prevalence among adults in the United States. J Am Acad Dermatol. 2014;70(3):512–6.
5. Stern RS, Nijsten T, Feldman SR, Margolis DJ, Rolstad T. Psoriasis is common, carries a substantial burden even when not extensive, and is associated with widespread treatment dissatisfaction. J Investig Dermatol Symp Proc. 2004;9:136–9.
6. Lowes MA, Bowcock AM, Krueger JG. Pathogenesis and therapy of psoriasis. Nature. 2007;445(7130):866–73.
7. Dhar S, Banerjee R, Agrawal N, Chatterjee S, Malakar R. Psoriasis in children: an insight. Indian J Dermatol. 2011;56(3):262.
8. Gottlieb SL, Gilleaudeau P, Johnson R, Estes L, Woodworth TG, Gottlieb AB, Krueger JG. Response of psoriasis to a lymphocyte-selective toxin (DAB389IL-2) suggests a primary immune, but not keratinocyte, pathogenic basis. Nat Med. 1995;1(5):442–7.
9. Ritchlin C. Psoriatic disease—from skin to bone. Nat Clin Pract Rheumatol. 2007;3(12):698–706.
10. Ainsworth C. Immunology: a many layered thing. Nature. 2012;492(7429):S52–4.
11. Kolls JK, Lindén A. Interleukin-17 family members and inflammation. Immunity. 2004;21(4):467–76.
12. Zhao JX, Wang Y, Di TT, Liu X, Li P. The IL-23/IL-17 axis in the immunopathogenesis of psoriasis. Basic Clin Med. 2012;4:027.
13. Dolgin E. New anti-IL-23 drugs raise hopes for psoriasis plaque clearance. London: Nature Publishing Group; 2016.
14. McKenzie BS, Kastelein RA, Cua DJ. Understanding the IL-23–IL-17 immune pathway. Trends Immunol. 2006;27(1):17–23.
15. Kauffman CL, Aria N, Toichi E, McCormick TS, Cooper KD, Gottlieb AB, Everitt DE, Frederick B, Zhu Y, Graham MA. A phase I study evaluating the safety, pharmacokinetics, and clinical response of a human IL-12 p40 antibody in subjects with plaque psoriasis. J Investig Dermatol. 2004;123(6):1037–44.
16. van der Fits L, Mourits S, Voerman JS, Kant M, Boon L, Laman JD, Cornelissen F, Mus A-M, Florencia E, Prens EP. Imiquimod-induced psoriasis-like

17. skin inflammation in mice is mediated via the IL-23/IL-17 axis. J Immunol. 2009;182(9):5836–45.
18. Lillis JV, Guo C-S, Lee JJ, Blauvelt A. Increased IL-23 expression in palmoplantar psoriasis and hyperkeratotic hand dermatitis. Arch Dermatol. 2010;146(8):918–35.
18. Harper EG, Guo C, Rizzo H, Lillis JV, Kurtz SE, Skorcheva I, Purdy D, Fitch E, Iordanov M, Blauvelt A. Th17 cytokines stimulate CCL20 expression in keratinocytes in vitro and in vivo: implications for psoriasis pathogenesis. J Investig Dermatol. 2009;129(9):2175–83.
19. Woo YR, Cho DH, Park HJ. Molecular mechanisms and management of a cutaneous inflammatory disorder: psoriasis. Int J Mol Sci. 2017;18(12):2684.
20. Kim J, Krueger JG: Psoriasis and other skin inflammatory diseases. Inflammation: from molecular and cellular mechanisms to the clinic; 2018. p. 1091–1104.
21. Crow JM. Psoriasis uncovered. Nature. 2012;492(7429):S50.
22. Crow JM. Therapeutics: silencing psoriasis. Nature. 2012;492(7429):S58–9.
23. Rizvi S, Chaudhari K, Syed BA. The psoriasis drugs market. Nat Rev Drug Discovery. 2015;14(11):745–6.
24. branch CSoDP. Chinese psoriasis treatment experts consensus (2014 Edition). Chin J Dermatol. 2014;47(3):3.
25. Mrowietz U, Kragballe K, Reich K, Spuls P, Griffiths C, Nast A, Franke J, Antoniou C, Arenberger P, Balieva F. Definition of treatment goals for moderate to severe psoriasis: a European consensus. Arch Dermatol Res. 2011;303(1):1–10.
26. Griffiths G, Clark C, Chalmers R, Li Wan Po A, Williams H. A systematic review of treatments for severe psoriasis. Health Technol Assess. 2000;4:1–125.
27. Colao R, Yanofsky VR, Lebwohl MG. Successful treatment of palmoplantar psoriasis using combination acitretin and apremilast: a case report. J Psoriasis Psoriatic Arthritis. 2016;1(2):66–9.
28. AbuHilal Md, Walsh S, Shear N. Use of apremilast in combination with other therapies for treatment of chronic plaque psoriasis: a retrospective study. J Cutan Med Surg. 2016;20(4):313–6.
29. Lapteva M, Mondon K, Möller M, Gurny R, Kalia YN. Polymeric micelle nanocarriers for the cutaneous delivery of tacrolimus: a targeted approach for the treatment of psoriasis. Mol Pharm. 2014;11(9):2989–3001.
30. Chao Y. General treatise on the cause and symptoms of diseases. Beijing: People's Medical Publishing House; 1955.
31. Wu Q. The golden mirror of medicine. Beijing: People's Medical Publishing House; 1973.
32. Zhao B. Zhao Bingnan clinical experience set. Beijing: People's Medical Publishing House; 1975.
33. Bingnan Zhao ZZ. Concise dermatology of traditional Chinese medicine. Beijing: China outlook press; 1983.
34. Song P, Li B. Sharing the methods of "Treated form blood differentiation"—experiences of Renkang Zhu in treating psoriasis. Chin J Tradit Chin west Med. 2004;01:1–2.
35. Qifeng Jin DZ. Dermatology of TCM. Beijing: Beijing China Medical Science and Technology Press; 2001.
36. Wang P, Zhang P, Deng B, Sun L. TCM syndrome differentiation and psoriasis treatment of Zhili Zhang. Chin J Tradit Chin West Med. 2004;04:191–3.
37. Xu Y. Dermatology TCM diagnosis and treatment. Beijing: People's Medical Publishing House; 1997.
38. Ma S, Li Y. Report of 312 cases of psoriasis treated by syndrome differentiation. Hunan Guiding J TCMP. 1999;07:21.
39. Bingxu DC, Chunyan J, Ping W. The rule of distribution and development of TCM syndromes of psoriasis. J Tradit Chin Med. 2006;47:770–2.
40. Li J, Xu L, Zhou F, Jiang Y, Zhang T, Li D, Zheng D. Study on the distribution of TCM syndrome of psoriasis in central China. Chin J Tradit Chin West Med. 2011;01:8–12.
41. Zhang G, Wang P, Wang J, Jiang C, Deng B, Li P, Zhang Y, Liu W, Qu X, Chen W, et al. The distribution of syndrome manifestations and evolvement rules on 2651 psoriasis vulgaris cases. J Tradit Chin Med. 2008;10:894–6.
42. Wang M, Wang Y, Zhao J, Di T, Meng Y, Xie X, Zhai C, Li P. The application of regulating-blood Chinese traditional medicine in treating psoriasis. World Chin Med. 2017;09:2263–8.
43. Min W, Shupeng S, Yun GA, Yuhua G, Zhong KX. Efficacy of Yinxieling ointment on 675 cases. Chin Tradit Patent Med. 1990;11:21.

44. Shi Q, Shengshun T, Zhiping S, An ZJ, Yi YJ, Ping L. Clinical study on Huox-uesanyu xiaoyin decoction for treating psoriasis vulgaris with blood stasis syndrome. J Chin Med Mater. 2005;05:442–4.

45. Wei ZH, Xi ZY. Clinical research on JiaWeiHuangLianJieD decoction for treatment of psoriasis vulgaris. Chin J Inf Tradit Chin Med. 2010;04:65–6.

46. Baohua Y, Yong X, Guorong S. Clinical research on Tuiyintang combined with NB-UVB for psoriasis vulgaris. LiShizhen Med Mater Med Res. 2014;01:125–7.

47. Yao D-N, Lu C-J, Wen Z-H, Yan Y-H, Xuan M-L, Li X-Y, Li G, He Z-H, Xie X-L, Deng J-W. Oral PSORI-CM01, a Chinese herbal formula, plus topi-cal sequential therapy for moderate-to-severe psoriasis vulgaris: pilot study for a double-blind, randomized, placebo-controlled trial. Trials. 2016;17(1):140.

48. Feng YH, Ning G, Fen TA. The clinical curative effect of dampness Kushen decoction in the treatment of psoriasis vulgaris with damp heat syn-drome. Chin J Biochem Pharm. 2017;05:209–10.

49. Lin YK, Yen HR, Wong WR, Yang SH, Pang JHS. Successful treatment of pediatric psoriasis with Indigo naturalis composite ointment. Pediatr Dermatol. 2006;23(5):507–10.

50. Zhou N, Bai YP, Man XH, Zhang YB, Kong YH, Ju H, Chang M. Effect of new Pulian Ointment () in treating psoriasis of blood-heat syndrome: a randomized controlled trial. Chin J Integr Med. 2009;15(6):409–14.

51. Yuqi TT. Review of a treatment for psoriasis using herose, a botanical formula. J Dermatol. 2005;32(12):940–5.

52. Chen HXJ, Zhang Y. Effects of curcuma on expression of CD45RO, VEGF and iNOS in psoriatic lesions. Chin J Dermato Venerol Integ Trad W Med. 2004;3(4):198–201.

53. Cho J-W, Lee K-S, Kim C-W. Curcumin attenuates the expression of IL-1β, IL-6, and TNF-α as well as cyclin E in TNF-α-treated HaCaT cells; NF-κB and MAPKs as potential upstream targets. Int J Mol Med. 2007;19(3):469–74.

54. Kurd SK, Smith N, VanVoorhees A, Troxel AB, Badmaev V, Seykora JT, Gelfand JM. Oral curcumin in the treatment of moderate to severe psoriasis vulgaris: a prospective clinical trial. J Am Acad Dermatol. 2008;58(4):625–31.

55. Yingbiao T, Zehui C, Qin Y, Limei Y, Hong Z, Min W. Effect of compound curcuma oil cream on psoriasis—like animal model. Pharmacol Clin Chin Mater Med. 2009;03:57–9.

56. Fuchang L, Jinqi L. Study on prevention and treatment of psoriasis by curcumol ethanol cream and its action mechanism. Pharmacol Clin Chin Mater Med. 2016;03:95–8.

57. Ali MS, Alam MS, Imam FI, Siddiqui MR. Topical nanoemulsion of turmeric oil for psoriasis: characterization, ex vivo and in vivo assessment. Int J Drug Deliv. 2012;4(2):184.

58. Sun L, Liu Z, Wang L, Cun D, Tong HH, Yan R, Chen X, Wang R, Zheng Y. Enhanced topical penetration, system exposure and anti-psoriasis activity of two particle-sized, curcumin-loaded PLGA nanoparticles in hydrogel. J Control Release. 2017;254:44–54.

59. Xie X. Effects of Liangxuejiedu formula and indigo on the activation of KC/γδT involved CCL20 in psoriasis model. Master. Beijing University of Chinese Medicine; 2017.

60. Zhao J, Di T, Wang Y, Wang Y, Liu X, Liang D, Li P. Paeoniflorin inhibits imiquimod-induced psoriasis in mice by regulating Th17 cell response and cytokine secretion. Eur J Pharmacol. 2016;772:131–43.

61. Di T-T, Ruan Z-T, Zhao J-X, Wang Y, Liu X, Wang Y, Li P. Astilbin inhibits Th17 cell differentiation and ameliorates imiquimod-induced psoriasis-like skin lesions in BALB/c mice via Jak3/Stat3 signaling pathway. Int Immunop-harmacol. 2016;32:32–8.

62. Zhao J, Di T, Wang Y, Liu X, Liang D, Zhang G, Li P. Multi-glycoside of Trip-terygium wilfordii Hook. f. ameliorates imiquimod-induced skin lesions through a STAT3-dependent mechanism involving the inhibition of Th17-mediated inflammatory responses. Int J Mol Med. 2016;38(3):747–57.

63. Wang Y, Zhao J, Zhang L, Di T, Liu X, Lin Y, Zeng Z, Li P. Suppressive effect of β, β-dimethylacryloyl alkannin on activated dendritic cells in an imiquimod-induced psoriasis mouse model. Int J Clin Exp Pathol. 2015;8(6):6665.

64. Wang Y, Zhao J, Di T, Wang M, Ruan Z, Zhang L, Xie X, Meng Y, Lin Y, Liu X. Suppressive effect of β, β-dimethylacryloyl alkannin on activated dendritic cells in psoriasis by the TLR7/8 pathway. Int Immunopharmacol. 2016;40:410–8.

14

Shuganyin decoction improves the intestinal barrier function in a rat model of irritable bowel syndrome induced by water-avoidance stress

Lu Lu[1†], Liang Yan[2†], Jianye Yuan[3], Qing Ye[4*] and Jiang Lin[1*]

Abstract

Background: To determine the effect of Shuganyin decoction (SGD) on the intestinal barrier function in an irritable bowel syndrome (IBS) rat model induced by water-avoidance stress.

Methods: Forty male Wistar rats were divided into control, water-avoidance stress (WAS) group, WAS plus Shuganyin decoction (SGD) group and WAS plus dicetel (Dicetel) group. IBS was induced in rats by subjecting them to water-avoidance stress for 7 days. On day 4 of the WAS protocol, the rats were treated for 7 consecutive days (days 4–11) with SGD, dicetel or a negative control (saline). The number of feces granules, histopathological changes of the intestine and mast cell (MC) morphometry were determined. Intestinal permeability was approximated by measuring the absorption of FITC-dextran 4400 (FD-4) from the lumen into the bloodstream in vivo and in vitro experiments. Also, the expression of protease active receptor-2 (PAR-2) and tumor necrosis factor-α (TNF-α) was estimated using immunohistochemical staining and ELISA, respectively. Tight junction (TJ) protein abundance was measured following a quantitative immunofluorescent analysis of intestinal sections and western blotting.

Results: In vivo, WAS elicited a significantly increase in the transfer of FD-4 from the intestine to blood about threefold in 30 min compared with control group. After treated with SGD, the intestinal permeability to FD-4 of WAS-induced rats was significantly attenuated ($P < 0.05$). In vitro, the permeability coefficient (Papp) values were measured for FD-4 absorption across the excised intestine. WAS was shown to increase the intestinal permeability to $(4.695 \pm 0.3629) \times 10^{-7}$ cm/s in 120 min, which was 2.6-fold higher than the control group. Rats treated with SGD showed a significant decrease in Papp values of FD-4 as compared to WAS group ($P < 0.05$). Furthermore, by immuno-fluorescent detection we found that WAS elicited the irregular distribution of TJ proteins. Using the quantitative analysis software of the medical image, the average optical density and protein abundance of TJ proteins was shown to be lower in the WAS group as compared to control group, ($P < 0.05$). SGD could attenuate this response and improve TJ distribution ($P < 0.05$). Western blot analysis confirmed that TJ protein abundance was significantly decreased in WAS group and that they could be returned to control levels following an SGD treatment. WAS also induced an increase in number of MCs, their area and diameter as compared to controls. These observations were attenuated with an SGD

---

*Correspondence: yeqing1982889@126.com; lin_jiang@hotmail.com
[†]Lu Lu and Liang Yan contributed equally to this work
[1] Department of Gastroenterology, Longhua Hospital Affiliated to Shanghai University of Traditional Chinese Medicine, Shanghai 200032, China
[4] Department of Neurology, Longhua Hospital Affiliated to Shanghai University of Traditional Chinese Medicine, Shanghai 200032, China

Shuganyin decoction improves the intestinal barrier function in a rat model of irritable bowel syndrome...

149

or dicetel treatment. Similarly, the expression of PAR-2 and TNF-α exceeded control values in the WAS group and were shown to be successfully attenuated with an SGD treatment.

Conclusion: WAS-induced IBS rat model exhibited intestinal barrier dysfunction, which was manifested as tight junction damage and structural rearrangements that increased the intestinal permeability. Under these conditions, MCs were activated and degranulated in the intestinal mucosa leading to the activation of PAR-2. Our data showed that SGD could inhibit the activation of MCs and down-regulate the expression of both PAR-2 and TNF-α. In turn, this was shown to improve the expression and structural arrangement of TJ proteins in the intestinal mucosa, thereby regulating the intestinal permeability. It was concluded that Shuganyin could protect the intestinal barrier.

Keywords: Shuganyin decoction, Water-avoidance stress, Intestinal barrier function, Mast cell, Protease activated preceptor-2, Rat model

Background

Irritable bowel syndrome (IBS) refers to a commonly seen functional bowel disorder with the features of chronic abdominal pain or discomfort and the change in bowel habits. IBS has a major influence on patients' life quality. In the past, most reports in the literature focused on the study of gastrointestinal motility disorders and visceral hypersensitivity. Motility disorders and hypersensitivity are the main pathophysiologic consequences of IBS [1, 2]. However, more recent studies show the innerconnection between intestinal barrier dysfunction and immune activation [3, 4]. Furthermore, according to existing data, IBS patients with predominant diarrhea have a higher degree of intestinal permeability [5–7]. The pathophysiological signals leading to the destruction of intestinal permeability in IBS are still unclear.

Mast cells (MCs) are important regulators of the immune response, especially in the gastro-intestinal tract. When pressure signals are conveyed through the brain–gut axis, MCs release proinflammatory mediators, including tryptase. In turn, these mediators stimulate nerve terminals and influence intestinal motility. Specifically, following their interaction with PAR-2 receptors on the epithelial cells, the TNF-α expression is increased and tight junction (TJ) proteins are modulated [8–11]. Ultimately, stress-induced changes to the brain–gut axis can result in intestinal hyperpermeability.

It is common knowledge that there is no standard therapeutic agent to cure IBS. Currently, the most frequently used therapeutic is dicetel. Dicetel is a calcium antagonist that acts as a gastrointestinal antispasmodic by inhibiting the calcium channels of the smooth muscle cells that line the intestinal wall, thus preventing excessive intestinal contraction. In addition, dicetel can block the expression of the nerve peptide, regulate the intestinal hypersensitivity and, thereby, improve abdominal pain and discomfort. Nevertheless, the therapeutic effects of dicetel have not been satisfactory. An alternative is Shuganyin, a traditional Chinese medicine that has gained some traction in the research community for the treatment of IBS.

Although its underlying mode of action remains to be elucidated, Shuganyin has been successful for the treatment of IBS patients with disharmony of liver and spleen. Compared to dicetel, Shuganyin has the advantage of overall regulation.

The first aim of this study was to characterize the changes that can be observed in water-avoidance stress-induced rat model of diarrhoea-IBS by measuring the number and degranulation of MCs, the expression of PAR-2 and TNF-α proteins, the intestinal permeability, and the reorganization and abundance of TJ proteins. Secondly, we tested the hypothesis that Shuganyin can alleviate intestinal barrier dysfunction through a mechanism mediating the interaction between MCs, PAR-2, and the intestinal epithelium. The effect of Shuganyin on WAS-induced IBS in rats was determined by measuring the intestinal permeability, the spatial organization and the expression of TJ, and MC morphometry. The effects of Shuganyin were compared to a positive control treatment with dicetel, a calcium antagonist commonly prescribed to treat IBS.

Methods

The Minimum Standards of Reporting Checklist contains details of the experimental design, and resources used in this study (Additional file 1).

Preparation of Shuganyin decoction

SGD is comprised of the following five herbs: white atractylodes rhizome (Baizhu), 9 g; Paeoniae Radix Alba (Baishao), 6 g; Tangerine Peel (Chengpi), 6 g; Radix Saposhnikovia (Fangfeng), 4.5 g; and Radix Bupleuri (Chaihu), 6 g. And the total mass used was 31.5 g which is the common dose for adult humans. All the herbs were purchased from Yanghetang Pharmacy (Shanghai, China) as crude herbs. Dry powder of SGD's aqueous extract was made by Herbal Chemistry Labomouseory of Shanghai University of Traditional Chinese Medicine. SGD were prepared as follows: firstly, 31.5 g crude SGD were made into powder and put in 8 cups of water for 12 h, boiled for at least 2 h, and filtered. Then, the liquid was collected. Repeat such procedures. Put the liquid from two steps together, dry them in vacuum until there is no aqueous phase. When they are dried in a vacuum drying oven, 125 g of SGD powder can be obtained separately. The crude drugs were extracted twice and the filtrates were combined and vacuum dried to obtain a solid aqueous extract. Each final gram contained 3.36 g of the initial crude drugs. The aqueous extract was prepared at Shanghai University of Traditional Chinese Medicine. Previous pharmacodynamics performed by our team found that the effect of middle dose SGD on IBS model is the best. So, we selected the middle dose SGD directly in this study [12].

Animals water avoidance stress model

Male Wistar rats 250–280 g were purchased from Sino-British BK Lab Animal Ltd. (Shanghai, China) and acclimatized for 7 days after being delivered. All rats were allowed to get rodent chow and water and kept with 12 h light/dark cycle at 22 °C.

During the experiment, the rats were assigned to control ($n = 10$), WAS ($n = 10$), WAS plus dicetel ($n = 10$) (positive control), and WAS plus SGD ($n = 10$) groups. IBS was induced in rats subjecting them to water avoidance stress for 1 h/day for 10 days as previously described [11]. Briefly, rats were weighed and placed on a platform (8×6 cm) affixed to the center of a plastic container (55×50 cm) which is filled with water to 1 cm below the platform. On day 8, after rats were anaesthetized, sections of terminal ileum were wiped out instantly, for in vitro measurements. Ileum samples were dissected and stored at $- 80$ °C for histological analysis. In addition, another set of experimental rats (n = 10 per group) was used for in vivo intestinal permeability measurements.

Animals drug treatment

On day 4 of the WAS protocol, rats were treated (*i.g.*) daily, 1 h before the stress for 7 consecutive days (days 4–10) with SGD, Dicetel or vehicle (saline). The conversion of the human dose to that used in rats was calculated based on body surface. Rats in the control and WAS groups were given saline (1.0 ml/200 g). Rats in the WAS plus SGD group were administered the Shuganyin decoction, that was prepared by mixing solid aqueous extract in distilled water (196.9 mg/ml), and administering a dose of 1.0 ml/200 g body weight. Rats in the Dicetel group received Pinaverium bromide (Pinaverium bromide, Lot Number: H20120127, Abbott Products SAS, Solvay Pharmaceuticals, France) that was ground into fine powder, dissolved in distilled water (4.2 mg/ml), and administered at a dose of 1.0 ml/200 g.

In vivo measurement of intestinal permeability

Rats were anaesthetized with nembutal (45 mg/kg, i.p.) and cannulated via the jugular vein for blood collection. A midline abdominal incision was performed and the distal ileum was ligated and catheterized for administration of FD-4. Before closing the abdominal wall by suture, renal pedicles should be ligated. The intestinal mucosal permeability was evaluated by measuring the lumen-to-plasma entrance of FD-4. Tyrode's solution (in mmol/l: NaCl 137, KCl 2.7, $CaCl_2$ 1.8, $MgCl_2$ 1.0, $NaHCO_3$ 12, NaH_2PO_4 0.4, glucose 5.5, PH 7.4) containing FD-4 (0.4 mg/ml) was injected into the intestinal (50 ml/kg), and blood samples (80 µl) were subsequently collected at 0, 15, 30, 60, 90 and 120 min. A fluorometer (485 nm excitation, 530 nm emission) was used to detect the FD-4 concentration in blood [13].

In vitro mucosal permeability measurement

Rats were all anaesthetized and then euthanized, a section of distal ileum was immediately removed, washed, and then placed in oxygenated Krebs, then stripped of muscle layers gently. The mucosa layer was then mounted in a Ussing chamber (Physiology Instruments, San Diego, CA). The chamber opening exposed 0.5 cm^2 of tissue surface area to 5 ml of circulating oxygenated Krebs buffer (in mmol/l: NaCl 107, KCl 4.5, $NaHCO_3$ 25, NaH_2PO_4 0.2, Na_2HPO_4 1.8, $CaCl_2$ 1.2, $MgSO_4$ 1.0, glucose 12, PH 7.4) at 37 °C. Intestinal regions with visible damage were excluded from the studies. After the preparation had maintained stable for at least 30 min, FD-4 (0.1 mg/ml) was dropped in the mucosal reservoir. Samples (200 µl) were removed and supplied with identical volumes of fresh buffer at 0, 15, 30, 60, 90 and 120 min from the serosal side. The mucosal permeability was assessed by measuring transepithelial flux of FD-4, and was evaluated by apparent permeability (Papp) in cm/s as the equation: Papp = dQ/dt/AC. dQ/dt is FD-4 appeared in the membrane part. A is the tissue's surface part, and C is the original compound concentration in the mucosal compartment [14].

Immunohistochemistry

The intestines were washed out and tissue samples were kept in phosphate-buffered saline (PBS) containing 4% paraformaldehyde and 2 mM egtazic acid (EGTA). These tissue samples were then rinsed and agitated in PBS containing EGTA and sucrose before incubating them overnight at 4 °C. Tissues were embedded in optimum cutting temperature compound and cryostat sections (5 µm) were mounted on poly-L-lysine coated slides with acetone for 10 min at $- 20$ °C and rinsed in PBS-EGTA [15].

For the immunohistochemical staining of PAR-2, paraffin sections were dewaxed to water using standard procedures and the samples were rinsed three times with PBS. Then the tissue slides were incubated with the primary goat-anti-mouse PAR-2 antibody (Boster-Biological Technology, Wuhan, China) at 4 °C overnight. The tissues were incubated with second antibodies at room temperature for 20 min, after washed with PBS for five times. Following *Dolichos biflorus* agglutinin reaction, positive cells displayed brown–yellow particles in the cytoplasm. Digital images were collected from at least three random high power fields for further analysis.

For the immunohistochemical staining of TJ proteins ZO-1 and occludin, samples were labeled with either rabbit polyclonal C terminal anti-occludin antibody (rabbit polyclonal anti-ZO-1) or anti-occludin antibody raised against a 69 kDa fusion protein (Sigma, Shanghai, China) in a humidified chamber at 37 °C for 1 h. Samples were rinsed for three times with PBS and then embedded in PBS-glycerol. Approximately 20 tissue sections from each animal's intestine sample were analyzed and imaged with a fluorescence microscope in a darkroom [16]. For F-actin immunofluorescence, samples were rinsed in PBS containing 0.5 µg/ml of TRITC-conjugated phalloidin for 30 min at room temperature. After washing with PBS with EGTA, the samples were evaluated and imaged with a fluorescence microscope in a blinded fashion.

Optical density values and masculine area were analyzed from digital images using the Medical Image Quality Analyze System (MIQAS) (Qiuwei Biotechnological Co. Ltd., Shanghai, China). IHC = positive area × optical density/total area.

Histology
Full thickness segments of colon were fixed in paraformaldehyde, embedded in paraffin, and subsequently stained with toluidine blue (ECL, Beyotime, Nantong, China). Mast cells were counted at 400× magnification and non-overlapping areas above the muscularis mucosae were observed.

ELISA
Intestine segments were washed repeatedly with a saline solution and the mucosal layer was scraped off. Homogenised mucosa was subsequently centrifuged to collect and store the supernatant at − 80 °C. TNF-α protein abundance was determined with an ELISA kit (JingMei Biotech, Beijing, China), according to the manufacturer's protocol.

Toxicity
After 7 consecutive days treatment with SGD, segments of liver, kidney, and lung tissues were fixed in paraformaldehyde and embedded in paraffin. Hematoxylin and

eosin (H&E, Beyotime, Nantong, China) staining was used to observe the morphological changes in the liver, kidney and lung tissues at 200× magnification. Also, blood samples were taken from the abdominal aorta and centrifuged to obtain the serum. Levels of alanine aminotransferase (ALT), aspartate aminotransferase (AST), blood urea nitrogen (BUN), and creatinine (Cr) in the serum were estimated using biochemical kits (JingMei Biotech, Beijing, China).

Western blot
Briefly, intestine segments were harvested and extracted with RIPA lysis buffer with a protease inhibitor cocktail (Sigma, Shanghai, China) for 30 min at 4 °C. Forty micrograms on each lysate were separated by 10% SDS-PAGE and conveyed to polyvinylidene difluoride (PVDF) membranes (Sigma, Shanghai, China). After overnight blocking with 5% nonfat dry milk, blots were sequentially incubated with primary (Sigma, Shanghai, China) and secondary antibodies (Sigma, Shanghai, China) for 60 min at room temperature. β acting was used as a loading control. Membranes were washed four times with TBST and incubated with anti-rabbit secondary antibodies (Sigma, Shanghai, China) for 2 h. Quantitative results were revealed by using the ECL detection system (GE Health-care).

Statistical analysis
Results were expressed as the mean ± SD. One-way ANOVA was used for the determination of statistical significance as appropriate. For comparison of pathological scores, the Mann–Whitney rank sum test was used. P were considered as significance.

Results
SGD alleviated WAS-induced defecation
During the WAS protocol, the body weight of the rats was measured before and after each stress period. The number of fecal granules was recorded within 1 h. Rats in the control group were weighed and the number of fecal granules was recorded in the same timeframe. No difference in body weight was observed between the groups on day 1 ($P > 0.05$) and on days 6 and 10 (respectively 3 and 7 days after administering SGC or dicetel) (Fig. 1).

On day 3, prior to the administration of SGD or dicetel, the number of fecal granules collected from the WAS, SGD and Dicetel groups was increased above control levels ($P < 0.01$). Stool from the SGD and Dicetel groups appeared thin and soft. On days 6 and 10, at respectively 3 and 7 days after treatment with SGD or dicetel, the number of fecal granules for the SGD and Dicetel group rats was lower than for the WAS group (P < 0.01), but still higher than for controls ($P < 0.01$) (Fig. 2).

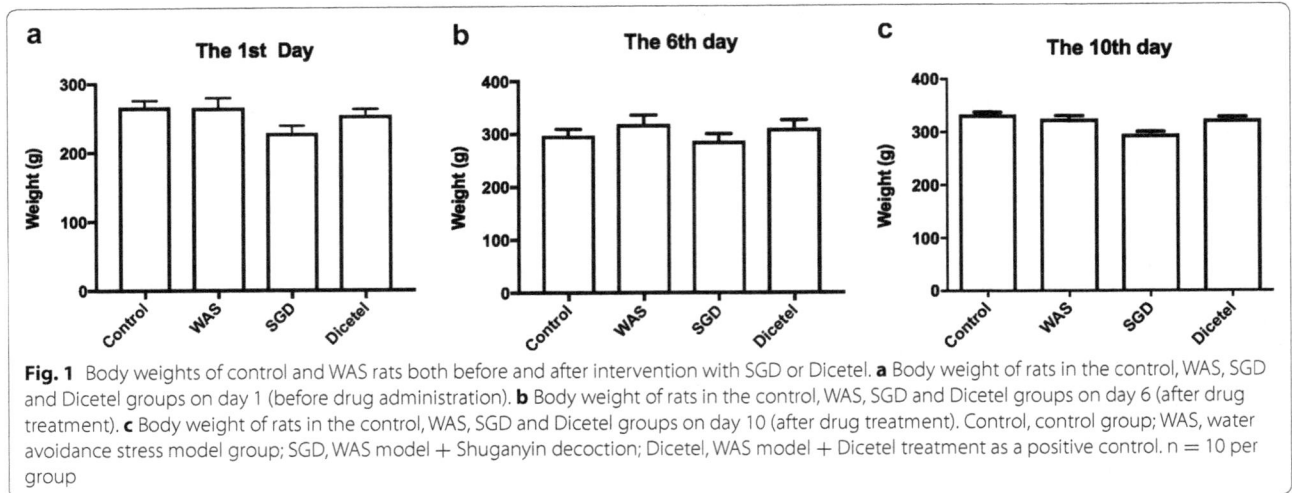

Fig. 1 Body weights of control and WAS rats both before and after intervention with SGD or Dicetel. **a** Body weight of rats in the control, WAS, SGD and Dicetel groups on day 1 (before drug administration). **b** Body weight of rats in the control, WAS, SGD and Dicetel groups on day 6 (after drug treatment). **c** Body weight of rats in the control, WAS, SGD and Dicetel groups on day 10 (after drug treatment). Control, control group; WAS, water avoidance stress model group; SGD, WAS model + Shuganyin decoction; Dicetel, WAS model + Dicetel treatment as a positive control. n = 10 per group

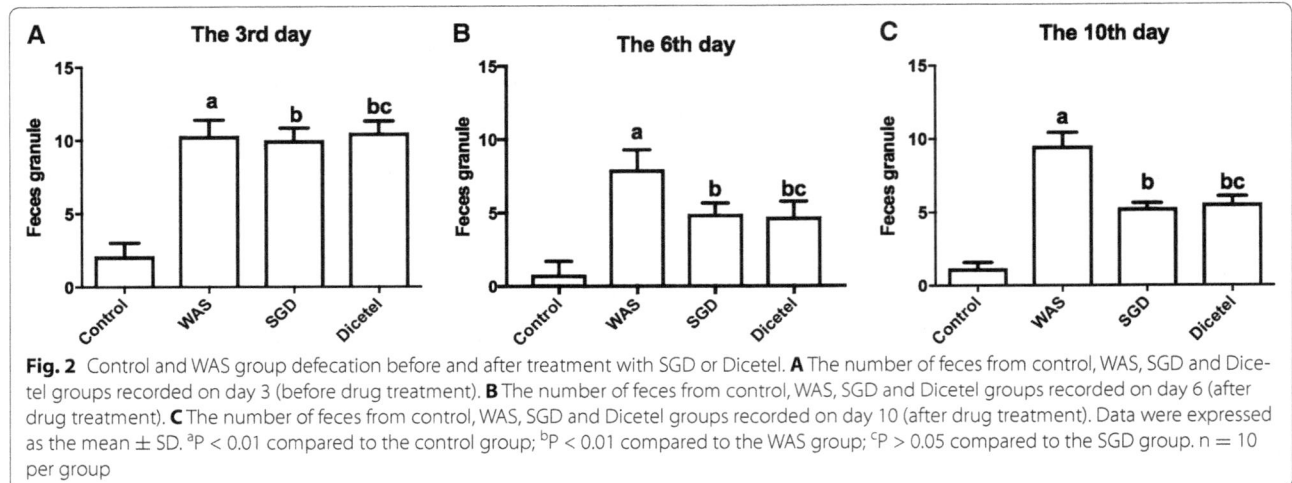

Fig. 2 Control and WAS group defecation before and after treatment with SGD or Dicetel. **A** The number of feces from control, WAS, SGD and Dicetel groups recorded on day 3 (before drug treatment). **B** The number of feces from control, WAS, SGD and Dicetel groups recorded on day 6 (after drug treatment). **C** The number of feces from control, WAS, SGD and Dicetel groups recorded on day 10 (after drug treatment). Data were expressed as the mean ± SD. [a]P < 0.01 compared to the control group; [b]P < 0.01 compared to the WAS group; [c]P > 0.05 compared to the SGD group. n = 10 per group

SGD attenuated the WAS-induced increase in intestinal permeability

Changes in intestine permeability were determined by measuring FD-4 absorption through the intestinal epithelium in vitro and in vivo. In vitro, apparent permeability (Papp) values were estimated across excised segments of intestine. The ileum from rats subjected to WAS displayed a 2.6-fold increase in intestinal permeability (WAS group, $4.695 \pm 0.363 \times 10^{-7}$ cm/s in 120 min) above control Papp values. Rats treated with SGD showed a significantly lower FD-4 Papp value than the WAS group (Fig. 3A, B). In vivo, FD-4 absorption was estimated based on the amount absorbed into the bloodstream 120 min after an intraluminal injection of FD-4. Relative to controls, WAS caused an approximately threefold increase in FD-4 absorption across the intestinal mucosa. After treating with SGD, the intestinal permeability to FD-4 could be significantly attenuated. Moreover, the intestinal permeability of WAS-induced rats treated with dicetel was equivalent to SGD (Fig. 3C). Our in vivo data corroborated the aforementioned in vitro permeability estimates.

WAS-induced ZO-1, occludin, and F-actin expression was reversed by SGD treatment

As shown in Figs. 4 and 5, ZO-1, occludin and F-actin protein levels were significantly lower in the intestinal mucosa from the WAS rats than controls. Interestingly, WAS elicited an apparent disruption and irregular distribution of ZO-1, occludin and F-actin staining. Using image analysis software assay, the average optical density of each of these TJ proteins was found to be lower than in the control group. While a treatment with SGD attenuated the disrupted pattern of the three TJ proteins and the expression of ZO-1 and occludin, the levels of F-actin were only partially restored by SGD treatment. Similar observations were made for the positive control treatment with dicetel.

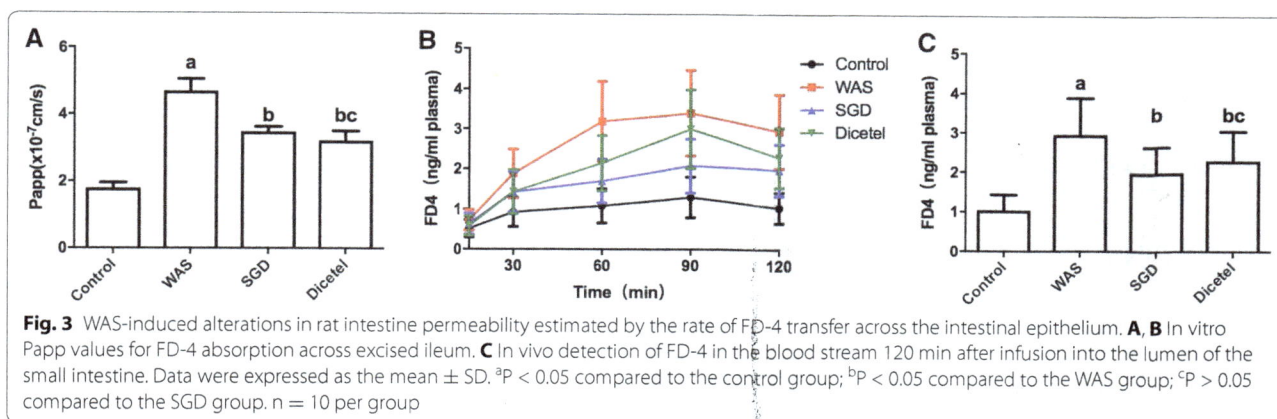

Fig. 3 WAS-induced alterations in rat intestine permeability estimated by the rate of FD-4 transfer across the intestinal epithelium. **A, B** In vitro Papp values for FD-4 absorption across excised ileum. **C** In vivo detection of FD-4 in the blood stream 120 min after infusion into the lumen of the small intestine. Data were expressed as the mean ± SD. [a]$P < 0.05$ compared to the control group; [b]$P < 0.05$ compared to the WAS group; [c]$P > 0.05$ compared to the SGD group. n = 10 per group

Western blot analysis showed that compared to the control group, protein abundance of the three TJ proteins was significantly decreased in the WAS group. Furthermore, SGD was shown to increase TJ protein abundance in WAS-induced rats.

SGD decreased WAS-induced increases in mast cell number and size

Microscopy of toluidine blue stained tissues revealed that the cytoplasm of MCs appeared granulated with coarse, violet–red pigments. Furthermore, the MCs were disseminated near small blood vessels in the mucosa and submucosa of the colon (Fig. 6A). MCs are characteristically round or spindle-shaped and have cytoplasmic membrane-bound granules. When the rats were subjected to WAS, MCs univocally appeared granulated, irregular in shape and unable to maintain plasma membrane integrity with granules leaking out of the cell. Treating these rats with SGD almost completely restored MC morphology. A similar observation was made when treating with dicetel. Also, the number, area and diameter of mast cells was calculated (Fig. 6B–D). The density, area, perimeter and diameter of the MCs were found to be significantly increased in the WAS group, compared to the control group. After treating with SGD or Dicetel, MC morphology returned to control appearance.

SGD decreased WAS-induced activation of PAR-2

Based on the immunohistochemical staining, PAR-2 was expressed in the colon tissue and distributed in the cytoplasm. Using image analysis software, the average optical density of the PAR-2 staining was found to be higher in WAS-induced rats than in controls. SGD was able to significantly attenuate the expression of PAR-2 in WAS-induced rats as compared to the untreated WAS group ($P < 0.05$; Fig. 7).

WAS-induced TNF-α expression was reversed by SGD treatment

Although H&E staining showed no inflammation in the colonic tissues, TNF-α abundance was higher in the WAS group than in the control group ($P < 0.05$). The previous was indicative of a low-grade mucosal inflammation in WAS-induced rat intestine. As for PAR-2, TNF-α expression in colonic tissue could be significantly reduced when treating the WAS-induced rats with SGD ($P < 0.05$; Fig. 8).

The toxicity evaluation of SGD

Chinese medicine formulae may induce unexpected toxicity in vivo, we, therefore, examined liver, kidney and lung tissue slices and measured the serum levels of several biomarkers after 7 consecutive days of Shuganyin treatment. As shown in Figs. 9 and 10, there is no

(See figure on next page.)
Fig. 4 Immunohistological detection of ZO-1, occludin and F-actin protein levels in intestinal mucosa. **A** Immunohistological detection ZO-1 protein in the intestinal mucosa of animals from control group (**a**), WAS group (**b**), SGD group (**c**) and Dicetel group (**d**), (×400); average optical density levels of ZO-1 protein in the different groups (right panel). **B** Immunohistological detection of occludin protein levels in intestinal mucosa of animals from control group (**a**), WAS group (**b**), SGD group (**c**) and Dicetel group (**d**), (×400); average optical density levels of occludin in different groups (right panel). **C** Immunohistological detection of F-actin protein level in intestinal mucosa of animals from control group (**a**), WAS group (**b**), SGD group (**c**) and Dicetel group (**d**), (×400); average optical density levels of F-actin in different groups (right panel). Data were expressed as the mean ± SD. [a]$P < 0.05$ compared to the control group; [b]$P < 0.05$ compared to the WAS group; [c]$P > 0.05$ compared to the SGD group. n = 10 per group

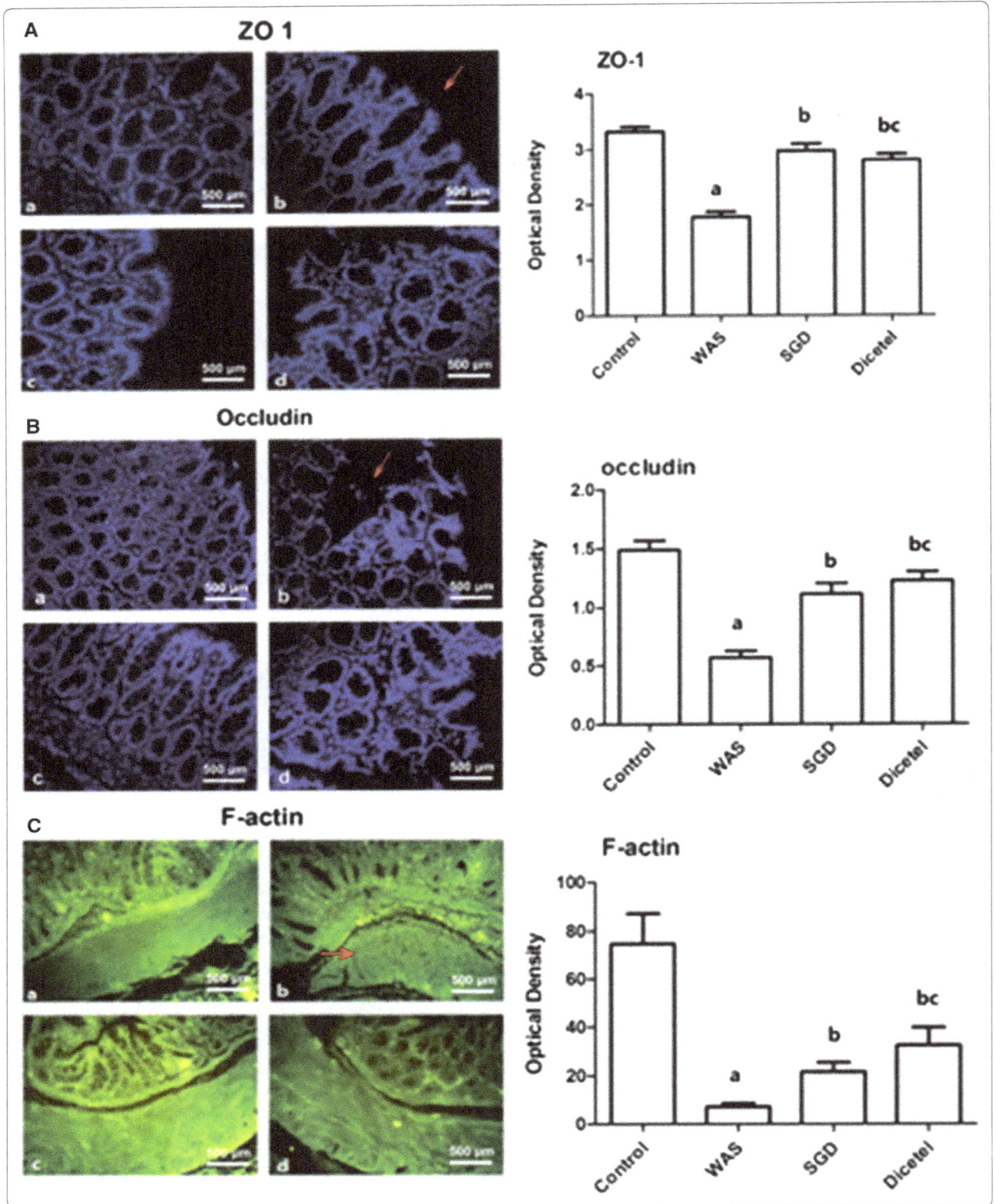

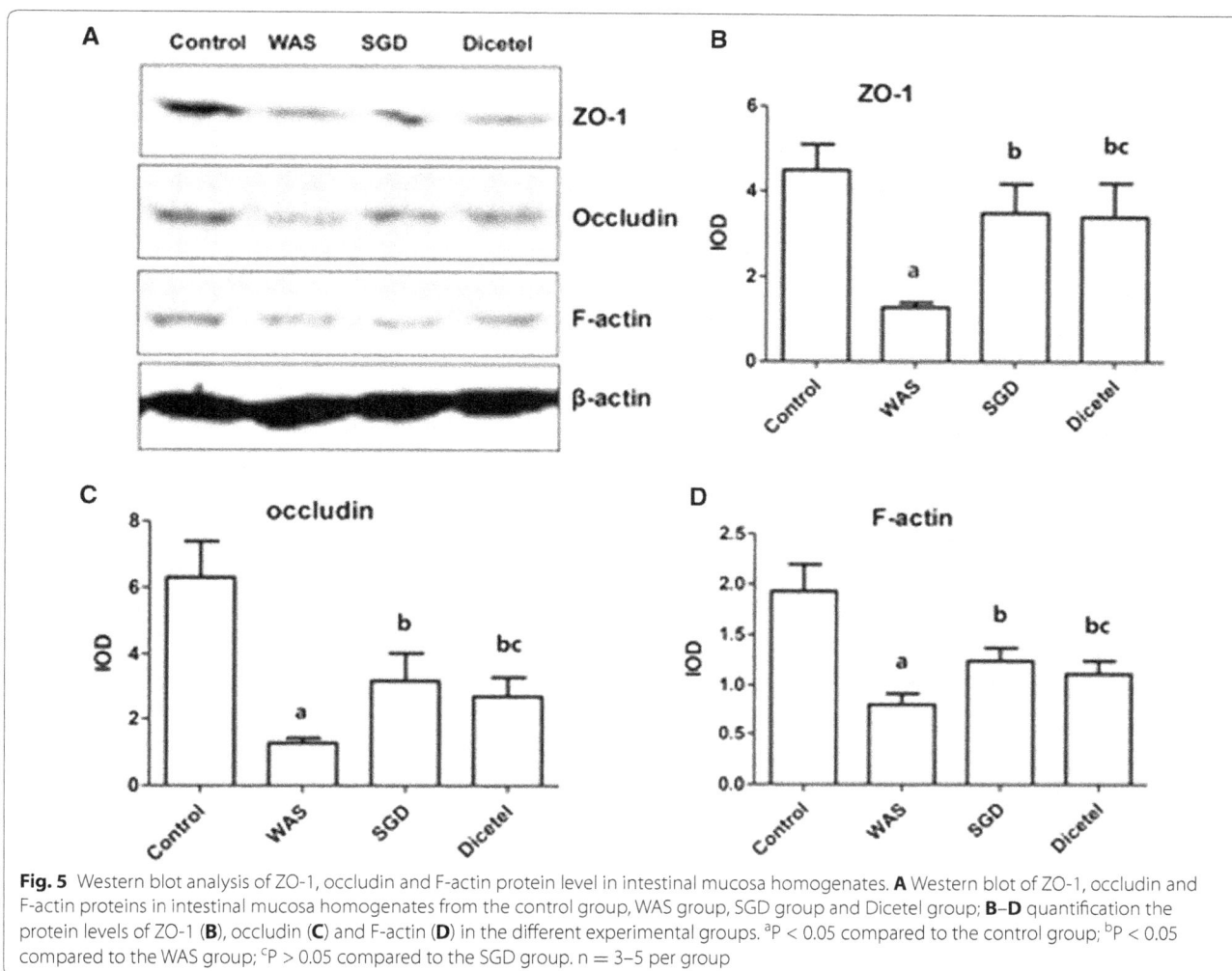

Fig. 5 Western blot analysis of ZO-1, occludin and F-actin protein level in intestinal mucosa homogenates. **A** Western blot of ZO-1, occludin and F-actin proteins in intestinal mucosa homogenates from the control group, WAS group, SGD group and Dicetel group; **B–D** quantification the protein levels of ZO-1 (**B**), occludin (**C**) and F-actin (**D**) in the different experimental groups. [a]$P < 0.05$ compared to the control group; [b]$P < 0.05$ compared to the WAS group; [c]$P > 0.05$ compared to the SGD group. n = 3–5 per group

significant adverse event or changes in histopathological and biochemical parameters were recorded ($P > 0.05$).

Discussion

IBS is usually considered as a disease of unknown cause, in addition to gastrointestinal motility disorders, visceral hypersensitivity, intestinal infections and brain–gut axis dysfunction, social background and psychological factors are considered to be closely related. Many reports have demonstrated that stress factors have a major impact on the epithelial cell permeability, however, whether psychological stress in patients with IBS would undermine the integrity of the intestinal barrier function remains unclear [17]. Currently, there are many views on the mechanism of intestinal barrier function changes under stress, including interaction between immune cells, intestinal neurons and epithelial cells mediated by corticotrophin-releasing hormone release, activation of the vagus nerve and mast cells secrete media [18–20].

Intestinal barrier function of intestinal epithelial means the inner partition intestine substance has the ability to prevent the pathogenic antigen intrusion. Intestinal barrier includes mechanical barrier, immunological barriers and bacteria barrier. Mechanical barrier is most important, which includes intestinal epithelial cells and the tight junction between cells. The so-called tight junction (TJ) locates between adjacent epithelial cells, which is the main connection between the intestinal epithelial cells, and plays a role in closing the gap cells within the intestine to prevent substance freely through the cell gap, through epithelial cell layer and regulating intestinal barrier permeability [21–23]. Tight junction contains a series of over 30 proteins [24], including blocking protein occludin and claudin, junction associated molecule (JAM) and other transmembrane proteins, cytosolic attachment protein ZO family (zonula occludens protein) and wire connected thereto actin-like protein. Among them, ZO-1 and occludin are most important. Filamentous actin

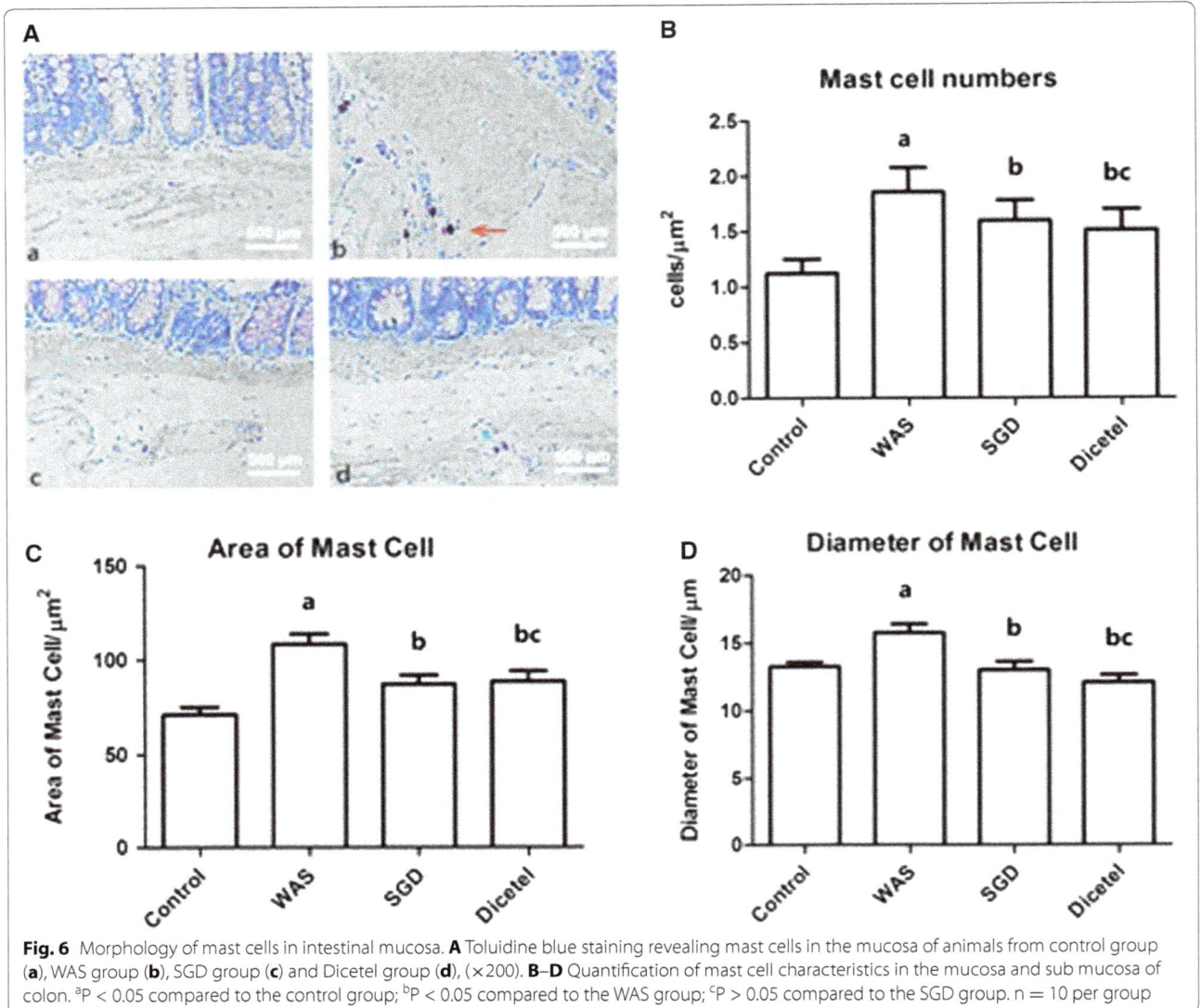

Fig. 6 Morphology of mast cells in intestinal mucosa. **A** Toluidine blue staining revealing mast cells in the mucosa of animals from control group (**a**), WAS group (**b**), SGD group (**c**) and Dicetel group (**d**), (×200). **B–D** Quantification of mast cell characteristics in the mucosa and sub mucosa of colon. [a]$P < 0.05$ compared to the control group; [b]$P < 0.05$ compared to the WAS group; [c]$P > 0.05$ compared to the SGD group. n = 10 per group

F-actin, appears in all eukaryotic cells, and is an important component of the cytoskeleton. F-actin was associated with tight junction through a manner of patchy dense, they function together to regulate inner and outer cellular signal transduction pathways, change actin contractility, affect the assembly and function of tight junction, and regulate the permeability. Our study found that water-avoidance stress method almost destroyed all the tight junctions of intestinal mucosa. Western blot results showed that ZO-1, occludin, F-actin expressions were significantly reduced. In addition, the combination use of in vivo and in vitro method, showed that results of diarrhea-predominant IBS ileum permeability strongly suggest that water-avoidance stress model in rats can increased intestinal permeability. Thus, we assumed that the main cause of intestinal barrier dysfunction is the expression of tight junctions between epithelial cells reduced which leads to destruction of epithelial cells dense structure, and finally leads to increased intestinal permeability.

Studies have shown that the activation of immune cells in the intestinal mucosa is related to intestinal mucosal barrier disruption. The cytokine TNF-α is mainly secreted by monocytes and macrophages and associated with a range of physiological and pathological responses. TNF-α is known to induce apoptosis of intestinal epithelial cells and change the assembly of intercellular TJ proteins [25]. Martinez et al. found that, compared with healthy controls, intestinal mast cell activation expression of tryptase increased significantly, while the

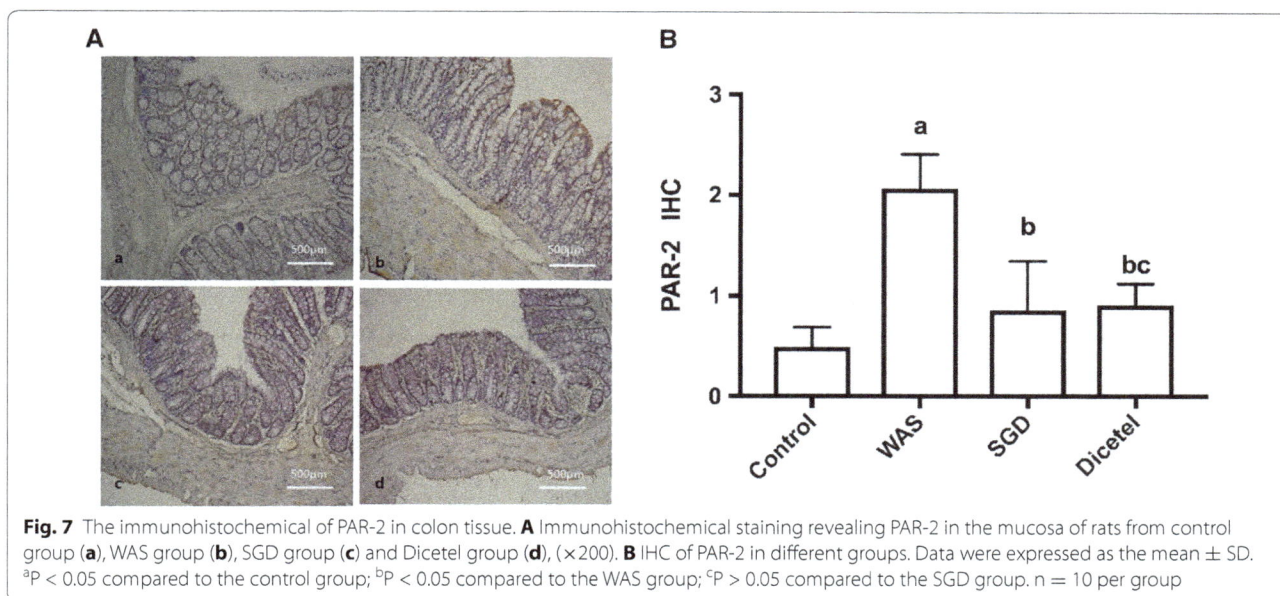

Fig. 7 The immunohistochemical of PAR-2 in colon tissue. **A** Immunohistochemical staining revealing PAR-2 in the mucosa of rats from control group (**a**), WAS group (**b**), SGD group (**c**) and Dicetel group (**d**), (×200). **B** IHC of PAR-2 in different groups. Data were expressed as the mean ± SD. [a]$P < 0.05$ compared to the control group; [b]$P < 0.05$ compared to the WAS group; [c]$P > 0.05$ compared to the SGD group. n = 10 per group

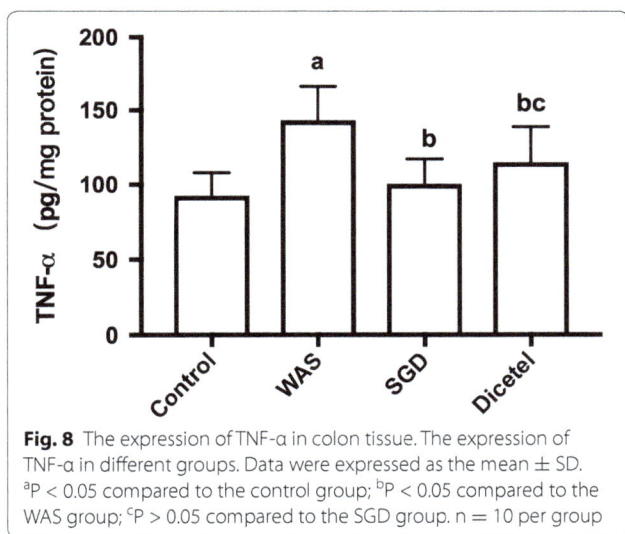

Fig. 8 The expression of TNF-α in colon tissue. The expression of TNF-α in different groups. Data were expressed as the mean ± SD. [a]$P < 0.05$ compared to the control group; [b]$P < 0.05$ compared to the WAS group; [c]$P > 0.05$ compared to the SGD group. n = 10 per group

intestinal mucosa ZO-1 and protein ZO-3 decreased significantly [26, 27]. MCs are located in the blood vessels, nerves and mucous membranes nearby lymph and they act as the main antigen receptors regulating the immune response of the intestinal mucosa. When a specific antigen stimulates the immune system, sensory nerve endings excite and induce the production of IgE antibody. Following an antigen–antibody interaction MCs can activate, degranulate, and release a variety of biologically active mediators, of which tryptase is closely related to intestinal permeability. As a serine protease enzyme, tryptase is a strong protease-activated receptor activator of PAR-2. Activation of PAR-2 can induce a rearrangement of intestinal epithelial TJ and the cytoskeleton. This, in turn, changes the intestinal barrier structure and increases the permeability of the intestinal mucosa [28–30]. The study presented herein reported the changes inflicted by WAS-induced IBS in rats with measurements

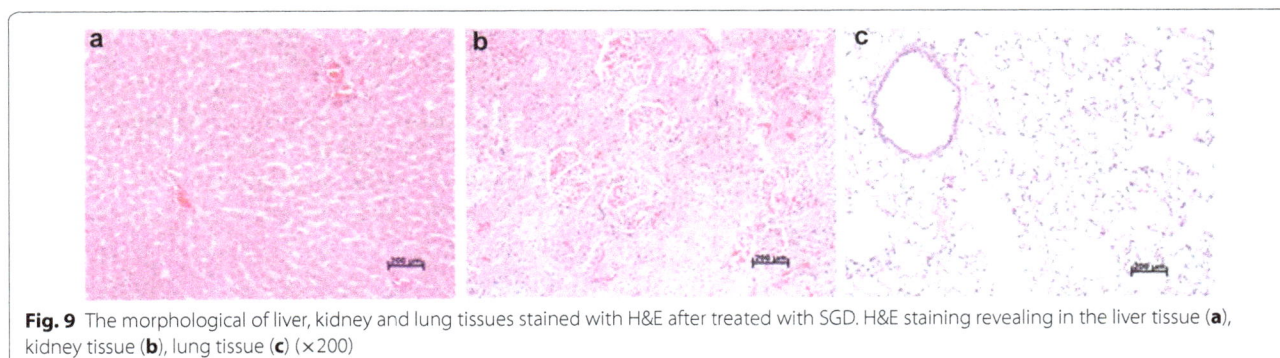

Fig. 9 The morphological of liver, kidney and lung tissues stained with H&E after treated with SGD. H&E staining revealing in the liver tissue (**a**), kidney tissue (**b**), lung tissue (**c**) (×200)

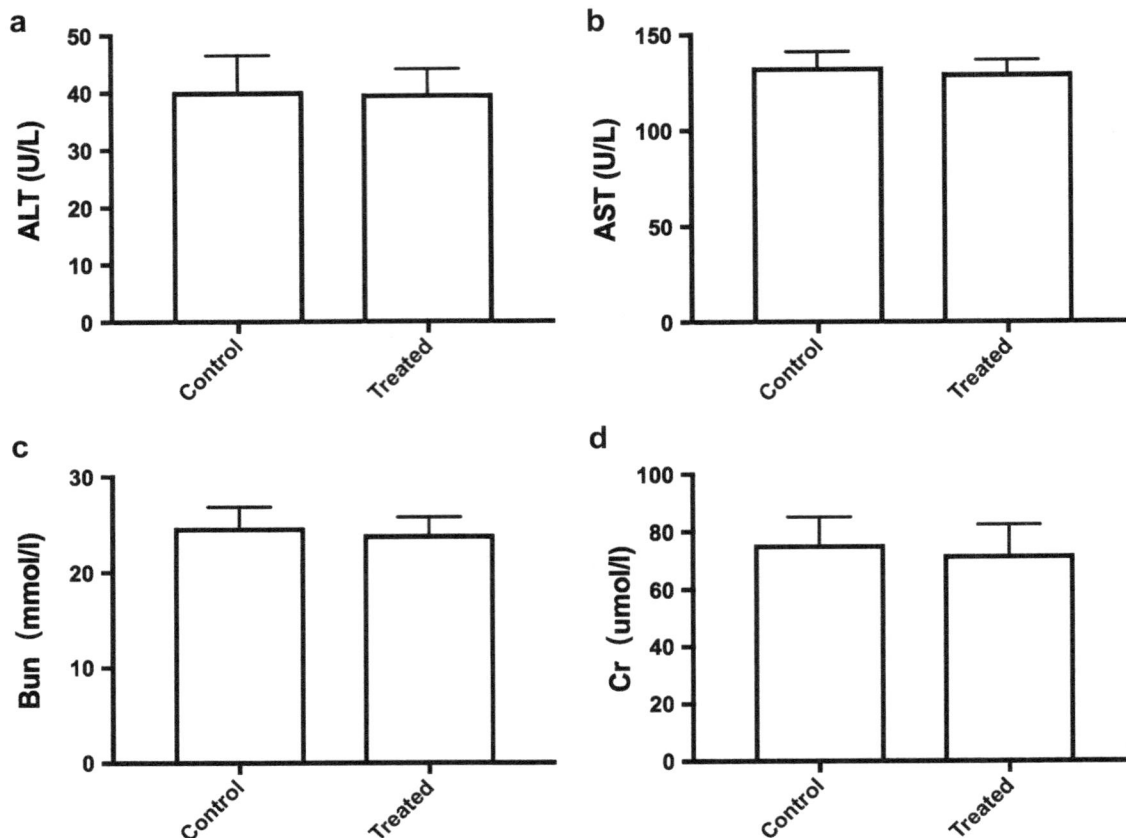

Fig. 10 The biochemical parameters of rats after treated with SGD. **a** The expression of ALT before and after treated with SGD; **b** The expression of AST before and after treated with SGD; **c** The expression of BUN before and after treated with SGD; **d** The expression of Cr before and after treated with SGD. Data were expressed as the mean ± SD. n = 10 per group

of including the intestinal mucosa PAR-2 expression, mast cells number, area, perimeter, roundness, and diameter. MCs were clearly activated because of the stress and some were even degranulating. The model was also used to test Shuganyin as a potential treatment of IBS and, indeed, following the treatment of WAS-induced rats with SGD, PAR-2 and intestinal TJ protein expressions were decreased to control levels. Also, the intestinal hyperpermeability due to the stress could be attenuated by SGD. Arguably, Shuganyin inhibits the activation and degranulation of mast cells. In turn, the release of biologically active mediators is reduced, inhibiting the rearrangement of intestinal epithelial TJs and thus reducing the permeability of the intestinal mucosa. Shuganyin is therefore believed to protect the intestinal barrier.

There were some limitations to the study as we did not use the PAR-2 high-pressure inhibitor GB88 [31]. A follow-up study using GB88 and an intestinal epithelial

PAR-2 pressure specific gene knockout animal model has already been planned.

Conclusions

The WAS-induced IBS rat model was shown to exhibit intestinal barrier dysfunction given the TJ damage and structural rearrangements that led to an increased intestinal permeability. Also, the activation and degranulation of MCs could be observed in their intestinal mucosa. When treated with Shuganyin, MC activation was inhibited and the expression of both PAR-2 and TNF-α was downregulated, whereas the expression of TJ proteins in the intestinal mucosa was increased. In addition, Shuganyin was shown to suppress the increase in intestinal permeability observed in rats subjected to WAS. It was concluded that Shuganyin can protect the intestinal barrier function.

Abbreviations

SGD: Shuganyin decoction; WAS: water-avoidance stress; PAR-2: protease active receptor-2; TNF-α: tumor necrosis factor-α; TJ: tight junction; FD-4: FITC-dextran 4400; IBS: irritable bowel syndrome; MC: mast cell; GI: gastrointestinal; BGA: brain–gut axis; TCM: traditional Chinese medicine; Papp: apparent permeability; MIQAS: Medical Image Quality Analyze System; PVDF: polyvinylidene difluoride.

Authors' contributions

LL participated in in vitro and in vivo mucosal permeability assay and drafted the manuscript. LY carried out the immunoassays. JYY performed the statistical analysis. JL participated in the design of the study. QY conceived of the study, and participated in its design and coordination and helped to draft the manuscript. All authors read and approved the final manuscript.

Author details

[1] Department of Gastroenterology, Longhua Hospital Affiliated to Shanghai University of Traditional Chinese Medicine, Shanghai 200032, China. [2] Department of General Surgery, Shuguang Hospital Affiliated to Shanghai University of Traditional Chinese Medicine, Shanghai 201203, China. [3] Research Institute of the Spleen and Stomach Disease, Longhua Hospital Affiliated to Shanghai University of Traditional Chinese Medicine, Shanghai 200032, China. [4] Department of Neurology, Longhua Hospital Affiliated to Shanghai University of Traditional Chinese Medicine, Shanghai 200032, China.

Acknowledgements
Not applicable.

Competing interests
The authors declare that they have no competing interests.

Consent for publication
Not applicable.

Funding
This manuscript was supported by Natural Science Foundation of China (Grant No. 81202665).

References

1. Longstreth GF, Thompson WG, Chey WD, Houghton LA, Mearin F, Spiller RC. Functional bowel disorders. Gastroenterology. 2006;130:1480–91.
2. Thompson WG, Longstreth GF, Drossman DA, Heaton KW, Irvine EJ, Muller-Lissner SA. Functional bowel disorders and functional abdominal pain. Gut. 1999;45(Suppl 2):II43–7.
3. Piche T, Barbara G, Aubert P, Bruley des Varannes S, Dainese R, Nano JL, et al. Impaired intestinal barrier integrity in the colon of patients with irritable bowel syndrome: involvement of soluble mediators. Gut. 2009;58:196–201.
4. Park JH, Park DI, Kim HJ, Cho YK, Sohn CI, Jeon WK, et al. The relationship between small-intestinal bacterial overgrowth and intestinal permeability in patients with irritable bowel syndrome. Gut Liver. 2009;3:174–9.
5. Dunlop SP, Hebden J, Campbell E, Naesdal J, Olbe L, Perkins AC, et al. Abnormal intestinal permeability in subgroups of diarrhea-predominant irritable bowel syndromes. Am J Gastroenterol. 2006;101:1288–94.
6. Zhou Q, Souba WW, Croce CM, Verne GN. MicroRNA-29a regulates intes-

tinal membrane permeability in patients with irritable bowel syndrome. Gut. 2010;59:775–84.
7. Zhou Q, Zhang B, Verne GN. Intestinal membrane permeability and hypersensitivity in the irritable bowel syndrome. Pain. 2009;146:41–6.
8. Halland M, Saito YA. Irritable bowel syndrome: new and emerging treatments. BMJ. 2015;18(350):h1622.
9. Gershon MD. Nerves, reflexes, and the enteric nervous system: pathogenesis of the irritable bowel syndrome. J Clin Gastroenterol. 2005;39:S184–93.
10. Barbara G, Stanghellini V, De Giorgio R, Corinaldesi R. Functional gastrointestinal disorders and mast cells: implications for therapy. Neurogastroenterol Motil. 2006;18:6–17.
11. Bradesi S, Schwetz I, Ennes HS, Lamy CM, Ohning G, Fanselow M, Pothoulakis C, McRoberts JA, Mayer EA. Repeated exposure to water avoidance stress in rats: a new model for sustained visceral hyperalgesia. Am J Physiol Gastrointest Liver Physiol. 2005;289:G42–53.
12. Shi HL, Liu CH, Ding LL, et al. Alterations in serotonin, transient receptor potential channels and protease-activated receptors in rats with irritable bowel syndrome attenuated by Shugan decoction. World J Gastroenterol. 2015;21(16):4852–63.
13. Xiao DT, Hong C, Xiao WQ, et al. Platelet-activating factor increases mucosal permeability in rat intestine via tyrosine phosphorylation of E-cadherin. Br J Pharmacol. 2000;129(7):1522–9.
14. Fan Y, Wu DZ, Gong YQ, et al. Effects of calycosin on the impairment of barrier function induced by hypoxia in human umbilical vein endothelial cells. Eur J Pharmacol. 2003;481(1):33–40.
15. Saunders PR, Santos J, Hanssen NP, Yates D, Groot JA, Perdue MH. Physical and psychological stress in rats enhances colonic epithelial permeability via peripheral CRH. Dig Dis Sci. 2002;47:208–15.
16. Kiliaan AJ, Saunders PR, Bijlsma PB, Berin MC, Taminiau JA, et al. Stress stimulates transepithelial macromolecular uptake in rat jejunum. Am J Physiol. 1998;275:G1037–44.
17. Collins SM, Piche T, Rampal P. The putative role of inflammation in the irritable bowel syndrome. Gut. 2001;49:743–5.
18. Piche T. Tight junctions and IBS—the link between epithelial permeability, low-grade inflammation, and symptom generation? Neurogastroenterol Motil. 2014;26:296–302.
19. Gassler N, Rohr C, Schneider A, Kartenbeck J, Bach A, et al. Inflammatory bowel disease is associated with changes of enterocytic junctions. Am J Physiol Gastrointest Liver Physiol. 2001;281:G216–28.
20. Vanuytsel T, van Wanrooy S, Vanheel H, Vanormelingen C, Verschueren S, Houben E, et al. Psychological stress and corticotropin-releasing hormone increase intestinal permeability in humans by a mast cell-dependent mechanism. Gut. 2014;63:1293–9.
21. Madara JL. Loosening tight junction lessons from the intestine. J Clin Invest. 1989;83(4):1089–94.
22. Ivanov AI, Nusrat A, Parkos CA. Endocytosis of the apical junctional complex: mechanisms and possible roles in regulation of epithelial barriers. BioEssays. 2005;27:356–65.
23. Usami Y, Chiba H, Nakayama F, Ueda J, Matsuda Y, Sawada N, Komori T, Ito A, Yokozaki H. Reduced expression of claudin-7 correlates with invasion and metastasis in squamous cell carcinoma of the esophagus. Hum Pathol. 2006;37:569–77.
24. Anderson JM, Van Itallie CM. Tight junctions and the molecular basis for regulation of paracellular permeability. Am J Physiol. 1995;269:467–75.
25. Ma TY, Iwamoto GK, Hoa NT, et al. TNF-alpha-induce increase in intestinal epithelial tight junction permeability requires NF-KappaB activation. Am J Physiol Gastrointest Liver Physiol. 2004;286:G367–76.
26. Martinez C, Lobo B, Pigrau M, Ramos L, Gonzalez-Castro AM, Alonso C, Guilarte M, Guila M, et al. Diarrhoea-predominant irritable bowel syndrome: an organic disorder with structural abnormalities in the jejunal epithelial barrier. Gut. 2013;62:1160–8.
27. Martinez C, Vicario M, Ramos L, Lobo B, Mosquera JL, Alonso C, Sanchez A, Guilarte M, et al. The jejunum of diarrhea-predominant irritable bowel syndrome shows molecular alterations in the tight junction signaling

pathway that are associated with mucosal pathobiology and clinical manifestations. Am J Gastroenterol. 2012;107:736–46.

28. Cenac N, Chin AC, Garcia-Villar R, Salvador-Cartier C, Ferrier L, Vergnolle N, Buret AG, Fioramonti J, Bueno L. PAR2 activation alters colonic paracellular permeability in mice via IFN-gamma-dependent and -independent pathways. J Physiol. 2004;558:913–25.

29. Anton PA. Stress and mind-body impact on the course of inflammatory bowel diseases. Semin Gastrointest Dis. 1999;10(1):14–9.

30. Levenstein S, Prantera C, Varvo V, Scribano ML, Andreoli A, Luzi C, Arca M, Berto E, Milite G, Marcheggiano A. Stress and exacerbation in ulcerative colitis: a prospective study of patients enrolled in remission. Am J Gastroenterol. 2000;95:1213–20.

31. Lohman RJ, Cotterell AJ, Suen J, et al. Antagonism of protease-activated receptor 2 protects against experimental colitis. J Pharmacol Exp Ther. 2012;340(2):256–65.

15

Effect of Da-Cheng-Qi decoction for treatment of acute kidney injury in rats with severe acute pancreatitis

Ling Yuan, Lv Zhu[†], Yumei Zhang[†], Huan Chen, Hongxin Kang, Juan Li, Xianlin Zhao, Meihua Wan, Yifan Miao and Wenfu Tang[*]

Abstract

Background: The traditional Chinese formula Da-Cheng-Qi-decoction (DCQD) has been used to treat acute pancreatitis for decades. DCQD could ameliorate the disease severity and the complications of organ injuries, including those of the liver and lungs. However, the pharmacological effects in the kidney, a target organ, are still unclear. This study aimed to investigate the herbal tissue pharmacology of DCQD for acute kidney injury (AKI) in rats with severe acute pancreatitis (SAP).

Methods: Rats were randomly divided into the sham-operation group (SG), the model group (MG) and the low-, medium- and high-dose treatment groups (LDG, MDG, and HDG, respectively). Sodium taurocholate (3.5%) was retrogradely perfused into the biliopancreatic duct to establish the model of SAP in rats. Different doses of DCQD were administered to the treatment groups 2 h after the induction of SAP. The major components of DCQD in kidney tissues were detected by HPLC–MS/MS. Inflammatory mediators in the kidney tissues, as well as serum creatinine (Scr), blood urea nitrogen (BUN) and pathologic scores, were also evaluated.

Results: Ten components of DCQD were detected in the kidneys of the treatment groups, and their concentrations increased dose-dependently. Compared with the SG, the levels of inflammatory mediators, Scr, BUN and pathological scores in the MG were obviously increased ($p < 0.05$). The high dose of DCQD showed a maximal effect in downregulating the pro-inflammatory mediators interleukin-6 (IL)-6 and tumour necrosis factor-α (TNF-α), upregulating anti-inflammatory mediators IL-4 and IL-10 in the kidney and alleviating the pathological damages. DCQD decreased the pancreas and kidney pathological scores of rats with SAP, especially in the HDG ($p < 0.05$). Compared with the MG, the level of Scr in the HDG was significantly decreased ($p < 0.05$).

Conclusions: DCQD ameliorated AKI in rats with SAP via regulating the inflammatory response, which might be closely related to the distribution of its components in the kidney.

Keywords: Da-Cheng-Qi decoction, Acute pancreatitis, Acute kidney injury, Tissue distribution, Inflammatory response

*Correspondence: hxtangwenfu@126.com
†Lv Zhu and Yumei Zhang contribute equally as co-first authors
Department of Integrative Medicine, West China Hospital, Sichuan University, Chengdu 610041, Sichuan, People's Republic of China

Background

Acute pancreatitis (AP) is commonly a self-limited inflammatory disease caused by abnormally activated pancreatic digestive enzymes [1]. However, approximately 20% of AP cases develop into severe acute pancreatitis (SAP), with high mortality characterized by systemic inflammatory response syndrome (SIRS) and multiple organ injuries and even failure at an early stage [2, 3], including acute respiratory distress syndrome, acute kidney injury (AKI) and acute liver injury. AKI is diagnosed by accumulations of serum creatinine (Scr) and blood urea nitrogen (BUN) or decreased urine output, which reflects a rapid loss of the kidney's excretory function [4]. AKI is one of the most common complications of SAP increasing the disease mortality [5, 6]. A retrospective and multi-centre study showed that nearly 69.3% of SAP patients developed AKI [5]. Acute renal failure used to be defined as the severe form of AKI [7], which leads to a drastic increase in the mortality of SAP [8–10]. Therefore, it is essential to ameliorate AKI with SAP as early as possible to decrease the mortality.

The mechanism of SAP resulting in AKI is complex. Available studies revealed that SAP-induced AKI is mainly related to SIRS [9], which involves various cytokines and inflammatory mediators, such as nuclear factor kappa B (NF-B), tumour necrosis factor (TNF)-α, interleukin (IL)-1β, IL-6, IL-10, and high mobility group box protein 1(HMGB1) [11]. Endotoxins, reactive oxygen species (ROS), phospholipase A_2 (PLA_2), hypoxemia, as well as a decrease in renal perfusion pressure due to abdominal compartment syndrome and an impairment of renal microcirculation for the release of pancreatic amylase, may also play important roles in the pathophysiology of SAP-induced AKI [12]. The mortality of SAP patients with AKI remains high regardless of the progress in intensive care treatment [9]. Although many worldwide guidelines have been established for AP [13, 14], there is still no exact drug protocol recommended [15] other than renal replacement therapy (RRT) for AKI with SAP [4, 9]. However, the application of RRT remains controversial in many aspects and has many potential complications [16]. A multicentre, multinational, prospective study showed that RRT practice did not align with the best evidence, and variations in practice may be responsible for substantial morbidity [17]. Hence, it is worthwhile to find new interventions for SAP-induced AKI and to explore the potential mechanism.

Da-Cheng-Qi decoction (DCQD), which is composed of *Rheum palmatum* L. (Dahuang), *Magnolia henryi* Dunn. (Houpu), *Citrus aurantium* L. (Zhishi) and *Natrii Sulphas* (Mangxiao), has been applied to treat AP effectively for decades in China [18]. We hypothesized that the concentration and distribution of the components of the herbal prescription in the target organs were related to its pharmacological effect. Based on this hypothesis, our previous studies have verified that DCQD could alleviate the injuries of the pancreas, lungs, liver and intestines by inhibiting the inflammatory response in rats with AP based on the distribution of its components in target tissues [19–22]. However, the pharmacological effects of DCQD in the kidney, a target organ, are still unclear. Herein, this study investigates the herbal tissue pharmacology of DCQD in the kidneys of rats with SAP after the administration of different doses of DCQD and explores the underlying mechanisms.

Methods

Information of experimental design and resources

The information regarding the experimental design, statistics, and resources used in this study are attached in the minimum standards of reporting checklist (Additional file 1).

Animals

Forty healthy, clean grade, male Sprague–Dawley rats (SD, 220 ± 15 g) were purchased from Chengdu Dashuo Bio-Technique Co. Ltd. (Chengdu, China). The experimental protocol was performed according to the Animal Ethics Committee Guidelines of our hospital (2016001A, Chengdu, China). One week after acclimation, the animals were fasted with free access to water for 24 h prior to the experiment.

Preparation of DCQD

The spray-dried drug powders were obtained from Chengdu Green Herbal Pharmaceutical Co. Ltd. (Chengdu, China). The processing procedure of the crude formula components has been previously described [22]. According to the *Treaties on Exogenous Febrile Disease*, the suggested dose of DCQD for a person weighting 60 kg is 57 g, composed of 12 g of Dahuang, 24 g of Houpu, 12 g of Zhishi and 9 g of Mangxiao. As we have mentioned [22], we chose 6 g/kg BW (0.6 g/100 g) as the lowest dose. The drug powders mixed at the ratio of 12:24:12:9, were reconstituted with sterile distilled water at different concentrations (0.6, 1.2 and 2.4 g/mL).

Induction of SAP and intervention

The rats were randomly divided into five groups and marked as the low-dose treatment group (LDG, 6 g/kg BW), the medium-dose treatment group (MDG, 12 g/kg BW), the high-dose treatment group (HDG, 24 g/kg BW), the sham-operation group (SG) and the model group (MG). The SAP model was induced via biliopancreatic duct injection of 3.5% sodium taurocholate (Sigma, St. Louis, MO, USA) with a micro-infusion pump at a rate of 0.2 mL/min (1 mL/kg body weight) [20]. The rats in the SG received saline instead of 3.5% sodium taurocholate. Two hours after the operation, the rats in the treatment groups were administered DCQD intragastrically at 1 mL/100 g BW, with 0.6 g/mL for the LDG, 1.2 g/mL for the MDG and 2.4 g/mL for the HDG while the rats in the SG and MG were administered an equal volume of saline.

Sample collections and measurements

Twenty-four hours after administration, all the rats were sacrificed, and arterial blood as well as kidney pancreas tissues were collected for measurement. Pancreas and kidney tissues were cut into slices and were fixed with 10% neutral formalin, embedded in paraffin, cut into sheets (at thickness of 5–7 μm) and then stained with haematoxylin and eosin. Pathological scores were blindly evaluated by two independent pathologists with a previously established scoring system [20, 22, 23]. The severity of edema, neutrophil infiltration, necrosis, and haemorrhage was represented on a scale of 0–4 (0 = 0%, none; 1 = 25%, mild; 2 = 26–50%, moderate; 3 = 51–75%, sever; 4 = 76%, severe).

Additional pancreas and kidney tissues were stored at −80 °C. High-performance liquid chromatography–tandem mass spectrometry (HPLC–MS/MS) was used to measure the major components of DCQD (emodin, rhein, aloe-emodin, chrysophanol, rheochrysidin, hesperidin, naringin, naringenin, magnolol and honokiol) in the kidney tissue homogenates (10%) [24]. As we detected previously, the average contents of rhein, emodin, aloe-emodin, chrysophanol, rheochrysidin, naringin, naringenin, hesperidin, magnolol, and honokiol in DCQD were 0.86, 2.48, 1.73, 0.55, 2.61, 3.83, 4.16, 11.06, 1.11, and 1.26 mg/g respectively [24].

The levels of IL-6, TNF-a, IL-10 and IL-4 in kidney tissue homogenate were measured by using the Milliplex MAP Rat Cytokine/Chemokine magnetic bead immunoassay kit (Millipore Corporation, Billerica, MA). The blood samples were centrifuged at 3000 rmp for 5 min and the serum was distracted for Scr and BUN. The concentrations of Scr and BUN were detected by an Automatic Biochemical Analyser (AU5400, SIEMENS, Munich, Germany).

Preparation of standard and quality control samples

The ten major components of DCQD from the previous study [21, 24] were detected in this study by HPLC–MS/MS. Quality control samples were prepared to obtain the following plasma concentrations: 120, 20, 5 and 1.25 ng/mL for rheochrysidin; 100, 25 and 6.25 ng/mL for emodin; 3750, 625, 156.25 and 39.06 ng/mL for rhein; and 600, 100, 25 and 6.25 ng/mL for aloe-emodin, naringin,

chrysophanol, hesperidin, magnolol, naringenin, and honokiol. The spiked plasma samples (standard and quality control) were pretreated and detected in each analytical batch along with the unknown samples [24]. The remainder of the detected DCQD was deposited in the Public Experiment Platform of our hospital (Chengdu, China).

Data collection, peak integration, and calibration were all calculated with Analyst 1.4.2 software. Calibration curves were plotted according to the peak ratio of analytes to internal standards (ibuprofen), and the linear regression between tissue concentrations and peak area ratios were determined by $1/\chi^2$. Concentrations of QC and unknown samples were measured by interpolation from the calibration curves [24].

Statistical analysis

The statistical analysis was performed with PEMS3.1 for Windows (Sichuan University, China). All the data were expressed as the mean ± standard deviation (mean ± SD). One-way repeated-measures ANOVA, followed by multiple pair-wise comparisons using the Student–Neuman–Keuls procedure, was applied to the analysis of multiple groups. The data was considered significantly different when $p < 0.05$.

Results

Ten components of DCQD detected in kidney tissues

The ten major components of DCQD were all detected in the kidney tissues. The concentrations of emodin, rhein, aloe-emodin, chrysophanol, rheochrysidin and magnolol increased with the DCQD dose and showed significant differences when compared to the other treatment groups. The concentrations of hesperidin, naringin, naringenin, and honokiol were not as closely related to the dose. Rhein and naringenin were relatively higher than the other compounds of DCQD in all the treatment groups (Fig. 1).

DCQD downregulated the pro-inflammatory mediators and upregulated the anti-inflammatory mediators in kidney tissues

The levels of pro-inflammatory mediators (IL-6 and TNF-α) and anti-inflammatory mediators (IL-4) in the MG were significantly increased compared to those in the SG ($p < 0.05$), but there was no change in IL-10. Compared to the MG, the pro-inflammatory mediators in all the treatment groups were downregulated ($p < 0.05$), while the anti-inflammatory mediators in all the treatment groups were upregulated obviously ($p < 0.05$). The lowest level of pro-inflammatory mediators and the highest level of anti-inflammatory mediators were both in the HDG (Fig. 2A, B).

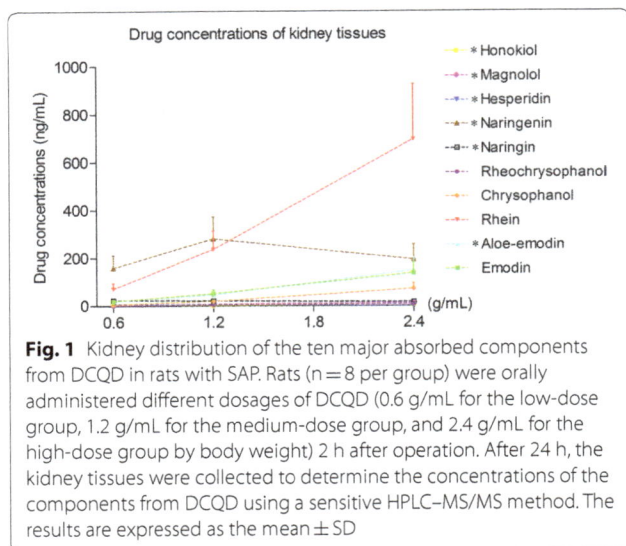

Fig. 1 Kidney distribution of the ten major absorbed components from DCQD in rats with SAP. Rats (n = 8 per group) were orally administered different dosages of DCQD (0.6 g/mL for the low-dose group, 1.2 g/mL for the medium-dose group, and 2.4 g/mL for the high-dose group by body weight) 2 h after operation. After 24 h, the kidney tissues were collected to determine the concentrations of the components from DCQD using a sensitive HPLC–MS/MS method. The results are expressed as the mean ± SD

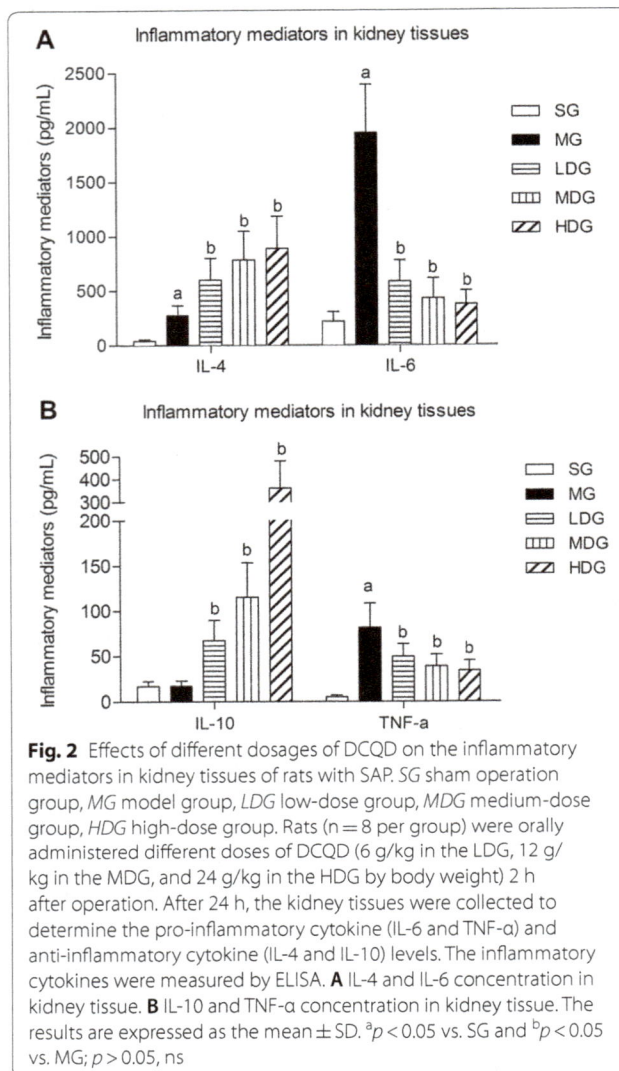

Fig. 2 Effects of different dosages of DCQD on the inflammatory mediators in kidney tissues of rats with SAP. SG sham operation group, MG model group, LDG low-dose group, MDG medium-dose group, HDG high-dose group. Rats (n = 8 per group) were orally administered different doses of DCQD (6 g/kg in the LDG, 12 g/kg in the MDG, and 24 g/kg in the HDG by body weight) 2 h after operation. After 24 h, the kidney tissues were collected to determine the pro-inflammatory cytokine (IL-6 and TNF-α) and anti-inflammatory cytokine (IL-4 and IL-10) levels. The inflammatory cytokines were measured by ELISA. **A** IL-4 and IL-6 concentration in kidney tissue. **B** IL-10 and TNF-α concentration in kidney tissue. The results are expressed as the mean ± SD. $^a p < 0.05$ vs. SG and $^b p < 0.05$ vs. MG; $p > 0.05$, ns

DCQD alleviated pathological damage in the kidney and pancreas

The pancreas of the SG rats showed slight edema, with no obvious inflammatory cell infiltration, haemorrhage or necrosis. Similar manifestations were shown in the kidneys of rats in the SG. In contrast, the pancreas in the MG displayed conspicuous interstitial edema, inflammatory cell infiltration, some spots of haemorrhage and signs of necrosis. The kidneys in the MG showed marked edema with inflammatory cell infiltration and haemorrhage. After giving DCQD, both the pancreas and kidneys in all the treatment groups had a significant reduction in interstitial edema, inflammatory cell infiltration, haemorrhage and necrosis, and the changes in the HDG were the most significant. DCQD reduced the pathological scores in the pancreas and kidneys of rats with SAP, especially in the HDG (Fig. 3A–C).

DCQD decreased the Scr levels

Based on the highest kidney distribution of DCQD and lowest kidney pathological scores in the HDG, we only detected Scr and BUN in the SG, MG and HDG. Compared with the SG, the Scr and BUN in the MG were obviously increased ($p < 0.05$). The level of Scr in the HDG was significantly lower than that in the MG ($p < 0.05$), without a difference in BUN (Fig. 4).

Discussion

The results demonstrated that major components of DCQD were detected in the kidneys and had protective effects of regulating the inflammatory response. The distributions of major components in kidneys with SAP

were similar to those in the serum, pancreas, intestine or liver [20, 22, 25]. However, there were still some differences in the kidney. The component with the highest concentration in the kidney of rats in HDG was rhein, which might be the most bioactive DCQD ingredient, even though it was less abundant than many compounds in DCQD [26], similar to that of plasma and the pancreas, emodin in lung and naringenin in intestine and liver [20, 22]. This finding once again confirms the hypothesis of the tissue pharmacology of the herbs recipe [27] and may be explained by the blood–tissue barriers in different tissues [20]. Our results showed that rhein and naringenin were relatively higher than the other compounds of DCQD in all the treatment groups. However, naringenin was the highest component in the LDG and MDG while rhein was the highest in the HDG. This phenomenon may result from the drug–drug interactions during

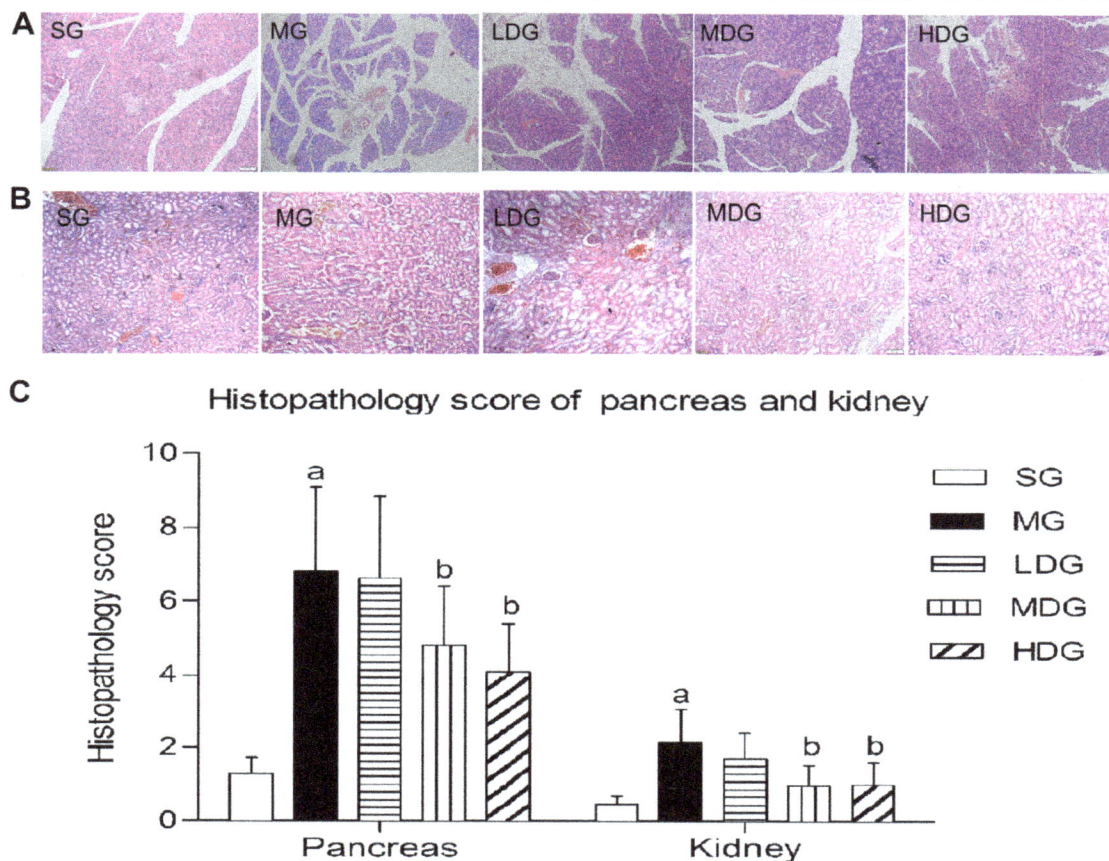

Fig. 3 DCQD alleviates pancreas and kidney pathological damages in rats with SAP. *SG* sham operation group, *MG* model group, *LDG* low-dose group, *MDG* medium-dose group, *HDG* high-dose group. Rats (n = 8 per group) were orally administered different doses of DCQD (6 g/kg in the LDG, 12 g/kg in the MDG, and 24 g/kg in the HDG by body weight) 2 h after operation. At 24 h after operation, the kidney samples were collected for pathological analysis and stained with hematoxylin and eosin (HE). **A** Pathological picture of pancreas (HE, ×200). **B** Pathological picture of kidney (HE, ×100). **C** Pathological scores of the pancreas and kidney. The results are expressed as the mean ± SD. $^{a}p < 0.05$ vs. SG and $^{b}p < 0.05$ vs. MG; $p > 0.05$, ns

absorption, distribution, metabolism, and excretion processes or from the procedure of decoction [28]. Zhang et al. [29] verified that Lidanpaidu prescription-a transformation of DCQD-could prevent LPS-induced AKI by restricting the NF-kB signaling pathway. Li et al. [30] proved that Huang-Lian-Jie-Du-decoction and its components had an effect on mitigating LPS-induced AKI by improving the disorder of oxidative stress and energy metabolism, preventing NF-κB and MAPK and activating the Akt/HO-1 pathway in mice. Cell research further confirmed that some single herbs were latently effective for AKI due to their ability to stop the activation of NGAL, HMGB1 and KIM-1 in an invitro AKI-mimicked condition [31]. Herein, Chinese herbs are a potentially effective treatment for AKI and are worth exploration.

AP begins with local inflammation in the pancreas, which often leads to SIRS and multiple organ failure, with high mortality [32]. The inflammatory cytokine response is initiated early and is sustained for several days in the systemic circulation during SAP [33]. The response is blamed for the systemic manifestations of AP and is related to distant organ dysfunction [34]. IL-6 is most credible in the appraisal of the severity of AP for predicting the risk for the occurrence of complications at early stages [35]. TNF-α can exert systemic effects on endothelial cells invivo that cause dystrophic changes to the tubular epithelial cells and cause damage to the peritubular and glomerular capillaries in the kidneys [36]. In contrast, the anti-inflammatory cytokines IL-4 and IL-10 act as potent suppressants to prevent the extracellular killing function of macrophages once activated [37]. IL-10 is likely a primary factor in the negative feedback system that hinders the production of pro-inflammatory cytokines and colony-stimulating factors in various cells

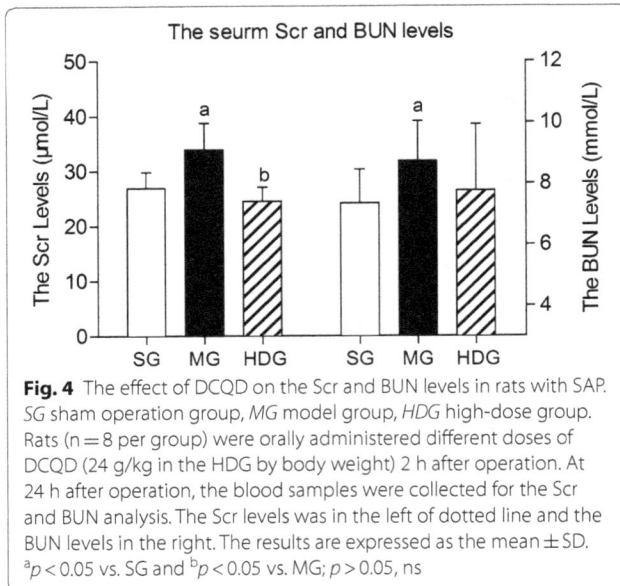

Fig. 4 The effect of DCQD on the Scr and BUN levels in rats with SAP. *SG* sham operation group, *MG* model group, *HDG* high-dose group. Rats (n = 8 per group) were orally administered different doses of DCQD (24 g/kg in the HDG by body weight) 2 h after operation. At 24 h after operation, the blood samples were collected for the Scr and BUN analysis. The Scr levels was in the left of dotted line and the BUN levels in the right. The results are expressed as the mean ± SD. [a]$p < 0.05$ vs. SG and [b]$p < 0.05$ vs. MG; $p > 0.05$, ns

[38]. Kusske et al. [39] found that IL-10 could inhibit the activation of macrophages and could alleviate inflammation by reducing the release of inflammatory cytokines and could eventually lower the death rate of SAP in mice.

In our study, we detected the levels of TNF-α, IL-4, IL-6, and IL-10 in kidney tissue to predict the inflammatory response after SAP modelling. The results showed that IL-6 was the highest mediators, and TNF-α was the lowest mediator, among those detected. Our finding echoed that IL-6 was the only significant parameter to predict a complicated AP [35]. After giving DCQD, the levels of pro-inflammatory mediators (TNF-α and IL-6) decreased and the anti-inflammatory mediators (IL-4 and IL-10) increased along with the dose. Moreover, the pathological scores of the kidneys and pancreas showed the same tendency. The highest dose of DCQD had the maximal effects in downregulating the pro-inflammatory mediators, upregulating anti-inflammatory mediators in the kidney and ameliorating pathological damage. The data demonstrated the regulatory effects of DCQD in the inflammatory response to ameliorate AKI with SAP and to eventually attenuate the severity of SAP. Our previous studies revealed a similar effect of DCQD on damage to the lungs, pancreas, intestine and liver [20–22]. Zhao et al. [21] reported that treatment with DCQD decreased the pathological scores of the lungs; increased the level of IL-10 mRNA and decreased the level of IL-6 mRNA in rats with SAP. Huang et al. [40] found that revised DCQD might reduce lung injury via inhibiting the induction of IL-6 and increasing the expression of HSP70 as well as

the concentration of IL-10. With the experimental progress of Chinese herbs, we found that it is essential to study DCQD on the molecular level [22]. As discussed above, rhein and naringenin were relatively higher and might be potentially effective components of DCQD for SAP-induced AKI. Rhein, one major component of Dahuang, bore comparison to the accredited painkiller ibuprofen with its anti-inflammatory effects in adjuvant-induced inflammation by ameliorating oxidative stress significantly [41]. Rhein induces a necrosis-apoptosis switch of damaged pancreatic acinar cells to ameliorate AP in a dose-dependent manner [42] and to prevent an endotoxin-induced AKI by inhibiting NF-κB activities [43]. The naringenin might be another effective component and was reported to alleviate acute inflammation by adjusting the degradation by intracellular cytokines [44] and to reduce kidney damage in diabetic nephropathy through Let-7a/transforming growth factor-β1 receptor (TGFBR1) signalling [45]. Li et al. concluded that emodin had an effect on the lipopolysaccharide-induced AKI by inhibiting the toll-like receptor 2 (TLR2) signalling pathway [46]. Future studies should focus on the relationship between the quantified molecules of DCQD and their pharmacological effects considering their target tissues in SAP.

In 1998, Zhao et al. [47] came to the conclusion that the effects of DCQD on the reduction of acute phase protein levels were dose-dependent in multiple organ disfunction syndrome. Our previous study proved that the concentrations of the ten major components of DCQD increased dose-dependently in the intestine after oral administration [20]. As shown above, the effects of DCQD in the treatment of the AKI with SAP was primarily dose-dependent by regulating the inflammatory response. Therefore, a dose–response for DCQD may exist for the treatment of SAP and needs further study. The HDG accounted for the highest kidney distribution of DCQD and the lowest kidney pathological scores. Therefore, we only detected the levels of Scr and BUN in the SG, MG and HDG. Compared with the MG, the level of Scr in the HDG decreased significantly, with no differences in the BUN. Argyri et al. discovered that BUN and Scr were increased 2–3 days after AKI occurred, when 50% of the renal function was lost, and early diagnosis and intervention reduced mortality [48]. However, we collected the samples nearly one day after successful modelling. This time period might be too short to display significant changes in BUN, which could be the reason for the change in BUN after giving DCQD. Hence, it is necessary to further study and apply more sensitive biomarkers for research and clinical interpretation.

Conclusions

In conclusion, most of the major components of DCQD were absorbed into the kidney of rats with SAP and their concentrations increased dose-dependently. Above all, DCQD ameliorated AKI in rats with SAP by regulating the inflammatory response, and it might be closely related to the intake dose.

Abbreviations

DCQD: Da-Cheng-Qi-decoction; AP: acute pancreatitis; SAP: severe acute pancreatitis; SIRS: systemic inflammatory response syndrome; AKI: acute kidney injury; Scr: serum creatinine; BUN: blood urea nitrogen; HPLC–MS/MS: high-performance liquid chromatography–tandem mass spectrometry; TNF-α: tumor necrosis factor α; IL-4: interleukin-4; IL-6: interleukin-6; IL-10: interleukin-10; RRT: renal replacement therapy.

Authors' contributions

LY, LZ and Y-mZ contribute equally to this work. W-fT designed the research. LY, LZ, HC, HK, JL and YM performed this study. Y-mZ, X-lZ, and M-hW analyzed the data. LY and LZ wrote the paper. W-fT was responsible for the critical revision of the paper. All authors read and approved the final manuscript.

Acknowledgements

Not applicable.

Competing interests

The authors declare that they have no competing interests.

Consent for publication

All authors have provided consent for publication in the journal of Chinese Medicine.

Funding

This work was supported by the National Natural Science Foundation of China, Nos. 81374042 and 81573857.

References

1. Forsmark CE, Vege SS, Wilcox CM. Acute pancreatitis. N Engl J Med. 2016;375(20):1972–81. https://doi.org/10.1056/NEJMra1505202.
2. Frossard JL, Steer ML, Pastor CM. Acute pancreatitis. Lancet. 2008;371(9607):143–52. https://doi.org/10.1016/S0140-6736(08)60107-5.
3. Buter A, Imrie CW, Carter CR, Evans S, McKay CJ. Dynamic nature of early organ dysfunction determines outcome in acute pancreatitis. Br J Surg. 2002;89(3):298–302. https://doi.org/10.1046/j.0007-1323.2001.02025.x.
4. Bellomo R, Kellum JA, Ronco C. Acute kidney injury. Lancet. 2012;380(9843):756–66. https://doi.org/10.1016/S0140-6736(11)61454-2.
5. Zhou J, Li Y, Tang Y, et al. Effect of acute kidney injury on mortality and hospital stay in patient with severe acute pancreatitis. Nephrology (Carlton). 2015;20(7):485–91. https://doi.org/10.1111/nep.12439.
6. Kumar R, Pahwa N, Jain N. Acute kidney injury in severe acute pancreatitis: an experience from a tertiary care center. Saudi J Kidney Dis Transpl. 2015;26(1): 56–60. http://www.sjkdt.org/text.asp?2015/26/1/56/148734
7. Bellomo R, Ronco C, Kellum JA, Mehta RL, Palevsky P. Acute renal failure—definition, outcome measures, animal models, fluid therapy and information technology needs: the Second International Consensus Conference of the Acute Dialysis Quality Initiative (ADQI) Group. Crit Care. 2004;8(4):R204–12. https://doi.org/10.1186/cc2872.
8. Herrera GME, Seller PG, de La Rubia De Gracia C, Chaparro SMJ, Nacle LB. Acute renal failure profile and prognostic value in severe acute pancreatitis. Med Clin (Barc). 2000;115(19):721–5. https://doi.org/10.1016/S0025-7753(00)71674-5.
9. Pupelis G. Renal failure in acute pancreatitis. Timing of dialysis and surgery. Przegl Lek. 2000;57(Suppl 5):29–31.
10. Li H, Qian Z, Liu Z, Liu X, Han X, Kang H. Risk factors and outcome of acute renal failure in patients with severe acute pancreatitis. J Crit Care. 2010;25(2):225–9. https://doi.org/10.1016/j.jcrc.2009.07.009.
11. Zhang XP, Wang L, Zhou YF. The pathogenic mechanism of severe acute pancreatitis complicated with renal injury: a review of current knowledge. Dig Dis Sci. 2008;53(2):297–306. https://doi.org/10.1007/s10620-007-9866-5.
12. Petejova N, Martinek A. Acute kidney injury following acute pancreatitis: a review. Biomed Pap Med Fac Univ Palacky Olomouc Czech Repub. 2013;157(2):105–13. https://doi.org/10.5507/bp.2013.048.
13. Banks PA, Freeman ML. Practice guidelines in acute pancreatitis. Am J Gastroenterol. 2006;101(10):2379–400. https://doi.org/10.1111/j.1572-0241.2006.00856.x.
14. IAP/APA. Evidence-based guidelines for the management of acute pancreatitis. Pancreatology. 2013;13(42):e1–15. https://doi.org/10.1016/j.pan.2013.07.063.
15. Yaklin KM. Acute kidney injury: an overview of pathophysiology and treatments. Nephrol Nurs J. 2011;38(1):13–8 **(quiz 19)**.
16. Ronco C, Ricci Z, De Backer D, et al. Renal replacement therapy in acute kidney injury: controversy and consensus. Crit Care. 2015;19:146. https://doi.org/10.1186/s13054-015-0850-8.
17. Uchino S. What is 'BEST' RRT practice. Contrib Nephrol. 2010;165:244–50. https://doi.org/10.1159/000313764.
18. Xia Q, Huang ZW, Jiang JM, Cheng GY, Yang XL, Tang WF. Yi-Huo-Qing-Xia method as the main therapy in integrated traditional Chinese and western medicine on severe acute pancreatitis: a report of 1161 cases. Chin J TCM WM Crit Care. 2006;13(3):131–4.
19. Zhao J, Zhong C, He Z, Chen G, Tang W. Effect of da-cheng-qi decoction on pancreatitis-associated intestinal dysmotility in patients and in rat models. Evid Based Complement Alternat Med. 2015;2015:895717. https://doi.org/10.1155/2015/895717.
20. Zhao X, Zhang Y, Li J, et al. Tissue pharmacology of Da-Cheng-Qi decoction in experimental acute pancreatitis in rats. Evid Based Complement Alternat Med. 2015;2015:283175. https://doi.org/10.1155/2015/283175.
21. Zhao J, Chen J, Tang W, Wan L, Xiong W, Zhou L. Effect of Da-Cheng-Qi decoction on pancreatitis-associated lung injury in patients and anti-inflammatory responses in rat models. Pharm Biol. 2011;49(10):1058–64. https://doi.org/10.3109/13880209.2011.565059.
22. Zhang YM, Ren HY, Zhao XL, et al. Pharmacokinetics and pharmacodynamics of Da-Cheng-Qi decoction in the liver of rats with severe acute pancreatitis. World J Gastroenterol. 2017;23(8):1367–74. https://doi.org/10.3748/wjg.v23.i8.1367.
23. Gibson-Corley KN, Olivier AK, Meyerholz DK. Principles for valid histopathologic scoring in research. Vet Pathol. 2013;50(6):1007–15. https://doi.org/10.1177/0300985813485099.
24. Tang W, Wan M, Zhu Z, Chen G, Huang X. Simultaneous determination of eight major bioactive compounds in Dachengqi Tang (DT) by high-performance liquid chromatography. Chin Med. 2008;3:5. https://doi.org/10.1186/1749-8546-3-5.
25. Gong HL, Tang WF, Yu Q, et al. Effect of severe acute pancreatitis on pharmacokinetics of Da-Cheng-Qi Decoction components. World J Gastroenterol. 2009;15(47):5992–9. https://doi.org/10.3748/wjg.15.5992.
26. Zhao J, Tang W, Wang J, Xiang J, Gong H, Chen G. Pharmacokinetic and pharmacodynamic studies of four major phytochemical components of Da-Cheng-Qi decoction to treat acute pancreatitis. J Pharmacol Sci. 2013;122(2):118–27. https://doi.org/10.1254/jphs.13037FP.
27. Tang WF, Wan MH, Huang X. Tissue pharmacology of recipe-A new hypothesis. Chin Tradit Herbal Drugs. 2005;36(1):1–3.
28. Xu F, Liu Y, Dong H, Song R, Zhang Z. Pharmacokinetic comparison in rats of six bioactive compounds between Da-Cheng-Qi decoction and its parent herbal medicines. Nat Prod Commun. 2010;5(5):795–800.

29. Zhang F, Lu S, Jin S, et al. Lidanpaidu prescription alleviates lipopol-ysaccharide-induced acute kidney injury by suppressing the NF-κB signaling pathway. Biomed Pharmacother. 2018;99:245–52. https://doi.org/10.1016/j.biopha.2018.01.059.

30. Li P, Liao ST, Wang JS, et al. Protection by Huang-Lian-Jie-Du decoction and its constituent herbs of lipopolysaccharide-induced acute kidney injury. FEBS Open Biol. 2017;7(2):221–36. https://doi.org/10.1002/2211-5463.12178.

31. Oh SM, Park G, Lee SH, Seo CS, Shin HK, Oh DS. Assessing the recovery from prerenal and renal acute kidney injury after treatment with single herbal medicine via activity of the biomarkers HMGB1, NGAL and KIM-1 in kidney proximal tubular cells treated by cisplatin with different doses and exposure times. BMC Complement Altern Med. 2017;17(1):544. https://doi.org/10.1186/s12906-017-2055-y.

32. Escobar J, Pereda J, Arduini A, et al. Role of redox signaling, protein phosphatases and histone acetylation in the inflammatory cascade in acute pancreatitis. Therapeutic implications. Inflamm Allergy Drug Targets. 2010;9(2):97–108. https://doi.org/10.2174/187152810791292773.

33. Brivet FG, Emilie D, Galanaud P. Pro- and anti-inflammatory cytokines during acute severe pancreatitis: an early and sustained response, although unpredictable of death. Parisian Study Group on Acute Pancreatitis. Crit Care Med. 1999;27(4):749–55.

34. Norman J. The role of cytokines in the pathogenesis of acute pancreatitis. Am J Surg. 1998;175(1):76–83. https://doi.org/10.1016/S0002-9610(97)00240-7.

35. Stimac D, Fisić E, Milić S, Bilić-Zulle L, Perić R. Prognostic values of IL-6, IL-8, and IL-10 in acute pancreatitis. J Clin Gastroenterol. 2006;40(3):209–12.

36. IuV P, Iul K, IuA B. The action of tumor necrosis factor on the microvascular endothelium and its role in the morphological changes in the internal organs. Biull Eksp Biol Med. 1991;111(3):294–7.

37. Oswald IP, Gazzinelli RT, Sher A, James SL. IL-10 synergizes with IL-4 and transforming growth factor-beta to inhibit macrophage cytotoxic activity. J Immunol. 1992;148(11):3578–82.

38. Geissler K. Current status of clinical development of interleukin-10. Curr Opin Hematol. 1996;3(3):203–8.

39. Kusske AM, Rongione AJ, Ashley SW, McFadden DW, Reber HA. Interleukin-10 prevents death in lethal necrotizng pancreatitis in mice. Surgery. 1996;120(2):284–8 **(discussion 289)**.

40. Huang L, Wang MH, Cheng ZY, et al. Effects of Chai-Qin-Cheng-Qi decoction () on acute pancreatitis-associated ung injury in mice with acute necrotizing pancreatitis. Chin J Integr Med. 2012. https://doi.org/10.1007/s11655-012-1207-7.

41. Cong XD, Ding MJ, Dai DZ, Wu Y, Zhang Y, Dai Y. ER stress, p66shc, and p-Akt/Akt mediate adjuvant-induced inflammation, which is blunted by argirein, a supermolecule and rhein in rats. Inflammation. 2012;35(3):1031–40. https://doi.org/10.1007/s10753-011-9407-4.

42. Zhao X, Li J, Zhu S, et al. Rhein induces a necrosis-apoptosis switch in pancreatic acinar cells. Evid Based Complement Alternat Med. 2014;2014:404853. https://doi.org/10.1155/2014/404853.

43. Yu C, Qi D, Sun JF, Li P, Fan HY. Rhein prevents endotoxin-induced acute kidney injury by inhibiting NF-κB activities. Sci Rep. 2015;5:11822. https://doi.org/10.1038/srep11822.

44. Jin L, Zeng W, Zhang F, Zhang C, Liang W. Naringenin ameliorates acute inflammation by regulating intracellular cytokine degradation. J Immunol. 2017;199(10):3466–77. https://doi.org/10.4049/jimmunol.1602016.

45. Yan N, Wen L, Peng R, et al. Naringenin ameliorated kidney injury through Let-7a/TGFBR1 signaling in diabetic nephropathy. J Diab Res. 2016;2016:8738760. https://doi.org/10.1155/2016/8738760.

46. Li Y, Xiong W, Yang J, et al. Attenuation of inflammation by emodin in lipopolysaccharide-induced acute kidney injury via inhibition of toll-like receptor 2 signal pathway. Iran J Kidney Dis. 2015;9(3):202–8.

47. Zhao Q, Cui N, Li J. Clinical and experimental study of effect on acute phase protein level of multiple organ dysfunction syndrome treated with dachengqi decoction. Zhongguo Zhong Xi Yi Jie He Za Zhi. 1998;18(8):453–6.

48. Argyri I, Xanthos T, Varsami M, et al. The role of novel biomarkers in early diagnosis and prognosis of acute kidney injury in newborns. Am J Perinatol. 2013;30(5):347–52. https://doi.org/10.1055/s-0032-1326985.

16

Ginsenoside G-Rh2 synergizes with SMI-4a in anti-melanoma activity through autophagic cell death

Da-lun Lv[1], Lei Chen[1], Wei Ding[1], Wei Zhang[1], He–li Wang[1], Shuai Wang[1] and Wen-bei Liu[2]* ⓘ

Abstract

Background: Melanoma is a leading cause of cancer death worldwide, and SMI-4a and G-Rh2 exert anti-tumor activity in multiple cancer. However, SMI-4a as well as a synergistic relationship between SMI-4a and G-Rh2 in anti-melanoma capacity are still unknown. Therefore, we investigated the effects of SMI-4a and combined SMI-4a with G-Rh2 on the viability, apoptosis and autophagy of melanoma, and to preliminarily explore the underlying mechanism of SMI-4a and combined SMI-4a with G-Rh2 in inhibiting tumor growth.

Methods: Cell viability was examined with cell counting Kit 8 assay and colony formation assay; Apoptosis was evaluated by flow cytometry and Caspase 3/7 activity assay; Western blotting was used to test proteins related to autophagy and the AKT/mammalian target of rapamycin (mTOR) signaling pathway; Tumor xenograft model in BALB/c nude mice was performed to evaluate the effects of SMI-4a and combined SMI-4a with G-Rh2 in anti-melanoma in vivo.

Results: SMI-4a, a pharmacological inhibitor of PIM-1, could decrease cell viability, induce apoptosis, and promote Caspase 3/7 activity in both A375 and G361 melanoma cells, and SMI-4a inhibited tumor growth by inducing autophagy via down-regulating AKT/mTOR axis in melanoma cells. Furthermore, G-Rh2 amplified the anti-tumor activity of SMI-4a in melanoma cells via strengthening autophagy.

Conclusions: Our results suggested that SMI-4a could enhance autophagy-inducing apoptosis by inhibiting AKT/mTOR signaling pathway in melanoma cells, and G-Rh2 could enhance the effects of SMI-4a against melanoma cancer via amplifying autophagy induction. This study demonstrates that combined SMI-4a and G-Rh2 might be a novel alternative strategy for melanoma treatment.

Keywords: SMI-4a, G-Rh$_2$, Apoptosis, Autophagy, Melanoma

Background

Melanoma is the highly aggressive skin cancer with mounting incidence over the past 30 years, which is associated with early metastasis, late diagnosis, and tolerance to chemotherapy in advanced stages [1]. The emergence of some novel therapies against melanoma such as genetically targeted therapies (e.g., BRAF inhibitors) and immunotherapies (e.g., PD-1/PD-L1 and CTLA-4 antibodies) has undoubtedly improved melanoma treatment, but the overall prognosis of patients remains poor [2, 3]. Therefore, it is urgently required to discover novel targets and develop more effective and lasting therapeutic strategies for melanoma.

PIM-1, a member of a newly defined class of serine/threonine kinases, has been showed to be overexpressed in multiple cancers such as prostate cancer and gastric carcinoma, and possesses oncogenic functions [4]. The overexpression of PIM-1 contributes to carcinogenesis by inhibiting apoptosis and promoting cell proliferation. Therefore, inhibition of PIM-1 activity is an emerging approach for cancer therapy. SMI-4a is a selective

*Correspondence: lwb0776@163.com
[2] Dermatological Department, First Affiliated Hospital of Wannan Medical College, Jinghu District, Wuhu 241000, Anhui, China

inhibitor of PIM-1 protein and exerts anti-tumor activity in chronic myeloid leukemia cells. In addition, PIM-1 could promote melanoma cells migration and invasion [5, 6]. However, whether SMI-4a is effective in melanoma has not been investigated.

Ginsenoside Rh2 (G-Rh2), a key bioactive component from roots of ginseng, have a wide variety of biological activities, such as anti-diabetes, anti-cancer and immune stimulation [7–9]. A recent report supported that G-Rh2 could inhibit the growth of human malignant melanoma cells by inducing apoptosis [10]. Also, G-Rh2 could inhibit hepatocellular carcinoma and cancer stem-like cells by increasing autophagy [11, 12]. Autophagy is a complex process that could degrade and recycle cellular compartments for survival during stress, whereas it may lead to cell death [13–15]. Moreover, autophagy could function as a tumor suppressor to suppress tumor growth by regulating cancer cell proliferation and apoptosis [16]. However, whether G-Rh2 could synergize with the other therapies (e.g., SMI-4a) to enhance their anti-melanoma function via inducing autophagy remains unknown.

Here, we demonstrated that SMI-4a had the anti-melanoma activity, and illustrated its potential mechanisms of activity, involving decreasing viability, enhancing apoptosis, strengthening Caspase 3/7 activity. In addition, SMI-4a inhibited the AKT/mTOR signaling axis to promote the apoptosis and autophagy. We further showed that G-Rh2 could synergize with SMI-4a in anti-melanoma capacity, possibly through enhancing autophagy both in vitro and in vivo.

Methods

The Minimum Standards of Reporting Checklist contains details of the experimental design, and statistics, and resources used in this study (Additional file 1).

Cell lines

Two human melanoma cell lines A375 and G361 were obtained from Cell Bank of Chinese Academy of Sciences (Shanghai, China), and propagated in DMEM supplemented with 10% heat-inactivated FBS, 100 units/ml penicillin and 0.1 mg/ml streptomycin. Both the cell lines were cultured 37 °C in a humidified atmosphere of 5% CO_2.

Cell viability analyses

Cell viability was tested by Cell Counting Kit-8 (CCK-8) assay (Beyotime, Shanghai, China) according to the manufacturer's instructions. Cells (6×10^3 cells/well) were treated with different concentrations of SMI-4a (0.625–10 µM) (Sigma-Aldrich, Merck KGaA, Darmstadt, Germany) or combination of G-Rh2 (Weikeqi Bioscience, China) and SMI-4a in 96-well plates for 24, 48 and 72 h,

respectively. After culture, cell viability was evaluated by CCK-8 assay.

Colony formation assays

6×10^2 cells per well were propagated into six-well plates and cultured with SMI-4a (0.3 and 1 µM) for 10 days, and cells were fixed with 3.7% formaldehyde after washing with cold PBS twice. Then cells were stained with 0.5% crystal violet in methanol, and the number of colony in each well was assessed.

Flow cytometry

Apoptosis was determined using Annexin-V-FITC/PI apoptosis detection kit (KGI Biotech, Nanjing, China) according to the manufacturer's protocol. After SMI-4a treatment for 48 h, cells were collected, re-suspended in 500 µl of binding buffer and stained with Annexin-V-FITC and PI. The signal cells were evaluated by a FAC-Scan (FACSCalibur, BD Biosciences, California, USA). For autophagic body production test, cells were incubated with SMI-4a (0.3, 1 and 3 µM). Cells were collected after treatment (48 h) and stained with 1 µg/ml acridine orange at room temperature (RT) for 15 min. The cells were re-suspended and analyzed by flow cytometry.

Caspase 3/7 activity assay

Cspase-3/7 activities were tested using the Caspase-Glo® 3/7 Assay kit (Promega Corporation, Madison, WI, USA) according to the manufacturer's protocol. In brief, cells were cultured in 96-well plates (5×10^3 cells/well) and treated with 1 µM SMI-4a, 3 µM G-Rh2 or combination of SMI-4a and G-Rh2 (1 + 3 µM) for 48 h. The reagent were added to cells for 1 h. At last, luminescence were measured by a microplate reader at a wavelength of 499 nm.

Western blotting

Cells were homogenized in RIPA lysis Buffer (CST, Danvers, MA, USA) on ice. The lysates were centrifuged at $14,000 \times g$ at 4 °C for 15 min. The concentration of protein was tested with BCA protein assay kit (EMD Millipore, Billerica, MA, USA). After mixing with 2× Laemmli buffer and boiled for 10 min, 50 µg protein was subjected to SDS polyacrylamide gel electrophoresis, and electro-transferred onto PVDF membranes. The signals were visualized by fluorography using RapidStep™ ECL Reagent (EMD Millipore) according to the manufacturer's directions. Antibodies recognizing GAPDH, LC3-II, Atg5, Beclin-1, AKT, p-AKT, mTOR, and p-mTOR were obtained from Cell Signalling Technology (Danvers, MA, USA).

Tumor xenograft

Female nude BALB/c mice (6-week-old) were obtained from Vital River Laboratory (Beijing, China). 3×10^6 A375 cells were injected subcutaneously into fossa axillaries of nude mice. Once the average tumor volume reached up to 200 mm³, the mice were randomized into four groups (n = 10) by random lottery: a control group (vehicle), a SMI-4a-treated group (15 mg/kg), an G-Rh2-treated group (30 mg/kg), and SMI-4a + G-Rh2-treated group (15 + 30 mg/kg). The tumor-bearing mice were injected intratumorally with SMI-4a, G-Rh2, or combination of SMI-4a and G-Rh2 every 2 days, and the tumor size was tested every 3 days by a caliper, and tumor volume was calculated using this formula: volume = (length × width²) × 1/2. We measured the tumor size and weighted the tumor samples at sacrifice. All animal protocols were performed in accordance with *the Guidelines for the care and Use of Laboratory Animals* published by the National Institutes of Health (NIH).

Statistical analysis

Data were plotted as the mean ± S.E.M. of at least triplicate independent samples. Differences between two groups or multiple groups were analyzed by the Student's t test or one-way ANOVA (Graphpad Prism 5). The difference was considered statistically significant when $p < 0.05$.

Results

SMI-4a suppressed cell growth in melanoma cells

To investigate the effect of SMI-4a on the inhibition of human melanoma cell growth, A375 and G361 cells were cultured with various concentrations of SMI-4a for 24, 48 and 72 h, respectively. As shown in Fig. 1a, SMI-4a markedly decreased cell viability of both A375 and G361 cells in a dose- and time-dependent fashion. Similarly, SMI-4a could also remarkably inhibit cell colony formation capacities of both A375 and G361 cells in a dose-dependent fashion ($p < 0.001$, Fig. 1b). Together, these data showed that SMI-4a could retard melanoma cell growth in vitro.

SMI-4a induced melanoma cells apoptosis

Next, we assessed whether SMI-4a induces cell apoptosis. The flow cytometry analysis suggested that SMI-4a could dramatically promote cell apoptosis in treated A375 and G361 cells compared with the control (Fig. 2a). To further confirm the pro-apoptotic effects of SIM-4a, we also examined the activity of caspase 3/7. As shown in Fig. 2b, SMI-4a significantly enhanced the activity of

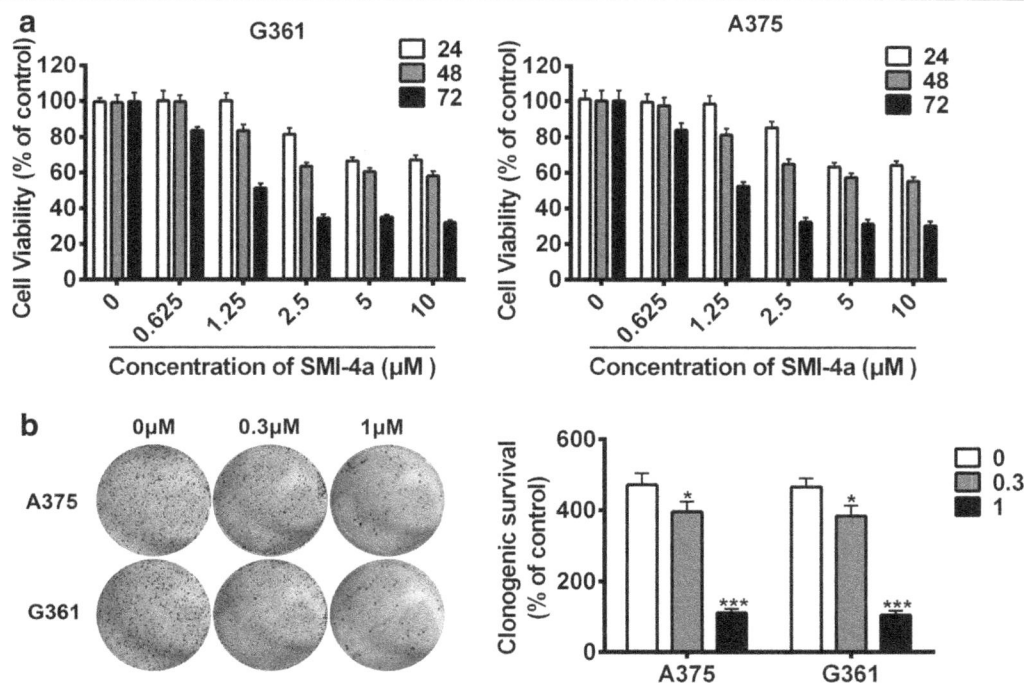

Fig. 1 SMI-4a inhibited melanoma cell growth. **a** Cells were incubated with various dose of SMI-4a (0.625–10 μM) for 24, 48 and 72 h, respectively, and and Cells viability was tested by CCK8 assay. The results were normalized to DMSO treated cells. **b** A375 and G361 cells were treated with SMI-4a (1 and 0.3 μM) for 10 days. Colonies were fixed, stained with crystal violet and quantified. The results are expressed as the mean ± SEM. *$p < 0.05$ and ***$p < 0.001$

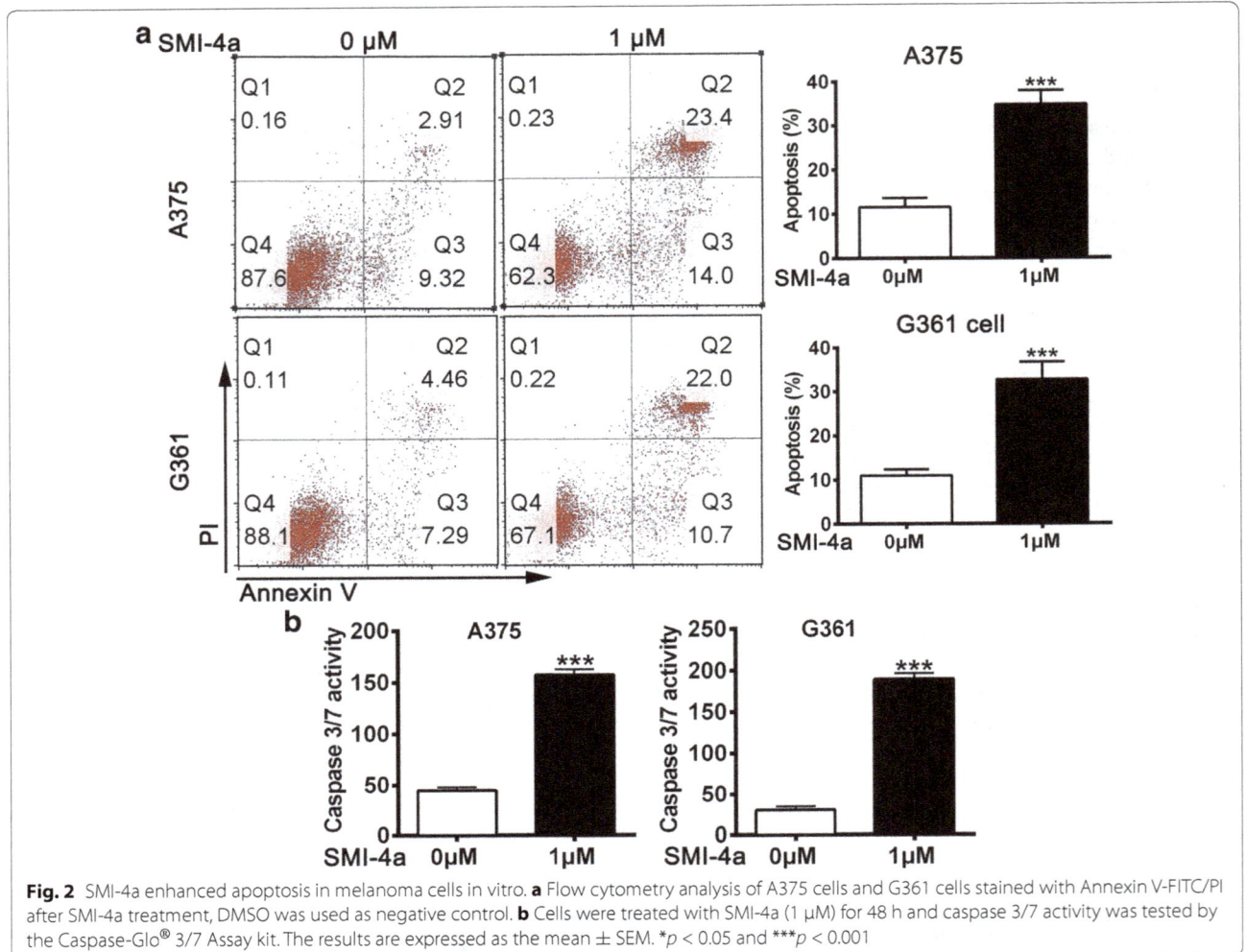

Fig. 2 SMI-4a enhanced apoptosis in melanoma cells in vitro. **a** Flow cytometry analysis of A375 cells and G361 cells stained with Annexin V-FITC/PI after SMI-4a treatment, DMSO was used as negative control. **b** Cells were treated with SMI-4a (1 μM) for 48 h and caspase 3/7 activity was tested by the Caspase-Glo® 3/7 Assay kit. The results are expressed as the mean ± SEM. *$p < 0.05$ and ***$p < 0.001$

caspase-3/7 in both A375 and G361 cells. These data indicate that SMI-4a could promote apoptosis of melanoma cells in vitro.

SMI-4a trigger autophagy through Akt/mTOR signaling pathway

To examine whether SMI-4a could induce autophagy to effect cell growth, we tested autophagic body production by acridine orange (AO) staining. Intriguingly, SMI-4a markedly promoted autophagic body formation in a dose-dependent fashion compared with the control group in melanoma cells (Fig. 3a). In addition, Western blotting assay also indicated that SMI-4a enhanced the protein levels of Atg5, LC3-II and Beclin1 in a dose-dependent manner in melanoma cells (Fig. 3b), indicating that SMI-4a could induce autophagy in melanoma cells.

Next, To investigate whether the potential underlying molecular mechanisms of SMI-4a-induced autophagy is related to AKT/mTOR pathway signaling, the expressions

of proteins associated with AKT/mTOR signaling were tested by western blot analysis. As shown in Fig. 3c, SMI-4a treatment decreased the phosphorylation level of Akt and mTOR without influencing the total protein amount in both A375 and G361 cells. Collectively, these data suggest that SMI-4a induces autophagy by inhibiting AKT/mTOR signaling, and consequently retards melanoma cells growth.

G-Rh2 sensitized SMI-4a-induced cell death via enhancing autophagy in vitro

Our results indicated that SMI-4a retarded cell growth by inducing autophagy, whereas G-Rh2 could also enhance autophagic flux. Therefore, we examined whether G-Rh2 could sensitize melanoma cells to SMI-4a-induced cell death. As shown in Fig. 4a, combination treatment with Rh2 and SMI-4a increased LC3-II protein expression, compared with Rh2 or SMI-4a treatment alone, suggesting that G-Rh2 may amplify the induction of autophagy

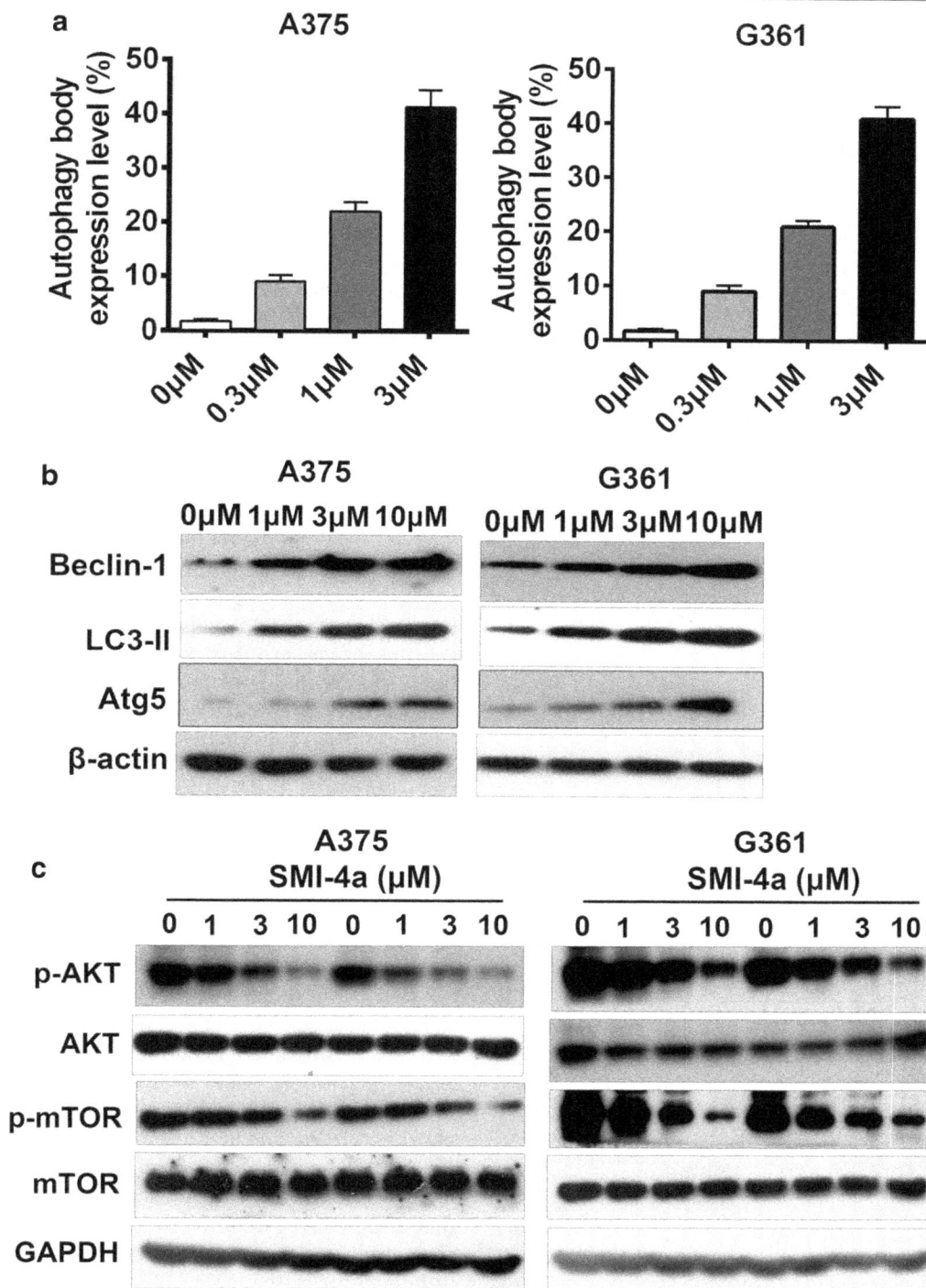

Fig. 3 SMI-4a induced autophagy via inhibiting AKT/mTOR signaling. **a** The autophagic body formation was tested by flow cytometry analysis through staining with acridine orange, after SMI-4a treatment for 48 h. **b** Cells were treated with various doses of SMI-4a for 24 h. The protein expression of Atg5, Beclin1 and LC3-II were evaluated by a western blotting assay. **c** The levels of total AKT (AKT), phosphorylated AKT (P-AKT), Total mTOR (mTOR), phosphorylated mTOR (P-mTOR) were tested by western blot. The results are expressed as the mean ± SEM. *$p < 0.05$; **$p < 0.01$; ***$p < 0.001$

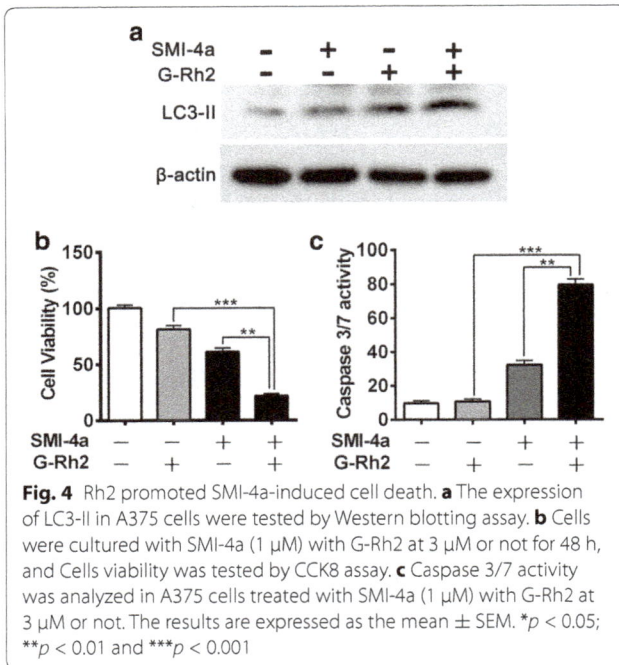

Fig. 4 Rh2 promoted SMI-4a-induced cell death. **a** The expression of LC3-II in A375 cells were tested by Western blotting assay. **b** Cells were cultured with SMI-4a (1 μM) with G-Rh2 at 3 μM or not for 48 h, and Cells viability was tested by CCK8 assay. **c** Caspase 3/7 activity was analyzed in A375 cells treated with SMI-4a (1 μM) with G-Rh2 at 3 μM or not. The results are expressed as the mean ± SEM. *$p < 0.05$; **$p < 0.01$ and ***$p < 0.001$

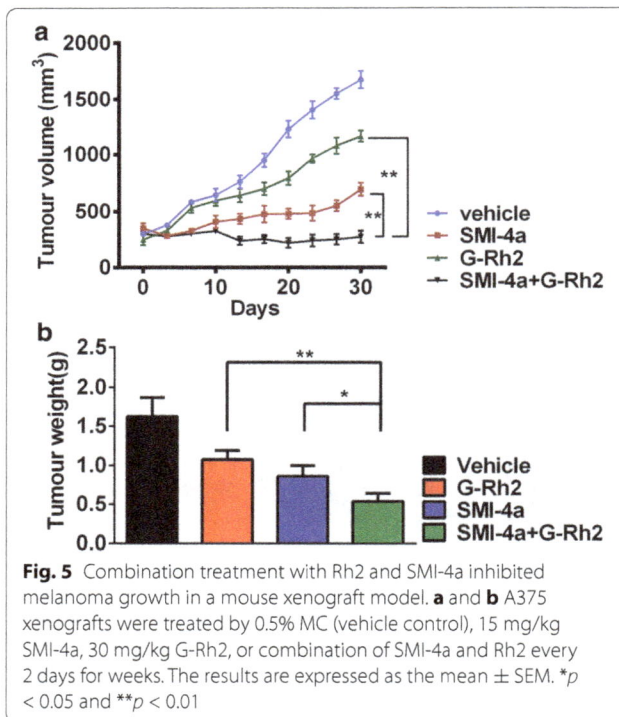

Fig. 5 Combination treatment with Rh2 and SMI-4a inhibited melanoma growth in a mouse xenograft model. **a** and **b** A375 xenografts were treated by 0.5% MC (vehicle control), 15 mg/kg SMI-4a, 30 mg/kg G-Rh2, or combination of SMI-4a and Rh2 every 2 days for weeks. The results are expressed as the mean ± SEM. *$p < 0.05$ and **$p < 0.01$

treatment versus SMI-4a alone, Fig. 4b). Furthermore, G-Rh2 also increased caspase3/7 activity by SMI-4a induction in melanoma cells ($p < 0.001$ for combination treatment versus SMI-4a alone, Fig. 4c). Together, these data suggest that Rh2 may contribute anti-tumor activity of SMI-4a in melanoma cells.

Combination of Rh2 and SMI-4a inhibited melanoma tumor growth in vivo

Subsequently, to investigate the synergistic anti-tumor capacity of Rh2 and SMI-4a in vivo, we established a tumor xenograft model by subcutaneously injecting A375 cells into athymic BALB/c nude mice. Rh2 or SMI-4a treatment alone had the capacity of inhibiting tumor growth at the doses used (Fig. 5a, b). However, combination treatment with Rh2 and SMI-4a markedly suppressed tumor growth of A375 xenografts, compared with Rh2 or SMI-4a treatment alone (Fig. 5a, b). These data demonstrated that treatment of combined Rh2 with SMI-4a significantly retards tumor growth in human melanoma tumor xenografts.

Discussion

Genetic changes of PIM-1 gene (e.g., amplifications, mutations, and deletions) are counted for about 8% of melanomas according to data of the Cancer Genome Atlas (TCGA). Silencing PIM-1 could inhibit the growth of melanoma cells [17]. In addition, SMI-4a could inhibit the growth of K562 and K562/G cells via enhancing the activity of GSK-3β [18, 19]. Similarly, in the current study we not only found that SMI-4a could dose- and time-dependently inhibit melanoma cell viability, but also dose-dependently decrease the number of colony formation in melanoma cells. Meanwhile, we also found that SMI-4a could promote cell death and increase caspase 3/7 activity in melanoma cells.

As is known to all, Akt/mTOR signaling pathway participates in multiple cellular functions, including cell survival, differentiation, and autophagy [20].The Akt/mTOR signaling pathway could negatively regulate autophagy through Akt phosphorylation, following by promoting phosphorylation and activation of mTOR [21, 22]. Notably, SMI-4a could down-regulate the phosphorylation level of Akt and mTOR. Accumulating evidence verifies that the selective inhibition of Akt/mTOR axis could suppress proliferation and invasion via enhancing autophagy in human melanoma cells [23]. Similarly, our data demonstrated that inhibition of Akt/mTOR pathway by SMI-4a markedly enhanced autophagic body formation and several key determinants of autophagy (e.g., LC3-II and Beclin-1) in a dose dependent fashion [24]. These results suggest that AKT/mTOR signaling pathway plays an important role in SMI-4a triggered autophagy in melanoma cells.

triggered by SMI-4a. When A375 cells were pre-cultured with G-Rh2 for 1 h following by a low concentration of SMI-4a of 24 h, cells underwent significant sensitization to SMI-4a-triggered cell death ($p < 0.001$ for combination

Autophagy play a complicated role in tumorigenesis, and is considered to appositive roles, pro-tumor and anti-tumor, depending on tumor cellular context. Cancer cells could utilize autophagy as a survival approach to supplement essential nutrient substances that are required for cell viability under stress. However, autophagy could not only maintain cell survival, but also may lead to cell death. Enhancing autophagy may substantially retard cancer cell growth [25–27]. Thus, SMI-4a has its inhibitory effect on melanoma cells through enhancing autophagy.

To date, many natural extracts, such as Hinokitiol and mountain tea extracts, have been shown to trigger autophagy that retard growth. Additionally, some natural extracts could synergize with some chemotherapeutic agents to eliminate cancer [28, 29]. This point was also supported in our findings showing that combined G-Rh2 with SMI-4a could markedly decrease cell viability, promote caspase 3/7 activity, and inhibit melanoma growth over their treatment alone via synergistic effects on autophagy induction, indicating that Rh2 has a synergistic effects on SMI-4a-induced anti-tumor capacity in vitro and in vivo.

Conclusions

In short, we found that SMI-4a could decrease cell viability, promote their apoptosis in melanoma cells. We also confirmed that inhibiting Akt/mTOR signaling axis to trigger autophagy is required for SMI-4a-inducing apoptosis. Moreover, G-Rh2 could assist SMI-4a to enhance its anti-melanoma activity via strengthening autophagy-induced apoptosis in vitro and in vivo. Taken together, our results suggest that combined SMI-4a with G-Rh2 might be a novel alternative approach for melanoma treatment.

Abbreviations
CCK-8: cell counting Kit 8; mTOR: mammalian target of rapamycin; P-mTOR: phosphorylated mammalian target of rapamycin; G-Rh2: ginsenoside Rh2; P-Akt: phosphorylated protein kinase B; Akt: protein kinase B; TCGA: the Cancer Genome Atlas.

Authors' contributions
DL, WL and LC designed all the experiments and revised the paper. WD and WZ performed the experiments, HW, SW and LC performed data analysis and wrote the paper. All authors read and approved the final manuscript.

Author details
¹ Department of Burn and Plastic Surgery, First Affiliated Hospital of Wannan Medical College, Jinghu District, Wuhu 241000, Anhui, China. ² Dermatological Department, First Affiliated Hospital of Wannan Medical College, Jinghu District, Wuhu 241000, Anhui, China.

Acknowledgements
Not applicable.

Competing interests
The authors declare that they have no competing interests.

Funding
This study was supported by the Natural science Foundation of the Higher Education Institutions of Anhui province (KJ2017A273).

References
1. Wu X, Yan J, Dai J, Ma M, Tang H, Yu J, Xu T, Yu H, Si L, Chi Z, et al. Mutations in BRAF codons 594 and 596 predict good prognosis in melanoma. Oncol Lett. 2017;14(3):3601–5.
2. Liu F, Jiang CC, Yan GX, Tseng HY, Wang CY, Zhang YY, Yari H, La T, Farrelly M, Guo ST, et al. BRAF/MEK inhibitors promote CD47 expression that is reversible by ERK inhibition in melanoma. Oncotarget. 2017;8(41):69477–92.
3. Brault L, Gasser C, Bracher F, Huber K, Knapp S, Schwaller J. PIM serine/threonine kinases in the pathogenesis and therapy of hematologic malignancies and solid cancers. Haematologica. 2010;95(6):1004–15.
4. Narlik-Grassow M, Blanco-Aparicio C, Carnero A. The PIM family of serine/threonine kinases in cancer. Med Res Rev. 2014;34(1):136–59.
5. van Lohuizen M, Verbeek S, Krimpenfort P, Domen J, Saris C, Radaszkiewicz T, Berns A. Predisposition to lymphomagenesis in pim-1 transgenic mice: cooperation with c-myc and N-myc in murine leukemia virus-induced tumors. Cell. 1989;56(4):673–82.
6. Rang Z, Yang G, Wang YW, Cui F. miR-542-3p suppresses invasion and metastasis by targeting the proto-oncogene serine/threonine protein kinase, PIM1, in melanoma. Biochem Biophys Res Commun. 2016;474(2):315–20.
7. Wu H, Chen J, Wang Q, Jia X, Song S, Yuan P, Liu K, Liu L, Zhang Y, Zhou A, Wei W. Ginsenoside metabolite compound K attenuates inflammatory responses of adjuvant-induced arthritis rats. Immunopharmacol Immunotoxicol. 2014;36(2):124–9.
8. Liu KK, Wang QT, Yang SM, Chen JY, Wu HX, Wei W. Ginsenoside compound K suppresses the abnormal activation of T lymphocytes in mice with collagen-induced arthritis. Acta Pharmacol Sin. 2014;35(5):599–612.
9. Chen J, Wu H, Wang Q, Chang Y, Liu K, Song S, Yuan P, Fu J, Sun W, Huang Q, et al. Ginsenoside metabolite compound k alleviates adjuvant-induced arthritis by suppressing T cell activation. Inflammation. 2014;37(5):1608–15.
10. Wang M, Yan SJ, Zhang HT, Li N, Liu T, Zhang YL, Li XX, Ma Q, Qiu XC, Fan QY, Ma BA. Ginsenoside Rh2 enhances the antitumor immunological response of a melanoma mice model. Oncol Lett. 2017;13(2):681–5.
11. Shi Q, Li J, Feng Z, Zhao L, Luo L, You Z, Li D, Xia J, Zuo G, Chen D. Effect of ginsenoside Rh2 on the migratory ability of HepG2 liver carcinoma cells: Recruiting histone deacetylase and inhibiting activator protein 1 transcription factors. Mol Med Rep. 2014;10(4):1779–85.
12. Wu R, Ru Q, Chen L, Ma B, Li C. Stereospecificity of ginsenoside Rg3 in the promotion of cellular immunity in hepatoma H22-bearing mice. J Food Sci. 2014;79(7):H1430–5.
13. Jardon MA, Rothe K, Bortnik S, et al. Autophagy: from structure to metabolism to therapeutic regulation. Autophagy. 2013;9(12):2180–2.
14. Tan W, Lu J, Huang M, Li Y, Chen M, Wu G, Gong J, Zhong Z, Xu Z, Dang Y, Guo J, Chen X, Wang Y. Anti-cancer natural products isolated from chinese medicinal herbs. Chin Med. 2011;6(1):27.
15. Zhang Y, Liang Y, He C. Anticancer activities and mechanisms of heat-clearing and detoxicating traditional Chinese herbal medicine. Chin Med. 2017;12:20.

16. Liang XH, Jackson S, Seaman M, et al. Induction of autophagy and inhibition of tumorigenesis by beclin 1. Nature. 1999;402(6762):672–6.
17. Shannan B, Watters A, Chen Q, Mollin S, Dörr M, Meggers E, Xu X, Gimotty PA, Perego M, Li L. PIM kinases as therapeutic targets against advanced melanoma. Oncotarget. 2016;7(34):54897–912.
18. Lin YW, Beharry ZM, Hill EG, Song JH, Wang W, Xia Z, Zhang Z, Aplan PD, Aster JC, Smith CD, Kraft AS. A small molecule inhibitor of Pim protein kinases blocks the growth of precursor T-cell lymphoblastic leukemia/lymphoma. Blood. 2010;115(4):824–33.
19. Fan RF, Lu Y, Fang ZG, Guo XY, Chen YX, Xu YC, Lei YM, Liu KF, Lin DJ, Liu LL, Liu XF. PIM-1 kinase inhibitor SMI-4a exerts antitumor effects in chronic myeloid leukemia cells by enhancing the activity of glycogen synthase kinase 3β. Mol Med Rep. 2017;16(4):4603–12.
20. Guo YQ, Sun HY, Chan CO, Liu BB, Wu JH, Chan SW, Mok DK, Tse AK, Yu ZL, Chen SB. Centipeda minima (Ebushicao) extract inhibits PI3K-Akt-mTOR signaling in nasopharyngeal carcinoma CNE-1 cells. Chin Med. 2015;10:26.
21. Heras-Sandoval D, Pérez-Rojas JM, Hernández-Damián J, Pedraza-Chaverri J. The role of PI3 K/AKT/mTOR pathway in the modulation of autophagy and the clearance of protein aggregates in neurodegeneration. Cell Signal. 2014;26(12):2694–701.
22. Mabuchi S, Kuroda H, Takahashi R, Sasano T. The PI3K/AKT/mTOR pathway as a therapeutic target in ovarian cancer. Gynecol Oncol. 2015;137(1):173–9.
23. Roy B, Pattanaik AK, Das J, Bhutia SK, Behera B, Singh P, Maiti TK. Role of PI3K/Akt/mTOR and MEK/ERK pathway in concanavalin A induced autophagy in HeLa cells. Chem Biol Interact. 2014;210:96–102.
24. Kim YC, Guan KL. mTOR: a pharmacologic target for autophagy regulation. J Clin Invest. 2015;125(1):25–32.
25. Liu L, Liao JZ, He XX, Li PY. The role of autophagy in hepatocellular carcinoma: friend or foe. Oncotarget. 2017;8(34):57707–22.
26. Mathiassen SG, de Zio D, Cecconi F. Autophagy and the cell cycle: a complex landscape. Front Oncol. 2017;7:51.
27. Gao L, Jauregui CE, Teng Y. Targeting autophagy as a strategy for drug discovery and therapeutic modulation. Fut Med Chem. 2017;9(3):335–45.
28. Kaushal GP, Kaushal V, Herzog C, Yang C. Autophagy delays apoptosis in renal tubular epithelial cells in cisplatin cytotoxicity. Autophagy. 2008;4(5):710–2.
29. Su Z, Li G, Liu C, Ren S, Deng T, Zhang S, Tian Y, Liu Y, Qiu Y. Autophagy inhibition impairs the epithelial-mesenchymal transition and enhances cisplatin sensitivity in nasopharyngeal carcinoma. Oncol Lett. 2017;13(6):4147–54.

17

Cardiac function evaluation for a novel one-step detoxification product of *Aconiti Lateralis Radix Praeparata*

Ya-nan He[1†], Ding-kun Zhang[1,2†] ⓘ, Jun-zhi Lin[3], Xue Han[1], Ya-ming Zhang[4], Hai-zhu Zhang[5], Jin Pei[1,2], Ming Yang[6*] and Jia-bo Wang[4*]

Abstract

Background: *Aconiti Lateralis Radix Praeparata* has been used as the first cardiac drug over a 1000 years in Asian countries. Although most detoxification products are confirmed to be safe, the effect is not potent as desired. In previous study, we designed a one-step detoxification product by fresh cutting and continuously dried, which preserved more water-soluble alkaloids while eliminating toxicity. It is thus necessary to find more in vivo evidence to support its industrial development.

Methods: Initially, network pharmacology was applied to analyze the related pathways of candidate components acting on heart failure diseases. Then, two heart failure models that were induced by propafenone hydrochloride and nimodipine (v/v, 1:1) and were given doxorubicin were carried out to test the cardiac activity. Moreover, the effect on mitochondrial energy metabolism was further assessed.

Results: Network pharmacology results indicated that *Aconiti Lateralis Radix Praeparata* treated heart failure through cAMP signaling pathway, calcium signaling pathway, adrenergic signaling in cardiomyocytes and so on. These pathways were highly correlated with myocardial contractility and mitochondrial energy metabolism. Trials on heart failure rats demonstrated that the novel processed-product could produce a stronger positive inotropic action and increase more Na^+–K^+–ATPase and Ca^{2+}–Mg^{2+}–ATPase than Heishunpian. Pathological results also revealed the novel one could better restore the morphology of cardiomyocytes and reduce vacuolar lesions. It also could inspire more energy with a lower concentration.

Conclusions: This study provides scientific evidence for the clinical application of new products. It is of great benefit to innovate the industrial detoxification process of Aconitum.

Keywords: *Aconiti Lateralis Radix Praeparata*, Detoxification approach, Mitochondrial energy metabolism, Cardiac function, Network pharmacology

Background

Heart failure (HF) is the ultimate destination of most cardiovascular diseases. Its mortality is gradually increasing with ageing. It has been one of the serious problems affecting global health [1]. In 2004, Van et al. proposed

*Correspondence: yangming16@126.com; pharm_sci@126.com
†Ya-nan He and Ding-kun Zhang contributed equally to this study
⁴ China Military Institute of Chinese Medicine, 302 Military Hospital, No. 100 Xisihuan, Beijing 100039, People's Republic of China⁶ Jiangxi University of Traditional Chinese Medicine, No. 18 Yunwan Avenue, Nanchang 330004, People's Republic of China

the concept of remodeling myocardial metabolic, and believed that energy metabolism disorder was one of the key mechanisms of HF [2]. At present, classical drugs for treating HF are neuroendocrine system inhibitors, such as angiotensin converting enzyme inhibitors, cardiac glycoside, β-receptor blockers, and aldosterone antagonists [3]. Although these drugs significantly improve the pathological symptoms, the mortality rate is still high. Traditional Chinese medicine plays an important role in complementary and alternative therapies, especially in cardiovascular disease and cancers [4–6].

Aconiti Lateralis Radix Praeparata (ALRP) is the daughter root of *Aconitum carmichaelii* Debx. It is regarded as a magic drug for its severe cardiotoxicity and great cardiac effect. How to achieve the dual purpose of toxicity elimination and efficacy preservation is always a bottleneck of industrial development. Traditional detoxification methods are extremely complicated and time-consuming, such as burning, grilling, baking, boiling, soaking, steaming, and so on [7, 8]. What are worse, over 90% alkaloids lost during the process due to unclear understanding of toxic and active ingredients [9]. Official quality standards of Heishunpian (HSP), Baifupian, Danfupian, Paofupian are cases. From the present perspective, aconitine, mesaconitine, and hypaconitine belong to the hypertoxic main components. When these ones are hydrolyzed under heating conditions, the hydrolysates are converted into possible energy metabolism promoters, including benzoylaconitine, benzoylmesaconitine, and benzoylhypaconitine [10]. Other water-soluble alkaloids, such as higenamine and salsolinol [11, 12], are considered to be crucial substances in enhancing myocardial contractility by activating β receptors [13]. Interestingly, both benzoyl alkaloids and water-soluble alkaloids have good water solubility and are easy to flow away.

According to the principle above, we have designed a novel detoxification approach by fresh cutting and continuously dried in 100 °C oven for 10 h [14]. In the previous study, this new method has been confirmed to achieve the same detoxification effect as traditional methods, and the loss of alkaloids dropped from 85.2 to 30% [14]. The crucial innovation has granted by Chinese patents (No. 201510347673.9). However, there is no direct evidence that the increase of alkaloid retention in vitro would lead to enhancing the effect in vivo. It is unknown whether the novel ALRP processed product (NAP) has a better efficacy on cardiac.

In this manuscript, in order to explore the mechanism of cardiac by ALRP, the methods and ideas of network pharmacology were applied. HSP was the most widely used ALRP detoxification product at present. To evaluate the clinical application advantages of NAP, cardiac activity experiment and mitochondrial promotion experiment were carried out. This study is expected to reveal the cardiac mechanism of ALRP and to facilitate the clinical application of NAP. It is also very important for scientific design of detoxification technology and efficient utilization of ALRP resources.

Methods
Materials
HSP and ALRP were provided by *Sichuan Jiangyou Zhongba Fuzi Science and Technology Development Co., LTD*. All samples, identified by Professor Xiaohe Xiao, were deposited at the Chengdu University of TCM, Chengdu, China. NAP was prepared by the one-step detoxification approach. In detail, fresh ALRP were cutting into particles with the size of 5*5*5 mm, and then dried in 100 °C oven for 10 h [14]. The information regarding the experimental design, statistics, and resources used in this study are attached in the minimum standards of reporting checklist (Additional file 1).

Chemicals
Coomassie (Bradford) Protein Assay Kit was purchased from Nanjing Jiancheng Bioengineering Institute (A045-2, China). Sucrose was purchased from BeijingYilijingxi Co., Ltd (20071227). Tris–HCl was purchased from BIOPCR (ZH136590). Na_2EDTA (20100512) and PBS (20150712) were purchased from Solarbio. Bovine serum albumin was purchased from Sigma (#SLBL5598V). Hepes was purchased from Hotaibio (H0070). Propafenone Hydrochloride Injection (PHI) was purchased from Guangzhou Baiyun Shan Ming Xing Pharmaceutical Co., Ltd., and the specification was 10 ml: 35 mg. Nimodipine Injection (NI) was purchased from Bayer Schering Pharma, and the specification was 50 ml: 10 mg. Normal saline (NS) was got from Shijiazhuang No. 4 Pharmaceutical, and the specification was 500 ml: 4.5 g. Adriamycin was purchased from Shenzhen Wanle Pharmaceutical Co., Ltd. and the specification was 10 ml: 20 mg. The ultrapure water used in the experiments was prepared using a Milli-Q Ultrapure water purification system (Millipore, Bedford, MA, USA).

Animals
Male Sprague–Dawley (SD) rats weighing 180–200 g were obtained from the Laboratory Animal Center of the Military Medical Science Academy of the PLA (Permit No. SCXK-(A) 2012-0004). The animals were maintained under controlled conditions of temperature 20 ± 0.5 °C, humidity $55 \pm 5\%$, and with 12 h light and 12 h dark cycles. Before experiments, they were fasting for 24 h with free access to water.

Network pharmacology analysis
Collect predicted targets of ALRP and known targets of heart failure
Benzoylaconitine, benzoylmesaconitine, benzoylhypaconitine, higenamine and salsoline were selected to explore the information of predicted targets. Information was obtained from BATMAN-TCM [15, 16]. Score cutoff >20 and P<0.05 were used as screening parameters to find potential targets of five components [15]. Known therapeutic targets for the treatment of heart failure were obtained from two resources. The first one was the Human Phenotype Ontology (HPO) database [17, 18], and the

second one was Therapeutic Target Database (TTD) [19, 20].

Protein–protein interaction (PPI) data and Network construction

PPI data were imported from String database [21, 22]. Then gave a score for each PPI data. In the analysis, homo species were chosen. To ensure the reliability, the one with a score of over 0.7 was considered acceptable [23]. Based on PPI data results, Cytoscape software (Version 3.5.1) was applied to visualize the interaction network. Network Analyzer, a plug-in for Cytoscape, was also used to calculate the topological properties [24], and construct an interaction network map of "drug target-disease target" with the target over the median of degrees, betweenness, and closeness.

Pathway enrichment analysis for candidate targets

DAVID Bioinformatics Resources 6.8 [25, 26] and KOBAS 3.0 were applied for pathway enrichment analysis [27, 28].

Effect on an acute heart failure model induced by Propafenone hydrochloride and nimodipine injection
Extraction of sample

200 g NAP or HSP were extracted 1 time with 10-fold the amount of water and 1 h each time. The extracted solution was cooled, contributing to weight loss during the extraction procedure, and then centrifuged 10 min with a speed of 5000 rpm min^{-1} to yield the sample solution.

Determination method

Eighteen male SD rats were divided into three groups consisting of six animals in each. They were control group, NAP group and HSP group, respectively. Rats were anesthetized using 20% urethane solution through intraperitoneal injection. Rats were placed in dorsal recumbency and a longitudinal midline incision was made in the neck. The right common carotid artery was isolated, and an arterial canal processed by heparin was inserted into the left ventricle. It could monitor the change of left ventricular maximum pressure rising rate (+dp/dtmax). A small incision was cut on the vein, and a venous cannula was inserted. The model drug and extraction were injected into the rats via it. All signals were synchronously recorded on the four-channel physiological recorder (RM6240BD, Chengdu instrument factory). Before the experiment, it was required to correct the pressure transducer using the sphygmomanometer. When measuring the left ventricular pressure, it should turn the three-way valve and close the duct to link the transducer and the atmospheric, after a fast zero correction, we can record data. Propafenone hydrochloride

and nimodipine injection (v/v, 1:1) were injected into rats at a constant speed of 4 ml h^{-1}. When the +dp/dtmax dropped more than 50%, the injection was stopped. If the value of +dp/dtmax did not rise in 5 min, the model was considered successful. At this time, the extraction of NAP or HSP was given at a constant speed of 10 ml h^{-1}. And the rise of +dp/dtmax within 15 min were figured out to evaluate the cardiac effect.

Effect on a heart failure model induced by Adriamycin
Extraction of sample

200 g NAP or HSP were extracted 2 times with 10-fold the amount of water, 1 h each time. The extraction was filtered through a qualitative filter paper and then the filtrate was concentrated to 1 g/ml at 60 °C.

Determination method

Twenty-four male SD rats were divided into four groups consisting of six animals in each. They were normal group, model group, NAP group and HSP group, respectively.

Each group was administered continuously for 5 days. Dose volume of 10 ml kg^{-1} extracts was given orally one time each day, while normal group and model group were given the same amount of water. On the sixth day, in addition to the normal group, the other four groups received 10 mg kg^{-1} Adriamycin through single intraperitoneal injection to copy heart failure model [29].

24 h after modeling, rats were anesthetized using 20% urethane solution through intraperitoneal injection. Rats were placed in dorsal recumbency and a longitudinal midline incision was made in the neck. The right common carotid artery was isolated, and an arterial canal processed by heparin was inserted into the left ventricle. After stable 20 min, a polygraph (RM6240BD, Chengdu instrument factory) was used to record left ventricular systolic pressure (LVSP), +dp/dtmax, and heart rate (HR). After the determination of cardiac function, hearts were removed and washed with cold saline water immediately. The contents of Na^{+}–K^{+}–ATPase and Ca^{2+}–Mg^{2+}–ATPase were determined after homogenization. The protein was quantitatively used in coomassie brilliant blue. This part was commissioned by Google biotechnology limited company.

The left ventricular myocardium was obtained by fixation with 10% formalin fixation fluid. Then it was prepared into a conventional tissue section and the pathological observation was performed after staining HE. This part was commissioned by Pathology Department of 302 Military Hospital.

All values were expressed as mean ± SD. The results were analyzed by one-way analysis of variance (ANOVA) using SPSS 22.0 software. A value of $p < 0.01$ was considered statistically significant.

Effect on the mitochondrial energy metabolism
Instrument
Microcalorimetry (TAM AIR 3114 Bioactivity monitor, Sweden) was utilized to measure the power–time curves of metabolic heat release of mitochondria. The baseline fluctuation was less than 20 µW over 24 h. The high-speed refrigerated centrifuge Sigma 3–18 k (Sigma, Germany) and Homogenizer machine T10 Basic (IKA, Germany) were applied in this research. For details of the performance and structure of the instrument, please see the instruction and Ref [30].

Test solution preparation
Buffer A was a mixture of 68.5 g sucrose, 3 g Tris–HCl, 0.18 g Na_2EDTA, and 0.5 g bovine serum albumin and diluted to 500 ml. Buffer B was a solution of 51.3 g sucrose, 1.2 g Tris–HCl, and 0.1 g Hepes and diluted to 500 ml and sterilized under high temperature and pressure. All chemicals were of analytical grade.

Sample preparation
10 g NAP or HSP were extracted 2 times with 10-fold the amount of water and 1 h each time. The extraction was filtered through a qualitative filter paper. The filtrate was prepared to a final concentration of 50 µg ml^{-1} with Buffer B as a solvent.

Mitochondria isolation
Mitochondria were isolated from the liver of SD rats killed by exsanguination and cut into small pieces and washed with PBS and Buffer A. Then, the liver tissues were homogenized by homogenizer aseptically. The homogenate was centrifuged at 5000 r min^{-1} for 15 min at 4 °C, and the sediment was discarded. The supernatant was centrifuged at 10,000 r min^{-1} for 20 min at 4 °C, then the sediment was kept. Finally, the sediment was re-suspended with Buffer B to form the mitochondria suspension. The isolated mitochondria were stored at 4 °C, and the concentration was quantified by Coomassie (Bradford) Protein Assay Kit [10].

Microcalorimetric measurement
The metabolic heat generation of isolated mitochondria and the thermal effects of NAP and HSP were determined using TAM Air Isothermal Microcalorimetry. The penicillin bottle was processed by strong acid, washed with ultrapure water, and sterilized at 37 °C. Ten milliliters of Buffer B was added into one penicillin bottle as the sterile control group (Ch 1). The same volume of mitochondria suspension was added into the rest seven penicillin bottles, including one blank control group (Ch 2) and five administered groups (Ch 3–7) at different concentrations of NAP or HSP extraction. The information of added solutions of each group was shown in Table 1.

Then, the bottles were sealed and put into the TAM Air Isothermal Microcalorimetry. The heat flow curves of each channel were recorded until they returned to a steady state. All data were collected by a dedicated software package in a real-time manner [10]. Principal component analysis (PCA) was performed on the quantitative thermokinetic parameters which were obtained by analyzing the power–time curves of rat liver mitochondria growth affected by NAP and HSP using SPSS 22.0 statistics software (SPSS Inc., Chicago, IL, USA).

The Minimum Standards of Reporting Checklist contains details of the experimental design, and statistics, and resources used in this study.

Results
Network pharmacology analysis
Network construction
124 predictive targets were obtained from BATMAN-TCM database. There were 212 related-targets of heart failure collected from HPO database. The interaction between drug targets and heart failure disease was constructed by String database and Cytoscape v3.5.1 (showed in Fig. 1). A total of 42 targets for anti-heart failure were found. The target was represented by a round node whose size represented degree (the number of interacting proteins in the network). In other words, the larger the node was, the more important it was to play a role in anti-heart failure networks. The top 10 targets for degree were CASR, ADCY5, CXCL12, CHRM2, AGTR1, DRD4, ADRB2, DRD2, OPRL1 and HTR2C. Among them, CHRM2 was the target of benzoylaconine, benzoylhypaconine, benzoylmesaconine and higenamine. DRD4, DRD2 and ADRB2 were the targets of higenamine and salsolinol.

Pathway enrichment analysis
There were eight main biological signal pathways obtained by pathway enrichment analysis of cardiac candidate targets. According to the p-value, it was cAMP signaling pathway

Table 1 Reagent addition to ampoule of each channel (mL)

Channel no	Mitochondria suspension/mL	Buffer B, solution/mL	Sample, solution/mL
Ch 1	0	10	0
Ch 2	6	4	0
Ch 3	6	3.95	0.05
Ch 4	6	3.9	0.1
Ch 5	6	3.8	0.2
Ch 6	6	3.6	0.4
Ch 7	6	3	1

$(p=1.41\times10^{-13})$, Renin secretion $(p=1.02\times10^{-10})$, Calcium signaling pathway $(p=8.87\times10^{-10})$, Dopaminergic synapse $(p=5.80\times10^{-9})$ and Adrenergic signaling in cardiomyocytes $(p=1.27\times10^{-8})$, respectively. The smaller the p value was, the higher the correlation was.

Based on the analysis above, it was found that the pathways significantly influenced myocardial contraction and energy metabolism. In detail, cAMP signaling pathway, Dopaminergic synapse, Adrenergic signaling in cardiomyocytes, Calcium signaling pathway were closely related to myocardial contractility. cAMP signaling pathway and Calcium signaling pathway also affected mitochondrial energy metabolism. Therefore, the experimental study of NAP or HSP on heart function mainly focused on myocardial contractility and energy metabolism.

Cardiac effect analysis on an acute heart failure model

Figure 2 indicated that +dp/dtmax of rats was rapidly decreased after injecting the mixture of propafenone hydrochloride and nimodipine. Combined use of both could cause a rapid inhibition of cardiac function in a very short time. At 7–8 min, +dp/dtmax dropped more than 50% and the injection was stopped. The value did not rise significantly in 5 min, so the model was considered successful. After giving NS, it was clear that the value did not increase (Fig. 2a), which meant the damaged myocardial contractility did not recover. However, the value of +dp/dtmax climbed immediately when the extraction of NAP or HSP was given (Fig. 2b, c). The most amazing result was NAP almost restored the severely impaired myocardial contractility to normal level, while HSP only made it return to the level of 70–80%. These results fairly proved the superiority of NAP in an acute heart failure model.

Cardiac effect analysis on an Adriamycin heart failure model

The effect of NAP and HSP on heart function indexes of rats was listed in Fig. 3. Comparing with normal group, LVSP, +dp/dtmax, and HR of model group rats were significantly dropped $(p<0.01)$ after continuous administration of Adriamycin, which indicated that cardiac function of rats was obviously inhibited. When given the extraction of NAP or HSP, LVSP, +dp/dtmax, and HR of rats increased greatly $(p<0.01)$, which meant the cardiac function improved dramatically. Overall, NAP showed a stronger cardiac function recovery than HSP.

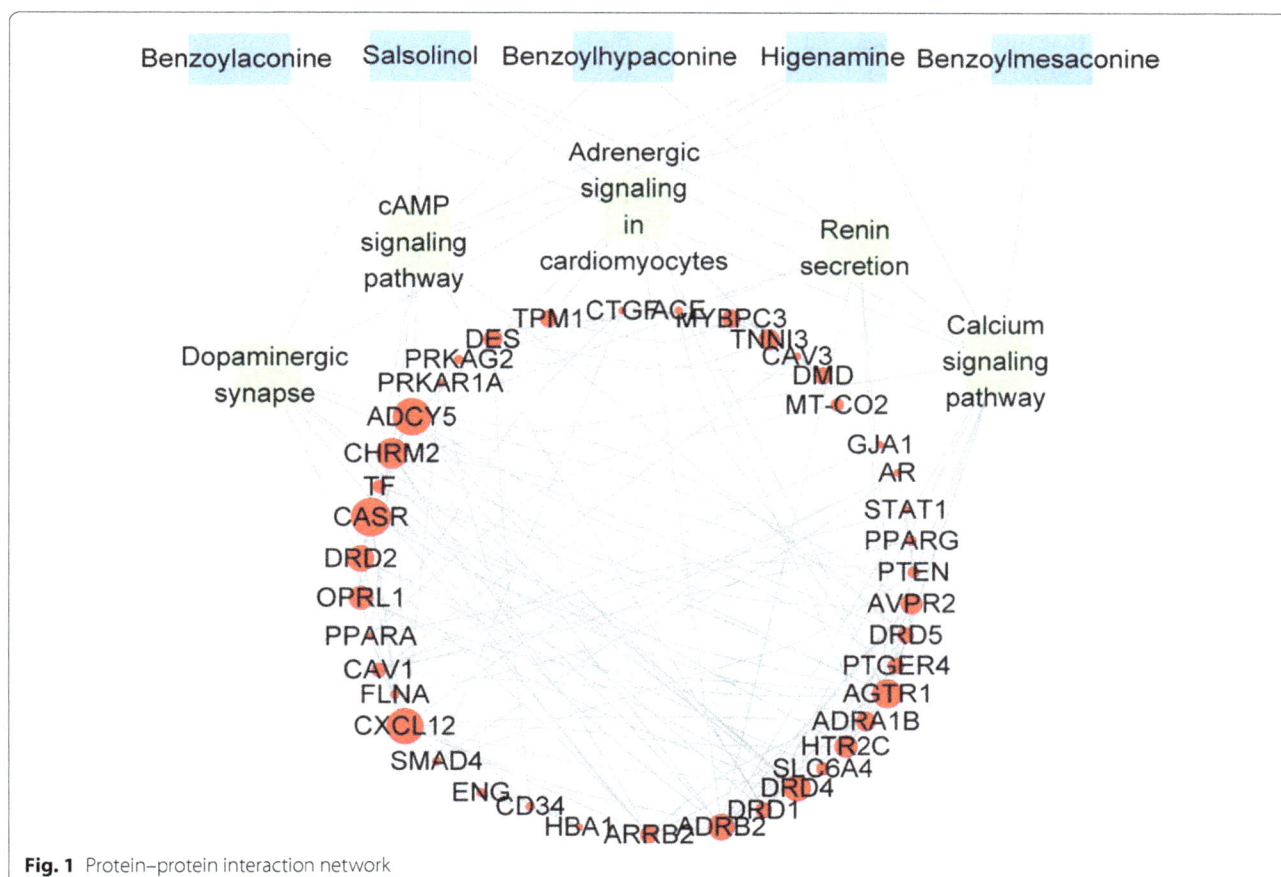

Fig. 1 Protein–protein interaction network

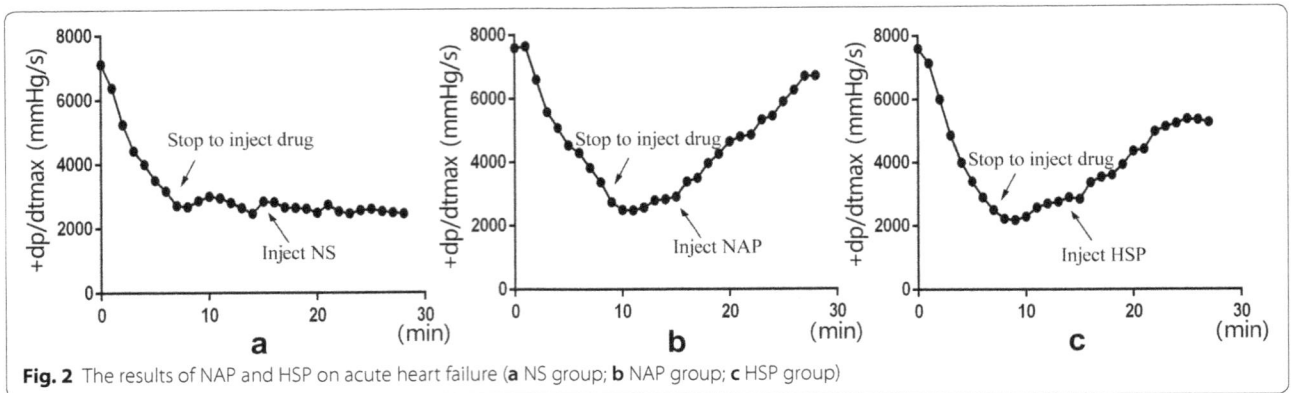

Fig. 2 The results of NAP and HSP on acute heart failure (**a** NS group; **b** NAP group; **c** HSP group)

Results of myocardial tissue ATPase and myocardial cell morphology

The effect of NAP and HSP on ATPase content in rat myocardial tissues was shown in Fig. 4a. Comparing with normal group, the content of $Na^+-k^+-ATPase$ and $Ca^{2+}-Mg^{2+}-ATPase$ in model group went down significantly (p < 0.05). After giving NAP or HSP for 5 days, the content of $Na^+-k^+-ATPase$ and $Ca^{2+}-Mg^{2+}-ATPase$ went up sharply. Totally speaking, HSP group was near to the normal one, while NAP even exceeded the normal one.

Pathological analysis results were showed in Fig. 4b. It demonstrated that normal myocardial cells were arranged in order without deformation, necrotic cells or inflammatory cell infiltration. After Adriamycin administration, myocardial cells injured obviously with myocardial fiber disorder, thinning, and dissolution fracture. Some ones were even interstitial edema, accompanied by vacuole-like changed. After giving NAP or HSP, myocardial cells could be recovered to a certain extent. The arrangement tended to be close and vacuolar changes decreased. In particular, the morphology of NAP group approached to the normal group, which suggested the protective effect of NAP on myocardium was quite excellent.

Quantitative thermo-kinetic parameters for mitochondria growth

As shown in Fig. 5, the power-time curves of heat generation of mitochondria in the absence or presence of different concentrations of NAP or HSP were recorded. It could be found that the shape of curves in the administered groups (Ch 2–7) changed when compared with the control group (Ch 1). With the rising of concentration, the curve shape changed more significantly. However, the variation trends of NAP and HSP were not exactly the same. In detail, low concentrations (0–1 µg ml^{-1}) in NAP group could promote the metabolism of mitochondria, while high concentrations (2–5 µg ml^{-1}) posed an inhibitory effect. From Table 2, the thermodynamic parameters also made a similar performance. Most ones reached their peaks at a concentration of 1 µg ml^{-1}, including k, P_{max}, Q and P_{av}. In HSP group, k, P_{max}, Q, P_{av}, T_{lag}, and P_{av} of samples all increased continuously within 0–2 µg ml^{-1}. When the applied concentration reached 5 µg ml^{-1}, the value of some parameters began to decrease. These results clearly showed that the extraction of ALRP had a complex regulating action on mitochondria metabolism. Energy metabolism could be promoted by low concentrations and inhibited by high concentration. Interestingly, NAP could achieve a higher promotion effect at a lower concentration range.

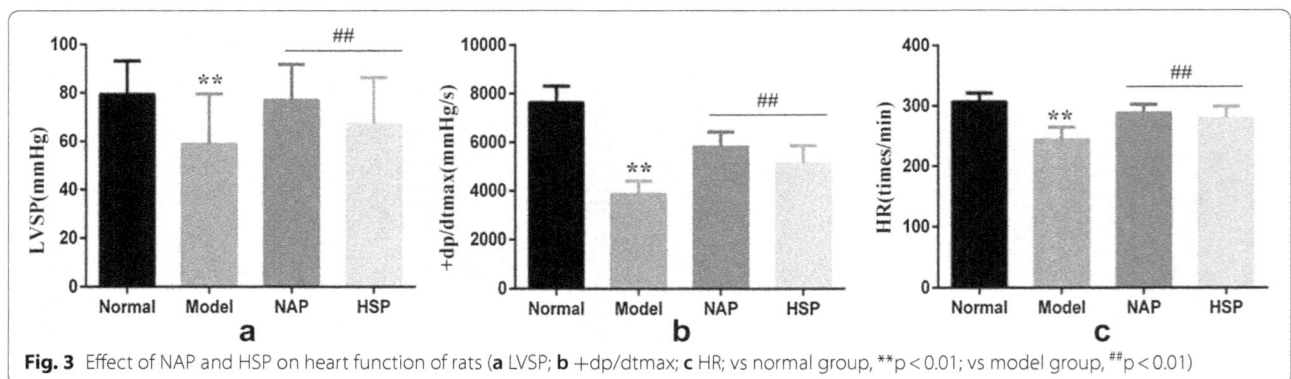

Fig. 3 Effect of NAP and HSP on heart function of rats (**a** LVSP; **b** +dp/dtmax; **c** HR; vs normal group, **p < 0.01; vs model group, ##p < 0.01)

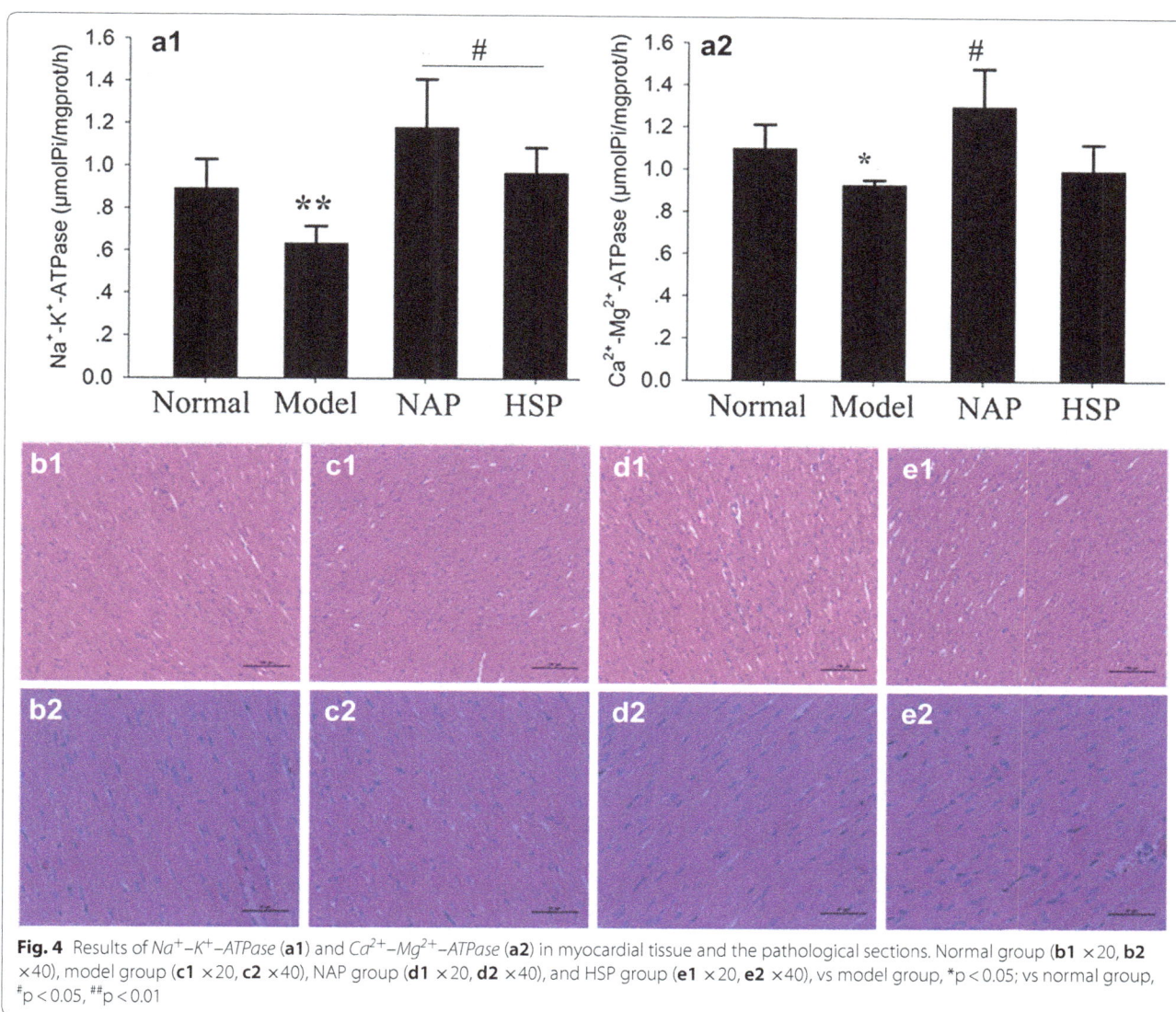

Fig. 4 Results of $Na^+–K^+–ATPase$ (**a1**) and $Ca^{2+}–Mg^{2+}–ATPase$ (**a2**) in myocardial tissue and the pathological sections. Normal group (**b1** ×20, **b2** ×40), model group (**c1** ×20, **c2** ×40), NAP group (**d1** ×20, **d2** ×40), and HSP group (**e1** ×20, **e2** ×40), vs model group, *p < 0.05; vs normal group, #p < 0.05, ##p < 0.01

Principal component analysis (PCA) results

The effects of various concentrations of NAP and HSP on mitochondrial energy metabolism differed greatly. It was difficult to objectively determine the thermodynamic parameters represent the eigenvalues. Therefore, PCA was introduced to extract the main parameters which could represent the main change rule of data after dimensionality reduction.

SPSS 22.0 statistical software was carried out PCA analysis on six parameters. Loadings plot (Fig. 5c) indicated that Q was the most important thermodynamic index to distinguish the difference of mitochondrial metabolism between NAP and HSP, for it was the longest point from the origin. Scores plot (Fig. 5d) suggested that there was a good separation between NAP and HSP, though a few overlaps existed. These results also revealed the action

diversity of two products. Through a visual analysis, total heat production of mitochondria peaked at 22.8 J when the concentration of NAP was 1 μg ml^{-1}, and then began to decline dramatically. That of HSP also peaked at 20.8 J at the concentration of 1 μg ml^{-1}, and then went down slowly. But the reduction speed was obviously lower. These results showed that the effect on promoting mitochondrial energy metabolism of NAP was better than HSP.

Discussions

The mechanism of heart failure is rather complex and has not yet been fully elucidated. The core pathogenesis is considered as the abnormal of systolic function. The basic determinants of myocardial contraction include myocardial contractile protein, energy metabolism and

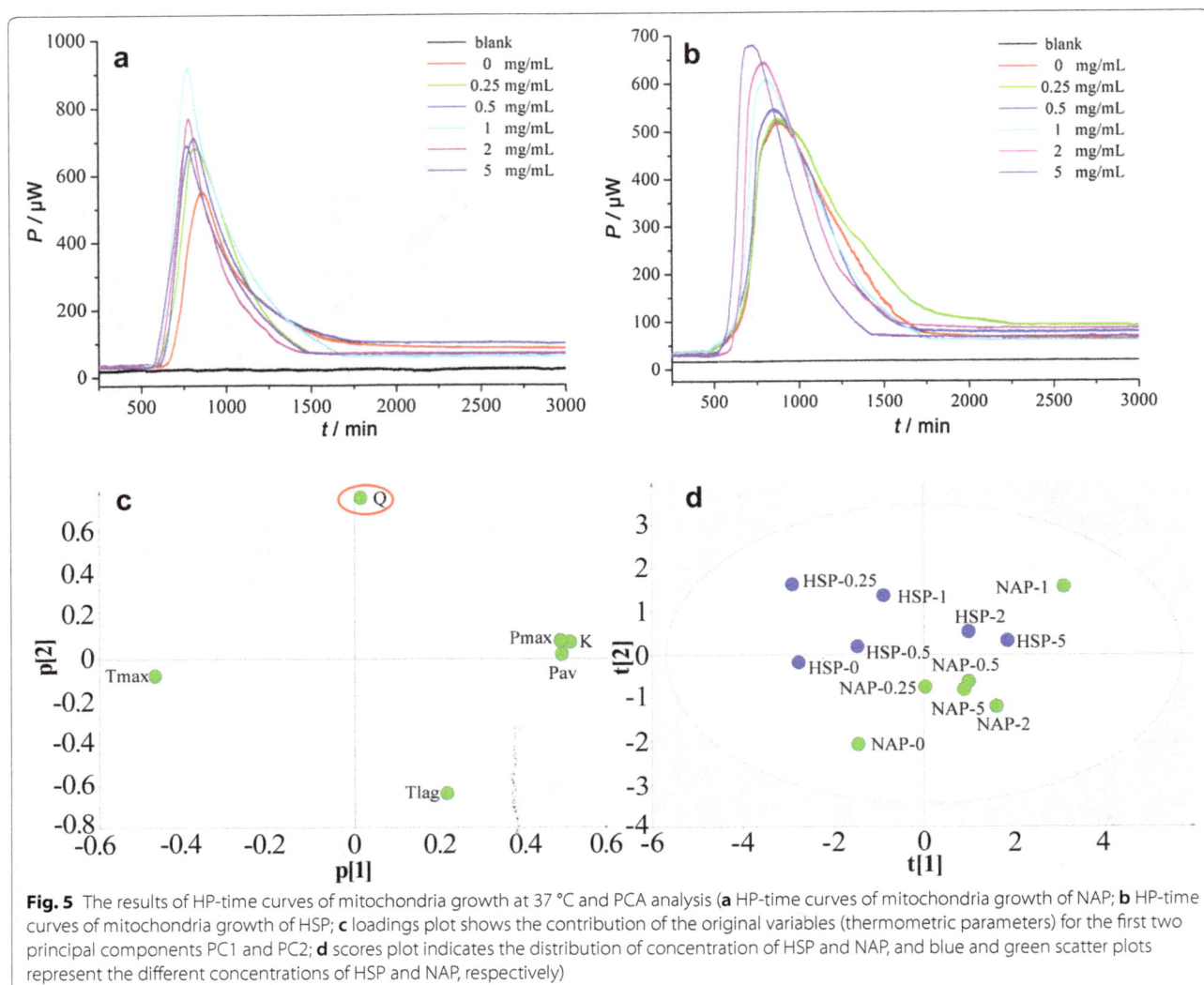

Fig. 5 The results of HP-time curves of mitochondria growth at 37 °C and PCA analysis (**a** HP-time curves of mitochondria growth of NAP; **b** HP-time curves of mitochondria growth of HSP; **c** loadings plot shows the contribution of the original variables (thermometric parameters) for the first two principal components PC1 and PC2; **d** scores plot indicates the distribution of concentration of HSP and NAP, and blue and green scatter plots represent the different concentrations of HSP and NAP, respectively)

Table 2 Quantitative thermo-kinetic parameters for mitochondria growth at 37 °C affected by NAP and HSP

Sample	$c/\mu g\ ml^{-1}$	$k/10^{-3}\ min^{-1}$	$P_{max}/\mu W$	T_{max}/min	Q/J	T_{lag}/min	$P_{av}/\mu W$
NAP	0	16.1	552.4	864.2	16.7	382.1	242.8
	0.25	17.6	680.7	824.3	17.2	294.1	299.3
	0.5	20.8	713.0	810.3	19.3	355.6	307.9
	1	28.5	919.8	775.5	22.8	291.9	331.6
	2	25.7	771.5	781.2	15.3	301.7	290.5
	5	21.1	690.6	771.3	16.6	294.2	293.1
HSP	0	14.2	522.7	884.2	17.2	211.5	229.5
	0.25	14.3	528.0	870.3	21.8	187.3	208.9
	0.5	15.4	547.8	847.2	19.0	244.8	274.7
	1	17.3	609.3	809.3	20.8	203.8	264.7
	2	23.0	645.9	799.0	20.1	274.5	326.3
	5	25.2	680.7	728.0	17.8	239.4	318.8

excitation–contraction coupling [31]. Any change of these factors can lead to heart failure. Adriamycin can cause serious myocardial toxicity, and the damage degree is highly correlated with dose [32]. The main poisoning mechanisms are oxidative stress and mitochondrial dysfunction [33]. It can induce lipid peroxidation injury, and produce malondialdehyde and other metabolites. These substances damage the integrity of the myocardial cell membrane and the mitochondrial membrane, and finally result in cell autolysis and the destruction of contractile protein [34]. Meanwhile, Adriamycin can inhibit the activity of $Na^+–K^+–ATPase$ in cell membranes and weaken the activity of $Ca^{2+}–ATPase$ in sarcoplasmic reticulum membranes. The direct result is that myosin does not decompose ATP normally [35]. Propafenone hydrochloride is a classic sodium channel blocker [36], while nimodipine blocks the calcium channels [37]. Their combination can not only interfere with the sodium influx during depolarization, but also block the calcium influx during the plateau, and contribute to the myocardial excitation–contraction coupling disorder. So these two models greatly reflect the basic pathogenesis of heart failure.

Multiple pathways found in network pharmacology analysis play an important role in the treatment of heart failure. The most impressive one is cAMP signaling pathway. When it works, adenylate cyclase is activated, and ATP is converted to cAMP [38]. It makes the receptor dependent calcium channel open and promote the increase of intracellular Ca^{2+} concentration [39]. This is an important mechanism to enhance myocardial contractility. It can also strengthen the beta oxidation of fatty acids and improve the energy metabolism of hypertrophic cardiomyocytes [40, 41]. In addition, this pathway can further pose an effect on the Renin pathway [42]. Another pathway to be mentioned is adrenergic signaling in cardiomyocytes. It also inspires adenylate cyclase and promotes ATP catabolism [43]. Calcium signaling pathway is a downstream one, which enables to boost the intracellular calcium concentration and act on the mitochondrial calcium uniporter [44]. When this network is activated by ALRP, myocardial contractility and energy metabolism should be improved comprehensively.

Higenamine and salsoline play a crucial role in the myocardial contractility. Higenamine is a full agonist of β-1 adrenergic receptor [45]. Meanwhile, it is confirmed to have β-2 adrenergic receptor agonist activity [46]. Salsolinol is a partial agonist for β-receptor [45]. According to our results, these two components in NAP were about 5–32 times as much as HSP (Additional file 2). The results of two animal experiments also proved the beneficial effects of the increase in components' contents on myocardial contractility. Monoester diterpenoid alkaloids are the key to energy metabolism of mitochondria [10, 47]. Previous study found that the abundance in NAP was 2–14 times over that of HSP, an Additional file shows this in more detail (see Additional file 2). Likewise, NAP performed a better effect on energy metabolism and produced more thermal energy in a lower concentration. Moreover, our tests also demonstrated the antagonistic effect of ALRP on Adriamycin induced myocardial injury. Although the effects and mechanisms are not yet clear, the increase in total alkaloids is benefit to enhance the therapeutic effect.

Conclusions
This study demonstrates the advantages of NAP with high alkaloid contents in treating heart failure, which provides sufficient scientific evidence for its industrial development.

Abbreviations
HF: heart failure; PHI: propafenone hydrochloride injection; NS: normal saline; NI: nimodipine injection; HR: heart rate; ALRP: Aconiti Lateralis Radix Praeparata; HSP: heishunpian; DDAs: diester diterpenoid alkaloids; MDAs: monoester diterpeniod alkaloids; LVSP: left ventricular systolic pressure; +dp/dtmax: left ventricular maximum pressure rising rate; NAP: a novel processed product of Aconiti Lateralis Radix Praeparata.

Authors' contributions
DZ, YH, MY, JP, and JW designed the study; DZ, YH, JL, XH, FW, and HZ performed experiments; DZ, YH, JP, and JW analyzed data; JP, and JW supplied materials and analytic tools; DZ, YH, and JW wrote the paper. All authors read and approved the final manuscript.

Author details
[1] State Key Laboratory Breeding Base of Systematic Research, Development and Utilization of Chinese Medicine Resources, Development and Utilization of Chinese Medicine Resources, Chengdu University of Traditional Chinese Medicine, Chengdu, People's Republic of China. [2] Sichuan Good Doctor Panxi Pharmaceutical Co., LTD, Xichang, China. [3] Central Laboratory, Teaching Hospital of Chengdu University of TCM, Chengdu, People's Republic of China. [4] China Military Institute of Chinese Medicine, 302 Military Hospital, No. 100 Xisihuan, Beijing 100039, People's Republic of China. [5] Department of Pharmacy and Chemistry, Dali University, Dali, People's Republic of China. [6] Jiangxi University of Traditional Chinese Medicine, No. 18 Yunwan Avenue, Nanchang 330004, People's Republic of China.

Acknowledgements
We thank 302 Military Hospital for providing an experimental platform.

Competing interests
The authors declare that they have no competing interests.

Consent for publication
The manuscript is approved by all authors for publication.

Funding
We are grateful to the support of National Key Research & Development Program - Modernization of Traditional Chinese Medicine (2018YFC1707200), National Natural Science Foundation Project (81503247), Sichuan Provincial

Administration of Traditional Chinese Medicine Research Project (2018NQ008), and Apricot Scholar Program of Chengdu University of Traditional Chinese Medicine (BSH 2018007).

References

1. Tanai E, Frantz S. Pathophysiology of heart failure. Compr Physiol. 2015;6:187–214.
2. van Bilsen M. "Energenetics" of heart failure. Ann N Y Acad Sci. 2004;1015:238–49.
3. Thorup L, Simonsen U, Grimm D, et al. Ivabradine: current and future treatment of heart failure. Basic Clin Pharmacol Toxicol. 2017;121:89–97.
4. Layne K, Ferro A. Traditional Chinese medicines in the management of cardiovascular diseases: a comprehensive systematic review. Br J Clin Pharmacol. 2017;83:20–32.
5. Wang M, Tao L, Xu H. Chinese herbal medicines as a source of molecules with anti-enterovirus 71 activity. Chin Med. 2016;11:2.
6. Zhang Y, Liang Y, He C. Anticancer activities and mechanisms of heat-clearing and detoxicating traditional Chinese herbal medicine. Chin Med. 2017;12:20.
7. Huang Q, Zhou Z, Wang J, et al. Investigation and collection development pattern for genuineness of Aconitum carmichali. China J Chin Mater Med. 2011;36:2599–601.
8. Wu X, Wang S, Lu J, et al. Seeing the unseen of Chinese herbal medicine processing (Paozhi): advances in new perspectives. Chin Med. 2018;13:4.
9. Zhou L, Li F, Ren Y, et al. Study on Amount variation of alkaloids components with marinated time in aconiti lateralis radix praeparata. Chin J Exp Tradit Med Formul. 2014;20:44–7.
10. Zhang DK, Yang ZR, Han X, et al. Microcalorimetric investigation of six alkaloids from Radix Aconite Lateralis Preparata (Fuzi) on the metabolic activity of mitochondria isolated from rat liver. J Therm Anal Calorim. 2017;130:1707–15.
11. Zhang N, Lian Z, Peng X, et al. Applications of Higenamine in pharmacology and medicine. J Ethnopharmacol. 2017;196:242–52.
12. Li Y, Li YX, Dang J, et al. Simultaneous determination and comparative pharmacokinetics of fuzi water-soluble alkaloids between normal and acute heart failure rats by ultra performance liquid chromatography method. J Chromatogr Sci. 2017;55:719–28.
13. Praman S, Mulvany MJ, Williams DE, et al. Hypotensive and cardio-chronotropic constituents of Tinospora crispa and mechanisms of action on the cardiovascular system in anesthetized rats. J Ethnopharmacol. 2012;140:166–78.
14. Zhang DK, Han X, Tan P, et al. Establishment of one-step approach to detoxification of hypertoxic aconite based on the evaluation of alkaloids contents and quality. Chin J Nat Med. 2017;15:49–61.
15. Liu Z, Guo F, Wang Y, et al. BATMAN-TCM: a bioinformatics analysis tool for molecular mechanism of traditional chinese medicine. Sci Rep. 2016;6:21146.
16. BATMAN-TCM. Beijing Proteome Research Center, Beijng. 2014. http://bionet.ncpsb.org/. Accessed Jan 2016.
17. Köhler S, Doelken SC, Mungall CJ, et al. The human phenotype ontology project: linking molecular biology and disease through phenotype data. Nucleic Acids Res. 2014;42:966–74.
18. Human Phenotype Ontology. The Jackson Laboratory for genomic medicine, Berlin. 2008. http://human-phenotype-ontology.github.io/. Accessed 9 Oct 2018.
19. Li YH, Yu CY, Li XX, et al. Therapeutic target database update 2018: enriched resource for facilitating bench-to-clinic research of targeted therapeutics. Nucleic Acids Res. 2017;46:1121–7.
20. Therapeutic Target Database. Bioinformatics & Drug Design group Singapore. 2002. https://db.idrblab.org/ttd/. Accessed 15 Sep 2017.
21. Szklarczyk D, Franceschini A, Wyder S, et al. STRING v10: protein–protein interaction networks, integrated over the tree of life. Nucleic Acids Res. 2015;43:447–52.
22. String database. the European Commission, Cambridgeshire. 2000. https://string-db.org/. Accessed 14 May 2017.
23. Zheng SC, Yan XY, Chen J, et al. Anti-inflammatory mechanism analysis of antirheumatic Chinese medicinal herb Aconiti Radix based on protein interaction network. China J Chin Mater Med. 2017;42:1747–51.
24. Smoot ME, Ono K, Ruscheinski J, et al. Cytoscape 2.8: new features for data integration and network visualization. Bioinformatics. 2011;27:431–2.
25. DAVID Bioinformatics Resources 6.8. Leidos Biomedical Research Inc., Frederick. 2002. https://david.ncifcrf.gov/home.jsp. Accessed March 2017.
26. Dennis G Jr, Sherman BT, Hosack DA, et al. DAVID: database for annotation, visualization, and integrated discovery. Genome Biol. 2003;4:3.
27. Xie C, Mao X, Huang J, et al. KOBAS 2.0: a web server for annotation and identification of enriched pathways and diseases. Nucleic Acids Res. 2011;39:W316–22.
28. KOBAS 3.0. Peking University, Beijing. 2005. http://kobas.cbi.pku.edu.cn/index.php. Accessed 22 Aug 2016.
29. Ma SF, Guan SD, Zhu Y. Effect of soybean isoflavones on heart function of rats with adriamycin-induced heart failure. J Chin Integr Med. 2004;2:278–80.
30. Kabanova N, Stulova I, Vilu R. Microcalorimetric study of the growth of bacterial colonies of Lactococcus lactis IL1403 in agar gels. Food Microbiol. 2012;29:67–79.
31. Braunwald E. Heart failure. JACC. 2013;1:1–20.
32. Shabalala S, Muller CJF, Louw J, et al. Polyphenols, autophagy and doxorubicin-induced cardiotoxicity. Life Sci. 2017;180:160–70.
33. Varga ZV, Ferdinandy P, Liaudet L, et al. Drug-induced mitochondrial dysfunction and cardiotoxicity. Am J Physiol. 2015;309:1453–67.
34. Renu K, Abilash VG, Pichiah PT, Arunachalam S, et al. Molecular mechanism of doxorubicin-induced cardiomyopathy—an update. Eur J Pharmacol. 2018;818:241–53.
35. Tacar O, Sriamornsak P, Dass CR. Doxorubicin: an update on anticancer molecular action, toxicity and novel drug delivery systems. J Pharm Pharmacol. 2013;65:157–70.
36. Sestito A, Molina E. Atrial fibrillation and the pharmacological treatment: the role of propafenone. Eur Rev Med Pharmacol Sci. 2012;16:242–53.
37. Dorhout Mees SM, Rinkel GJ, Feigin VL, et al. Calcium antagonists for aneurysmal subarachnoid haemorrhage. Cochrane Database Syst Rev. 2007;18:Cd000277.
38. Acin-Perez R, Russwurm M, Gunnewig K, et al. A phosphodiesterase 2A isoform localized to mitochondria regulates respiration. J Biol Chem. 2011;286:30423–32.
39. Wang Z, Liu D, Varin A, et al. A cardiac mitochondrial cAMP signaling pathway regulates calcium accumulation, permeability transition and cell death. Cell Death Dis. 2016;7:2198.
40. Ravnskjaer K, Madiraju A, Montminy M. Role of the cAMP pathway in glucose and lipid metabolism. Handb Exp Pharmacol. 2016;233:29–49.
41. Zhang F, Zhang L, Qi Y, et al. Mitochondrial cAMP signaling. Cell Mol Life Sci. 2016;73:4577–90.
42. Kim SM, Briggs JP, Schnermann J. Convergence of major physiological stimuli for renin release on the Gs-alpha/cyclic adenosine monophosphate signaling pathway. Clin Exp Nephrol. 2012;16:17–24.
43. Florea SM, Blatter LA. Regulation of cardiac alternans by beta-adrenergic signaling pathways. Am J Physiol Heart Circ Physiol. 2012;303:1047–56.
44. Chakraborti S, Das S, Kar P, et al. Calcium signaling phenomena in heart diseases: a perspective. Mol Cell Biochem. 2007;298:1–40.
45. Praman S, Mulvany MJ, Williams DE, et al. Crude extract and purified components isolated from the stems of Tinospora crispa exhibit positive inotropic effects on the isolated left atrium of rats. J Ethnopharmacol. 2013;149:123–32.
46. Kato E, Kimura S, Kawabata J. Ability of higenamine and related compounds to enhance glucose uptake in L6 cells. Bioorg Med Chem. 2017;25:6412–6.
47. Zhang DK, Han X, Zhou YF, et al. Development of Fuzi precision decoction pieces (PDP) (I): specification and quality uniformity. Chin J Chin Mater Med. 2015;40:3488–95.

PERMISSIONS

LIST OF CONTRIBUTORS

Haruka Fujinami
Department of Endoscopy, Toyama University Hospital, Toyama, Japan

Shinya Kajiura, Jun Nishikawa, Takayuki Ando and Toshiro Sugiyama
Department of Gastroenterology, Graduate School of Medicine and Pharmaceutical Science, University of Toyama, Sugitani 2630, Toyama City, Toyama 930-0194, Japan

Linlin Dong, Ruiyang Cheng, Lina Xiao, Guangfei Wei, Jiang Xu and Shilin Chen
Institute of Chinese Materia Medica, China Academy of Chinese Medical Sciences, Beijing 100700, China

Fugang Wei
Wenshan Miaoxaing Notoginseng Technology, Co., Ltd., Wenshan 663000, China

Yong Wang and Zhongjian Chen
Institute of Sanqi Research, Wenshan University, Wenshan 663000, China

Xiaotong Guo
College of Agriculture, Ludong University, Yantai 264025, China

Tao Huang, Ling Zhao, Zi-Wan Ning, Dong-Dong Hu and Ke Tian
Institute of Brain and Gut Research, School of Chinese Medicine, Hong Kong Baptist University, Room 307, Jockey Club School of Chinese Medicine, 7 Baptist University Road, Kowloon, Hong Kong, Hong Kong SAR, China

Linda L. D. Zhong and Zhao-Xiang Bian
Institute of Brain and Gut Research, School of Chinese Medicine, Hong Kong Baptist University, Room 307, Jockey Club School of Chinese Medicine, 7 Baptist University Road, Kowloon, Hong Kong, Hong Kong SAR, China
Hong Kong Chinese Medicine Clinical Study Centre, Hong Kong Baptist University, Room 307, Jockey Club School of Chinese Medicine, 7 Baptist University Road, Kowloon, Hong Kong, Hong Kong SAR, China

Chen-Yuan Lin
Institute of Brain and Gut Research, School of Chinese Medicine, Hong Kong Baptist University, Room 307, Jockey Club School of Chinese Medicine, 7 Baptist University Road, Kowloon, Hong Kong, Hong Kong SAR, China
YMU-HKBU Joint Laboratory of Traditional Natural Medicine, Yunnan Minzu University, Kunming 650500, China

Man Zhang
Institute of Brain and Gut Research, School of Chinese Medicine, Hong Kong Baptist University, Room 307, Jockey Club School of Chinese Medicine, 7 Baptist University Road, Kowloon, Hong Kong, Hong Kong SAR, China
Guangzhou Research Institute of Snake Venom, Guangzhou Medical University, Guangzhou 510000, China

Chung-Wah Cheng
Hong Kong Chinese Medicine Clinical Study Centre, Hong Kong Baptist University, Room 307, Jockey Club School of Chinese Medicine, 7 Baptist University Road, Kowloon, Hong Kong, Hong Kong SAR, China

Pengxin Dong
School of Pharmaceutical Sciences, Shandong University, Jinan, Shandong, China
International Research Center of Medical Administration, Peking University, Beijing, China

Shuwen Yu
School of Pharmaceutical Sciences, Shandong University, Jinan, Shandong, China
Shandong University Affiliated Jinan Central Hospital, Jinan, Shandong, China

Sheng Han
International Research Center of Medical Administration, Peking University, Beijing, China

Luwen Shi
International Research Center of Medical Administration, Peking University, Beijing, China
School of Pharmaceutical Science, Peking University Health Science Center, Beijing, China

Hao Hu and Carolina Oi Lam Ung
State Key Laboratory of Quality Research in Chinese Medicine, Institute of Chinese Medical Sciences, University of Macau, Taipa, Macao

Xiaodong Guan
School of Pharmaceutical Science, Peking University Health Science Center, Beijing, China

Chengliang Huang, Wenjun Wang, Fang Guo, Yuanyuan Chen, Bi Pan, Ming Zhang and Xianming Fan
Department of Respiratory Medicine II, The Affiliated Hospital of Southwest Medical University, Luzhou, Sichuan, China

Xu Wu
Laboratory of Molecular Pharmacology, Department of Pharmacology, School of Pharmacy, Southwest Medical University, Luzhou, Sichuan, China

Shengpeng Wang
State Key Laboratory of Quality Research in Chinese Medicine, Institute of Chinese Medical Sciences, University of Macau, Macao, China

Enliang Yan and Jialin Song
Institute of Electrical Engineering, Yanshan University, No. 438, Hebei Avenue, Qinhuangdao 066004, Hebei, People's Republic of China

Wenxue Hong
Institute of Electrical Engineering, Yanshan University, No. 438, Hebei Avenue, Qinhuangdao 066004, Hebei, People's Republic of China
Guangzhou University of Chinese Medicine, Guangzhou, Guangdong 510405, People's Republic of China

Chaonan Liu
Guangzhou University of Chinese Medicine, Guangzhou, Guangdong 510405, People's Republic of China

Ying-Jie Fu, Yu-Qi Yan, Hong-Qiong Qin, Sha Wu, Shan-Shan Shi, Xiao Zheng, Peng-Cheng Wang and Zhen-You Jiang
Department of Microbiology and Immunology, School of Basic Medical Sciences, Jinan University, Guangzhou 510632, Guangdong, China

Xiao-Yin Chen
College of Traditional Chinese Medicine, Jinan University, Guangzhou 510632, Guangdong, China

Xiao-Long Tang
Medical College, Anhui University of Science & Technology, Huainan 232001, Anhui, China

Yat-Tung Lo, Mavis Hong-Yu Yik and Pang-Chui Shaw
Li Dak Sum Yip Yio Chin R & D Centre for Chinese Medicine, State Key Laboratory of Phytochemistry and Plant Resources in West China (CUHK) and School of Life Sciences, The Chinese University of Hong Kong, Shatin, N.T., Hong Kong, China

Yan Zhang, Wei Li, Liang Zou and Hang Yang
School of Medicine, Chengdu University, No. 2025, Cheng Luo Road, Chengdu 610106, Sichuan, People's Republic of China

Yun Gong and Peng Zhang
Zhuzhou Qianjin Pharmaceutical Ltd. Co., No. 801 Zhuzhou Avenue, Tianyuan District, Zhuzhou 412000, Hunan, People's Republic of China

Shasha Xing
Drug Clinical Trial Center, Affiliated Hospital of Chengdu University, 2nd Ring Road, Jinniu District, Chengdu 610081, Sichuan, People's Republic of China

Xian-Qin Luo and Zhi Dong
Chongqing Key Laboratory of Biochemistry and Molecular Pharmacology, School of Pharmacy, Chongqing Medical University, Chongqing 400016, China

Ao Li and Xiao Xiao
College of Pharmacy and Bioengineering, Chongqing University of Technology, Chongqing 400054, China

Xue Yang, Tian-Wen Wang and Da-Jian Yang
Institute of Chinese Pharmacology and Toxicology, Chongqing Academy of Chinese Materia Medica, Chongqing 400065, China

Rong Hu
Drug Review Section, China Chongqing Technical Center for Drug Evaluation and Certification, Chongqing 400014, China

Xiao-Yun Dou
Institute of Life Sciences, Chongqing Medical University, Chongqing 400016, China

Wings Tjing Yung Loo, Lixing Lao, JieShu You, Feizhi Mo and Fei Gao
School of Chinese Medicine, The University of Hong Kong, Hong Kong, China

Xiao Zheng
School of Chinese Medicine, The University of Hong Kong, Hong Kong, China
Department of Dermatology, Guangzhou University of Chinese Medicine, Guangzhou 510020, China

Jianping Chen
School of Chinese Medicine, The University of Hong Kong, Hong Kong, China
Chengdu University of Traditional Chinese Medicine, Chengdu 510020, China

Ting Xie
Department of Dermatology, Guangzhou University of Chinese Medicine, Guangzhou 510020, China

Zhiyu Xia
School of Public Health, Peking University, Beijing, China

Kamchuen Tsui
The Hong Kong Associate of Chinese Medicine, Hong Kong, China

Jie Yang
Chengdu University of Traditional Chinese Medicine, Chengdu 510020, China

Li Duan and Chen-Meng Zhang
College of Chemistry and Material Science, Hebei Normal University, Shijiazhuang 050024, China

Lei Wang and Yu-Guang Zheng
School of Pharmacy, Hebei University of Chinese Medicine, Shijiazhuang 050200, China

Long Guo
School of Pharmacy, Hebei University of Chinese Medicine, Shijiazhuang 050200, China
Hebei Key Laboratory of Chinese Medicine Research on Cardio-cerebrovascular Disease, Hebei University of Chinese Medicine, Shijiazhuang 050200, China

E.-Hu Liu
State Key Laboratory of Natural Medicines, China Pharmaceutical University, Nanjing 210009, China

Qiang Yin
Department of Management, Xinjiang Uygur Pharmaceutical Co., Ltd., Wulumuqi 830001, China

Shikang Meng, Zibei Lin and Ying Zheng
State Key Laboratory of Quality Research in Chinese Medicine, Institute of Chinese Medical Science, University of Macau, Macau, China

Yan Wang
Beijing Hospital of Traditional Chinese Medicine, Affiliated with Capital Medical University, Beijing, China

Ping Li
Beijing Hospital of Traditional Chinese Medicine, Affiliated with Capital Medical University, Beijing, China
Department of Pathophysiology, Beijing Key Laboratory of Clinic and Basic Research with Traditional Chinese Medicine on Psoriasis, Beijing Institute of Traditional Chinese Medicine, 23 Meishuguan Back Street, Dongcheng, Beijing 100010, People's Republic of China

Zhenping Wang
Department of Dermatology, School of Medicine, University of California, San Diego, La Jolla, CA, USA

Lu Lu and Jiang Lin
Department of Gastroenterology, Longhua Hospital Affiliated to Shanghai University of Traditional Chinese Medicine, Shanghai 200032, China

Liang Yan
Department of General Surgery, Shuguang Hospital Affiliated to Shanghai University of Traditional Chinese Medicine, Shanghai 201203, China

Jianye Yuan
Research Institute of the Spleen and Stomach Disease, Longhua Hospital Affiliated to Shanghai University of Traditional Chinese Medicine, Shanghai 200032, China

Qing Ye
Department of Neurology, Longhua Hospital Affiliated to Shanghai University of Traditional Chinese Medicine, Shanghai 200032, China

Ling Yuan, Lv Zhu, Yumei Zhang, Huan Chen, Hongxin Kang, Juan Li, Xianlin Zhao, Meihua Wan, Yifan Miao and Wenfu Tang
Department of Integrative Medicine, West China Hospital, Sichuan University, Chengdu 610041, Sichuan, People's Republic of China

Da-lun Lv, Lei Chen, Wei Ding, Wei Zhang, He–li Wang and Shuai Wang
Department of Burn and Plastic Surgery, First Affiliated Hospital of Wannan Medical College, Jinghu District, Wuhu 241000, Anhui, China

Wen-bei Liu
Dermatological Department, First Affiliated Hospital of Wannan Medical College, Jinghu District, Wuhu 241000, Anhui, China

Ya-nan He and Xue Han
State Key Laboratory Breeding Base of Systematic Research, Development and Utilization of Chinese Medicine Resources, Development and Utilization of Chinese Medicine Resources, Chengdu University of Traditional Chinese Medicine, Chengdu, People's Republic of China

Ding-kun Zhang and Jin Pei
State Key Laboratory Breeding Base of Systematic Research, Development and Utilization of Chinese Medicine Resources, Development and Utilization of Chinese Medicine Resources, Chengdu University of Traditional Chinese Medicine, Chengdu, People's Republic of China
Sichuan Good Doctor Panxi Pharmaceutical Co., LTD, Xichang, China

Jun-zhi Lin
Central Laboratory, Teaching Hospital of Chengdu University of TCM, Chengdu, People's Republic of China

Ya-ming Zhang and Jia-bo Wang
China Military Institute of Chinese Medicine, 302 Military Hospital, No. 100 Xisihuan, Beijing 100039, People's Republic of China

Hai-zhu Zhang
Department of Pharmacy and Chemistry, Dali University, Dali, People's Republic of China

Ming Yang
Jiangxi University of Traditional Chinese Medicine, No. 18 Yunwan Avenue, Nanchang 330004, People's Republic of China

Index

www.ingramcontent.com/pod-product-compliance
Lightning Source LLC
Chambersburg PA
CBHW082012190326
41458CB00010B/3168